BioLogic REVELATION

The 10 Minute No-Sweat Anti-Aging Workout

WAYNE CAPARAS

WESTBOW PRESS®
A DIVISION OF THOMAS NELSON & ZONDERVAN

Endorsements and Testimonials

"A New Dawn in the way we need to work out. Forget your daily, hour long, sweaty, modestly effective exercise routine. You need quality, over quantity. There is a better, quicker, more effective way for better results based on solid scientific research. Personally, I modified my routine based on these well-researched facts and I am loving the results. A MUST READ!"

—Dr. Adrienne Denese, M.D.
New York Times Bestselling Author
Harvard Researcher, Anti-Aging Expert

"If you want to burn fat, build lean muscle, look younger and maintain youthful joints then I highly recommend Wayne's new book *BioLogic Revelation*. In this book Wayne unlocks the secrets to not only getting in the best shape of your life but also how to use fitness to help you slow the aging process. If you're ready to transform your health and fitness level with less effort then I highly recommend reading this book and implementing the cutting edge and science-backed workout routine Wayne has created."

—Dr. Josh Axe, Bestselling Author
Natural Health & Fitness Expert
Founder, DrAxe.com

"*BioLogic Revelation* is going to revolutionize the fitness industry with its heavily researched, time-proven body of work. Freedom from the bondage of punishing fitness trends is finally here! As a proponent of non-punishing fitness, I am relieved Wayne Caparas has written *BioLogic Revelation*. Now I have the resource to prove that more is not better, harder is not the answer, and proper form is always key to the results one needs and wants. Thanks to this groundbreaking book, undeniable proof is finally in black and white for all to see. Talk about a revelation!"

—Suzanne Bowen, Creator of *BarreAmped*
Internationally Renowned Fitness Expert
Founder, SuzanneBowenFitness.com

"Cutting-edge yet easy to read and understand, *Biologic Revelation* is a truly original work, rich with innovative exercise techniques, exhaustive research, nutrition advice, and motivational strategies—all delivered with the positive mental attitude that Wayne Caparas has always personified. It is a must-read for anyone serious about health, fitness, top performance, and longevity. Reading this book and following the program will change your life!"

—Dr. William Maguire, Jr., M.D.
Two-Time *Post and Courier* Golden Pen Winner

"If you're looking for the most effective and efficient workout program known to man, entirely based on the latest scientific research, then you have found it. The ten-minute, no-sweat, anti-aging workout taught in *BioLogic Revelation* is a game-changer. I've been using variations of BioLogic Workouts for nearly a decade and the results have been phenomenal. So much so, that I started teaching the protocols of the BioLogic Method to my patients six years ago and all who stay the course enjoy the full cascade of benefits detailed in *BioLogic Revelation.* As a researcher and teacher of natural health strategies, I can attest that the science Wayne Caparas teaches in this book is rock solid, and his Motivational Paradigm and words of encouragement are inspiring. Never again will I return to or promote hour-long sweat-drenching workouts that destroy precious muscle tissue and sabotage proper hormone production. A ten-minute stimulus is truly all it takes to accomplish all the highest goals of fitness. It may sound too good to be true to most exercise enthusiasts (and couch potatoes for that matter), but you can absolutely achieve superior increases in lean muscle mass (which is the single most effective predictor of longevity) and thereby burn more fat using the ten-minute BioLogic Method as compared to any of the traditional fitness programs you may have tried in the past. It's a remarkable revelation, and the news of this scientific breakthrough is long overdue."

—Dr. Ben M. Sweeney
Author, Natural Health & Healing Expert

"When I got pregnant and began losing all of my energy, even in my most lethargic state, I knew I could still adapt the entire BioLogic routine to take up just ten to twenty minutes, three days per week. So doable! Staying faithful to the BioLogic Method not only balanced my hormones during my pregnancy but also boosted my self-confidence by helping me keep a healthy weight despite my increased calorie intake. Even more, it gave me the core strength I needed to deliver my daughter naturally, the way I always dreamed. I am so excited that more moms and other young adults like me are going to reap the benefits of my father's professional life's work... the *BioLogic Revelation*!

—Amber Caparas Keeler
Producer, Lifestyle Writer, 2nd Degree Black Belt

WestBow Press books may be ordered through booksellers or by contacting:

WestBow Press
A Division of Thomas Nelson & Zondervan
1663 Liberty Drive
Bloomington, IN 47403
www.westbowpress.com
1 (866) 928-1240

ISBN: 978-1-5127-7564-8 (sc)
ISBN: 978-1-5127-7565-5 (hc)
ISBN: 978-1-5127-7563-1 (e)

Library of Congress Control Number: 2017902126

Print information available on the last page.

WestBow Press rev. date: 5/10/2017

TABLE OF CONTENTS

3. Fitness Defined

Section II: BioLogic Workouts and Protocols

4. BioLogic Workout Protocols 1 & 2

Appendix

FOREWORD

Dr. Kevin R. Baird

If you reviewed the expert endorsements, you already realize that this is not your typical health and fitness book. In fact, many of your presuppositions to fitness, eating, and exercise will be profoundly challenged. I encourage you to let that sink in. I had to do that very thing as I read the contents. There is a reason the word "revelation" is in the book's title. For many, this book will be what some call, "a light-bulb" moment. There may be an unveiling of understanding that you never before considered. You may have your own personal epiphany concerning health and fitness. I encourage you to be open to that possibility. We live in an era where people are increasingly health conscious and time sensitive. To be able to navigate both concerns with integrity would be a welcome relief to untold millions who are struggling to do one or the other. *BioLogic Revelation* offers that hope.

The natural response to that exhortation would be "why"? Why should the reader give this book a chance when we are inundated by media advertising promoting a plethora of dieting and exercise possibilities and programs? I can attest for my wife and myself, that we have purchased books, joined gyms, and hired professional trainers to assist us in our health and fitness needs and goals. While we were sincere in our pursuit of help, sincerity does not guarantee integrity. We received volumes of health, fitness, and exercise information—some of which contradicted simple common sense while others were simply gym gimmicks. I am empathetic to the discouragement the vast majority feel when it comes to straightforward information and realistic workouts. This book clearly addresses those challenges. Let me suggest four reasons for this belief that I identified while reading *BioLogic Revelation*.

1. Credibility—The author, Wayne Caparas, has spent a significant portion of his lifetime researching and implementing the precepts found in *BioLogic Revelation*. I know Wayne on a personal level, and had the joy of being a colleague and advisor for many years. I know most of his life journey. I know the ups and downs. I know the adversity and victories. I can attest to his character and diligence. He is the real deal. Wayne is not the stereotypical gym-junkie. Is he more athletic and fit than the vast majority of people over forty, despite being well into his fifties? Absolutely! However, he is also well-educated, well-read, and incredibly experienced. A simple perusal of the footnotes and his credentials leaves no question to his credibility and research.

2. Groundbreaking implications—Wayne is offering something new and fresh. What he is advocating is significantly different and— from my perspective—cutting-edge. He will challenge established fitness philosophy and back it up with solid scientific research. As I read his propositions it occurred to me that this area of fitness and exercise is not exempt from critical analysis or new breakthroughs. *BioLogic Revelation* has the potential to change the fitness landscape.

3. Compassion—Wayne understands people. All through the book you sense that he understands where the normal person lives and functions. *BioLogic Revelation* changes the mentality that a healthy lifestyle is simply unattainable for the normal person. How many of us have been overwhelmed by the thought of countless hours and energy that would have to be expended to attain a health or fitness goal? Wayne "gets" where most of us live and yet in that compassion will still challenge us to move purposefully where we need to be with regards to our health. As I write this foreword I am starting another new year with resolutions to pursue (once again) my health goals. *BioLogic Revelation* removes the feeling that I am circling the same mountain of fitness-frustration, as I now have the answers to remain encouraged as I take another run at it (no pun intended).

4. Comprehensive Perspective—I was impressed with the comprehensive approach of *BioLogic Revelation*. I suspect Wayne's deep faith and theological acumen guided him in his understanding that people are

more than just a pretty face and rockin' body. No one would disagree that a healthy, fit, body is a legitimate goal for every person, but Wayne underscores the place of the "mind" as well as the emotions in a successful fitness program. God created us with a mind, body, soul, and spirit and these four aspects of a human being's well-being permeate the writing of this book.

As I close, I am reminded that any "revelation" has as its purpose a reformation effect. Whether it be in the area of religion, technology, medicine, or health and fitness, the epiphany must lead to personal and corporate change. I can almost guarantee that as you read and reflect on what is shared in *BioLogic Revelation*, you will not escape the challenge to change. My hope is that you embrace that personal reformation. The greater question that will remain is whether the fitness industry will embrace the change. Time, I suppose, will decide that outcome. However, as it is with most reformations, industries and organizations react when people "see the light." *BioLogic Revelation* may well be that light.

Dr. Kevin R. Baird, D. Min.
Founder/Executive Director
The Bonhoeffer Institute

Scott Hasenbalg

Wayne Caparas recruited me straight out of college to work alongside him to lead the relatively large and diversified fitness operation that was his brainchild. I was a two-sport athlete from New York who wanted to start my career where I could help people, and Wayne's team was widely celebrated for launching new initiatives that empower people from all walks of life. It was a rare opportunity in a thriving fitness think tank, and the talent Wayne recruited before me was extraordinary, my older brother Michael (his V.P. of Operations) included. It was an exciting time in an important emerging industry, and we sincerely put our hearts into the way we cared for our members and the various communities we served. This was a core ethic of the organization, a direct reflection of its leader, and the primary reason I moved a thousand miles from home to start my professional life. Always the visionary, Wayne was a different kind of fitness innovator. He was very often one step ahead in recognizing future trends for both the members *and* the fitness industry at large. I saw thousands of lives changed in my time as Wayne's lieutenant, and I was well aware that his published works were reaching tens of thousands around the world. *BioLogic Revelation* is his greatest effort yet, and it should soon help millions more.

After several years in Wayne's camp, I went on to serve in a variety of Christian ministries. Most notably, I served alongside Mary Beth and Steven Curtis Chapman for twelve years as the Founding Executive Director of *Show Hope*—the orphan care and adoption ministry that is a most beautiful reflection of God's wisdom and love for the vulnerable. Serving alongside the Chapmans and the Show Hope team all those years grew my heart and expanded my discernment. Through my role with the Chapmans, I experienced time and again how God loves to use humble people who are dedicated to sharing their wisdom and insights for the betterment of others in the most miraculous ways. Wayne Caparas is one of those people, who through his dedication to gain wisdom and understanding, coupled with his love for people, has been used in remarkable ways. I was blessed to have gained the insights he imparted into me at the very beginning of my professional journey. They have served me well throughout my adult life, both as an advocate for the betterment of others and as the custodian of my personal health and the health of my family.

Upon reading *BioLogic Revelation,* though I was well-aware of Wayne's knack for breaking new ground, the book still took me by surprise with its countless new and exciting discoveries, all of which ring true. It is the harvest of two decades of research and investigation by a man of science and faith, and even the most educated fitness expert will learn from this book. *BioLogic Revelation* is a great work in every way. Within these pages you will find pathways long affirmed by the well-informed minority of the fitness industry. You'll also find brand new concepts that will inevitably disrupt the false and harmful thinking that exists in much of contemporary culture. It's another core ethic in all Wayne does. Wayne's writing style makes this information-rich text exceptionally colorful and enjoyable to read, so you should have no problem making sense of all the science and putting it into action. It is a rare text in that respect. As the husband to my wife Kerry and a father of four children, I truly care about active lifestyles for all of us, but I care even more about living in accordance with God's purpose for each day. This book epitomizes "proper balance" of these ideals. Read on, and be blessed.

Scott Hasenbalg, Family Advocate
President of Redemptive Ventures, LLC
Founding Executive Director of Show Hope

Dr. Michael A. Kollar

I have known Wayne Caparas for almost 30 years. At times, I have worked alongside Wayne as he was in the process of personally changing and altering the definitions of exercise, fitness, and aesthetics when it comes to deriving optimal benefits from "working out." As a psychologist, I know the positive effect exercise can have on one's emotional and psychological health. For this, I completed certification programs in group fitness and personal training. As a practitioner of both psychology and fitness, I firmly believe motivation and sustainability are the cornerstones of maintaining any fitness program. *Biologic Revelation* provides a mechanism for one to have joy and fun while participating in a fitness filled lifestyle. Starting on page 101 you will learn about "The Four Cornerstones of Motivation" which detail the importance of maintaining motivation in order to receive the tremendous benefits Wayne describes in his book.

Wayne has put together a primer that is easy to read and absorb and put into action. As you spend time going through each chapter, you will find many new breakthroughs that are based on current clinical and scientific research. Don't let any of the jargon get in the way of your finding the true meaning of *Biologic Revelation*.

I have been a fitness enthusiast my entire life and, like Wayne, grew up during a time when admitting pain or discomfort was considered a weakness, and finding pleasure or having fun as a result of exercising was discouraged. *Biologic Revelation* provides a mechanism for one to have joy and fun while participating in a fitness filled lifestyle, as Wayne has boldly yet subtly described the importance of finding joy and sincere care for oneself and others. Like many in Wayne's life, I am aware of how he has experienced physical and emotional pain and disappointments. What is unique about Wayne Caparas is that he discovers resources that propel him to recovery, and through *BioLogic Revelation*, he has found a way to show others how to do the same. Discovering the joy one feels as a result of feeling better both emotionally and physically is an ongoing and blessed accomplishment. *Biologic Revelation* provides the foundation for building that positive fitness mindset.

I know those in the fitness field will have difficulty upsetting their historic "apple carts." But if they can be open to new discoveries and the secrets revealed in *BioLogic Revelation*, many lives will be saved, and the joy for life will be multiplicatively enhanced. In closing, I deeply respect the person Wayne Caparas has become. I admire the dedication, servitude, and perseverance he has demonstrated by writing this landmark book.

Dr. Michael A. Kollar, Ed.D.
Outstanding Lifetime Contribution to Psychology Award
from the South Carolina Psychological Association

Dedicated to the beautiful, strong, and gifted women in my life—my gorgeous wife and partner Stacey, my vibrant mother Patricia, my multi-talented daughter Amber, and my spirited granddaughter Vienna. Thank you for your love, your inspiration, your commitment to real health, and—above all—your faith.

INTRODUCTION

Nothing But the Truth

The Jury Is In

Once the scientific community and common human genetics finally have their say, many millions of lives are going to change in an instant. *BioLogic Revelation* is a fitness breakthrough of the highest order, as every facet draws from an abundance of independent research performed by many of the world's leading biologists and physiologists. Together, these new discoveries have revealed a profoundly powerful link between specific muscle fiber activity over very short-durations and our ability to improve metabolic health, fight disease, and slow the aging process in incomparable fashion.[1] Though the revelation seemed paradoxical and *too good to be true* when it first came to light nearly twenty years ago, today it is scientifically clear and entirely logical. With more than two hundred peer-reviewed research studies and thirty years of success stories to support or prove our conclusions, the *BioLogic 10 Minute No-Sweat Anti-Aging Workout* is a fitness activity every man and woman alive should immediately adopt—or at very least adapt into their current regimen.

Likewise, the revelation leverages startling new research that exposes the destructive and often deadly results of long-term distance running and other forms of high-volume exercise.[2] I'll be introducing you to many of the scientists behind this groundbreaking research throughout the book. As you will soon see, one could hardly assemble a more highly-accomplished brain trust. Their studies have collectively demonstrated that the strength building, metabolism correcting, fat burning, heart strengthening, hormone balancing, diabetes destroying, immune system boosting, cancer-fighting, joint healing, body shaping benefits of BioLogic Workouts are rivaled only by their simplicity and ease—no matter your age or current shape.

I began testing the revelation back in the nineties while I was at the peak of my life as a fitness innovator and research journalist. Two decades later the scientific community has fully explained (down to the cellular level) the methods and protocols my like-minded colleagues and I began preaching to deaf ears far too long ago. Sadly, the news of this revolutionary research is still being suppressed and drowned out by the noise of establishment spin doctors, striving to protect their long-held narrative. So in all likelihood, you haven't heard a word about it . . . until now.

We finally have irrefutable scientific evidence that there is an amazingly easy, level path to achieve all of the highest goals of exercise. And unlike all the body-abusing, age-accelerating, time-wasting, and life-threatening approaches most enthusiasts are pitching, BioLogic Workouts truly heal and strengthen your body in very little time with no sweat required. We now know that fitness is not a function of the quantity of your work, but the quality of the stimuli you apply to specific muscle fibers in very small doses. This is the BioLogic Method. If you're in need of a fitness revelation or simply curious if such unprecedented claims could actually be true, I challenge you to test it out and judge for yourself.

Picture Yourself

We humans are visual creatures. For that, I'd like you to keep a simple visual in mind while reading through all the promises, warnings, and challenges I share in this book. There is an ideal version of your body hidden within the untapped potential of your most-neglected muscle cells, and in all likelihood—even if you're a lifelong fitness enthusiast—you don't yet know how to make it spring forth. Whether you're a couch potato, an avid runner, bodybuilder, professional athlete or anywhere in between, unless you've been applying the simple exercise stimuli and lifestyle advice I'll detail in this book, you're most likely heading in a far less favorable direction with your health and physical fitness—no matter how you look today. It will probably come as a shock to you that folks who have never worked out a day in their lives can more easily attain their ideal body than most enthusiasts who have been beating their bodies for decades. It's a scientifically sound fact. Stick with me and you'll soon see how this can be true.

Picture a professional marathon runner standing on the left, a massive bodybuilder on the right, and an Olympic sprinter in the middle. If you're a woman, you might want to replace the sprinter with a professional dancer, as their physiques are remarkably similar despite their very different training protocols. Male sprinters are widely recognized for having the ideal male physiques, and their female counterparts (dancers included) enjoy that same status. Likewise, they typically look much younger than their age and far younger than marathon runners and bodybuilders of the same age. The BioLogic Workout does not call for sprinting or dancing, so please bear with me. Now picture yourself in the condition of that sprinter or dancer in your visual. This picture is very close to the "you" that you were genetically designed to be, and we now know that achieving this physique has virtually nothing to do with the volume of sweaty work you perform or how well you can starve yourself. So you can get those myths out of your head right now.

If you know you're overweight it will obviously take you a bit longer to reach your present ideal, but you can clear any thoughts that crash diets or magic supplements play any role in the BioLogic lifestyle. Through the BioLogic Method, you will learn how to correctly perform a small number of very simple strength exercises through protocols that apply natural stimuli to very specific muscle fiber types in your body. These are stimuli that in just ten minutes will trigger an amazing metabolic domino effect of health benefits through every system in your body. Once combined with a more active lifestyle and proper nutrition, this metabolic cascade will put you on track to achieving your present ideal (your current potential for your own unique sprinter/dancer body), regardless of your age or current body weight.

I believe it's safe to assume that many of you are greatly intrigued by the fact that this stimulus can be applied in ten minutes or less. On the other hand, this revelation will likely prove to be a stumbling block for those who have been misled to believe that hours of body beating workouts every week are required to get in shape and to stay that way. My colleagues and I know that to be a lie, and key leaders in the medical community have finally proven exactly how this seemingly *too good to be true* revelation is scientific truth. So as you read on, remember that the BioLogic Method will lead you to hone the sprinter/dancer body for which you are genetically designed. Occasionally pause to take a mental glance back at the gaunt runner and the massive bodybuilder in our illustration, and be reminded where BioLogic Workouts will never lead you, as both are causing a great deal *more harm than good*. Then, if you stay on the straight and level path that is the BioLogic lifestyle, you will begin to make inroads toward a healthier, more youthful you in thirty days or less.

Whom Can We Believe?

It's tough enough getting through each day in this over-wired greed-inspired move-at-the-speed-of-light modern culture without all the confusion concerning what could and should be known as fundamental truth—especially concerning issues that truly matter, like life itself. The Internet allows us to access peer-reviewed research whenever we want, yet newly spun myths and hyped-up fabrications get most of our digital attention. Game-changing research is buried under stacks of fake news or hidden out of sight, especially when it discredits profitable establishment positions. The squeaky wheel still gets the grease even in the digital domain, and those with the most grease have mastered squeaking out their ear-tickling misinformation with such volume and fanaticism that there's little space left for the facts to enter into the discussion.

We often see this disheartening tactic play out in nearly every contentious debate in the global conversation. I believe most of you have realized long ago, deep in your gut, that there's something inherently wrong with the most popular approaches to getting fit. We simply aren't designed to waste so much time, energy, and life following the vanity-driven ways of beating our bodies. As you read on, I'm more than confident that you will find new inspiration to tune out the noise and recognize the truth while continuing with an open mind.

When I first received the BioLogic revelation, it was already scientifically valid to me due to a set of remarkable scientific theories that had been hidden away in plain sight by the vast majority of fitness writers, personal trainers, fitness fad-hucksters, snake oil peddlers, and their ilk. My personal research into these poorly-kept secrets was initiated by my need for a rehab workout that I could safely perform after one of my many sports related injuries. The results were profound, yet my peers generally dismissed my initial findings as being *too good to be true.* To this day, many industry pros are still operating as if the revelation has yet to reach their ears, as the table-flipping ramifications it could unleash on their business models is difficult to reconcile. Others are strangely unaware of the decades of scientific research, real world application, and undeniable logic that has been embraced by an enlightened minority for many years. Denial and silent rejection are normal human responses when one's belief system is staked on the shifting sands of long-held fallacies and misguided majority rule. So we shouldn't be surprised when we see the status quo holding firm. All these years later the excuses for ignorance have worn far too thin, and it's time for the fitness industry to embrace the good news—and grow up. I honestly didn't want to be the one to call them out in public, but so be it.

Sincerity Is No Excuse

Be reminded that in the not so distant past most people believed the world was flat, despite literature and logic revealing otherwise for many millennia beforehand. Even in my lifetime, people were once positively sure that cigarette smoking was mostly harmless, and that sugar-laden breakfast cereals made the ideal breakfast for kids. My favorites were Sugar Smacks and Sugar Frosted Flakes. I *dug'em* because they were *G-r-r-reat!* And God knows my parents thought their cigarettes were way *Kool*, no matter how many road trips were tainted by the drama of my hacking pleas for them to "roll down a window, for heaven's sake." My brother would often submissively (often violently) vomit in a bag, convinced by my ill-informed parents that their second-hand smoke had nothing to do with his chronic car sickness.

The masses of modern culture have always tended to blindly follow the most charming piper and move to the beat of the loudest drums no matter how badly it hurt, all the while tuning-out minority dissent—regardless of the evidence proving they're heading the wrong way. Many centuries of fear-based need for acceptance and misplaced trust in the powers-that-be are the two darkest forces behind our destructive tendency to be duped, and we're more confused today than ever. Like the crowds from the famous allegory, even when our gut instincts, logic, and visible observations are telling us otherwise, the masses simply don't want to admit they've invested so much time, money, and faith into just another emperor with no clothes, or just another path that leads to destruction.

Speaking of Emperors: Get Off Your Throne

We've all long known that sitting at a desk all day only to find ourselves sitting on the couch watching TV or surfing the web most of the evening is a slow road to an early death. Our national economic engines rely upon the majority of us sitting at desks or work benches or standing stationary at retail counters and assembly lines while heavy machinery or robotics do all the heavy lifting for us. If ever there was an era to envy skilled laborers and small family farmers, it's now. Yet year after year, the majority of Americans expend their lives like fuel for the furnace, burning up their candles at both ends while waiting for their employer, the government, their family doctor, or the major media to push them onto a healthier road before it's too late. Unfortunately, that cavalry is in no hurry to surge around that bend.

Despite the avalanche of published medical research that began pouring in during 2015 and 2016 from journals as diverse as *Experimental Physiology;* the *International Journal of Cancer; Creative Nursing;* the *Journal of Sports Sciences;* and the journal of *Ergonomics,* (to name a few), the mainstream media is turning a blind eye. Each study proved that those of us who sit for prolonged periods or live sedentary lifestyles suffer greater occurrence of premature death through early-onset cancer, heart disease, morbid obesity, metabolic dysfunction, venous and arterial disorders, and central nervous system breakdown.[3]

When all this concurring research was getting published, did you hear an outcry from the czars of information? Not so much, right? In 2016, the *President's Council on Fitness, Sports, & Nutrition* demonstrated that they were well aware of these horrifying trends, but you would have had to sift through their website for evidence. The *President's Council* reported that less than twenty percent of adults and adolescents met their minimal activity guidelines and that children spent more than seven and a half hours per day sitting on their butts with their eyes locked on a digital device or television screen[4] (big industries as you know). Yet the government and media remained mostly mum on these devastating trends, despite the fact that the numbers had been getting worse every year. It's well past time we all stop waiting for the government or media to educate us concerning health issues and start taking personal responsibility for our children's health and our own mortality.

A Word or Two for My Peers in the Business

Before I continue, I need to ensure you don't mistake my heavy criticisms of modern fitness as a blanket indictment against every program, facility, writer, or innovator in the industry. I believe it is crucial that you know exactly who is leading the vast majority of you down a path to destruction before you can understand the BioLogic revelation, but I need to ensure I don't hurt or diminish those who are doing good work. I also want to make clear that there are in fact other popular fitness programs that have proven fruitful (for a variety of reasons that I'll detail throughout the book) but be assured that they are very few.

You already know I have colleagues who teach their own versions of BioLogic-styled workouts, and if you're among their students you probably already realize I'm on their side. But there are also a handful of vastly different approaches that I can endorse for all the right reasons. Suzanne Bowen's *BarreAmped* is a graceful, functional workout that can give you a dancer's body minus all the joint stress. Drs. Josh and Chelsea Axe's *BurstFit* is a fun and effective example of *high-intensity interval training* (aka *HIIT*, which I'll discuss in Chapter 2). The renowned Billy Blanks' and his daughter Shellie's world famous *Tae Bo* is another example of functional training that can give you the strength and confidence to use several vital self-defense moves in a *fight or flight* situation. Some of my most memorable workouts occurred with that dynamic duo at the lead. My daughter (whom I raised up to be a 2nd-degree black belt in Taekwondo) is one of their instructors, so you know I value their role in the industry. The same is true for nearly all disciplines of the martial arts, and you'll soon understand why.

Likewise, many of the health clubs out there have great equipment and are owned and operated by folks who are doing a lot of very important work. The list of the good guys goes on, but as you'll soon see, they still collectively represent a tiny fraction of the industry. And though the folks I named above are now dear brothers and sisters of mine, that's not why I endorse their work. I love everything that is right about their programs, so for those of you who are growing healthier as a member of the close-knit communities of enthusiasts these experts have inspired, don't let me discourage you from breaking a good sweat with them. As discussed in Chapter 3, joy is an imperative motivator you must pursue if you hope to stay the course, and I know many thousands who enjoy these alternate approaches immensely. For you, the BioLogic Workout shouldn't be viewed as a replacement, but instead a quick ten-minute add-on, or maybe a once-per-week alternate workout. The same can be said for most low-volume high-intensity resistance training enthusiasts, as you are pretty much where I was before catching the revelation. You should be among the early adopters once you allow the overwhelming wealth of research to have its say. As you'll soon learn, only the BioLogic Method and others like it can deliver the unprecedented health, body-shaping, and anti-aging benefits I'll detail in *Section I*, so please stick with me. Now that I've delivered that important disclaimer, the remaining majority of fitness enthusiasts should brace yourselves for the alarming research I'm about to share.

In all my years as a trainer of trainers, I've seen many dozens of my students and clients become fitness experts in their own right. One of my struggles in finally writing this book was the impact it would have on several friends in the industry who have resisted change. With pure hearts, they have invested all they have into business models that promote one of the *more harm than good* approaches to fitness I'll expose throughout this book. Some are like family to me, and I pray they don't see this as an attack against their livelihood. Rather, it's my cry from the rooftop that they open their eyes to our culture's often destructive obsession with pseudo-fitness, just as I did two decades ago. When the BioLogic revelation was still new to me, I spoke of it with excitement but tamed my tongue when equally passionate colleagues pushed back with their "more is better" "no-pain no-gain" rationale.

Twenty years later, the bodily destruction and pre-aging I've witnessed among most of these friends have been heartbreaking, particularly among those who practiced long-duration endurance workouts. Today they're all approaching fifty or sixty, and nearly all look far more aged than their years. Even worse, the plethora of health scares and joint/spine injuries and absolute loss of youthful vigor (showing even in the pre-aging of their skin and hair) I've witnessed among the current generation of fitness gurus in their twenties and thirties is shocking. As you'll soon see, these fanatics have taken body abuse to an entirely insane level, typically for temporary carnal gains.

If we truly care about our friends and loved ones who are drinking their Kool-Aid, it's time to get the truth out there ASAP. Don't ever forget that those who control the message in the mainstream fitness industry have become exceptionally adept at selling and heralding the very few short-term positives their body abusive workouts offer—while entirely ignoring the startling long-term and short-term negatives. If you're among the victims of all the misinformation, please don't be discouraged. BioLogic Workouts can actually heal your body where damage has been done and even turn back the clock if you don't already have one foot in the grave. I'm living proof, and I'm certainly not alone.

Destroying Your Body?

I want to make sure I start uncorking the fitness industry's bottle of secrets in this introduction, and I'll expand on these particular topics as needed throughout the book. If you're anxious to learn about BioLogic Workouts and already know that endurance running and other forms of high-impact, long-duration training damage vital body systems and cause *more harm than good*, then feel free to jump ahead to the section titled "Hidden in Plain Sight" later in this Introduction. Otherwise, I compel you to read the next two sub-sections. The well-proven facts I'm about to share will be a hard pill for most exercise enthusiasts to swallow, but unless you want to become complicit in the ongoing cover-up, swallow you must.

Even if you've never considered the activities I'm about to expose, please read thoughtfully, as the research findings could help you liberate your friends or loved ones from irreparable damage, maybe even this very day. Whatever the case, please put aside your preconceptions for a moment and let the leading experts on these subjects finally have your ear. If you're not an exercise enthusiast, the overarching implications will likely come as no surprise to you; but if you're like most of my friends, the details of the latest research findings will alarm you.

Running to Your Funeral?

The running craze of the sixties pretty much gave birth to the modern fitness craze. Half a century later, running is in the midst of a second major boom, boasting more than sixty-million enthusiasts in America alone in 2016.[5] According to the National Sporting Goods Association, running/jogging participation has increased 70% since 2004; and of course the running gear industry could hardly be happier, as they enjoy upwards of three billion dollars annually (that's $3,000,000,000) in running shoe sales in the USA alone.[6] Sounds like evidence of a good thing, doesn't it? Now it's time for the proverbial "other shoe" to fall. Due to the universally destructive effect endurance running has on your body (especially on your heart), many medical research doctors don't even classify endurance running as a legitimate form of exercise, and my colleagues and I have wholeheartedly concurred for decades. Yes, depending on how you compartmentalize the facts, endurance running does offer a few benefits, but they are dwarfed by the potentially deadly health risks.

In a twelve-year mortality study published in 2015 by the *Journal of the American College of Cardiology*, researchers found that running enthusiasts suffer about the same risk of dying as those who sit on the couch most of their lives.[7] Even more disturbing, the study showed that casual runners who jog three times per week or less at a moderate pace for a total of 2.5 to 4 hours per week suffered an even higher mortality rate than the sedentary couch potatoes.[8] Please read that again, and let it set in. So much for the benefits of running ever outweighing the negatives; and by all indications, the same is true of most other forms of endurance training.

One would think such a landmark study would have been blasted across every major media outlet in the world, yet *Time Magazine* was the only significant news source to step up for "us." All this media silence despite decades of supporting research, and not one notable dissenting opinion from the medical community. It feels almost criminal to an activist like me. Lives are being put at risk by an industry we are encouraged to trust yet no one is talking about it. Even *Time Magazine* buried the story away in a subsection of their website, possibly tucked well behind many pages of running shoe ads. Did you hear the news when it broke? Considering my commentary above, we should all realize why your answer is probably "no."

Six years before this study broke, Dr. Doug McGuff and fitness journalist John Little published their trailblazing book *Body by Science.* They analyzed and reconciled more than thirty years of peer-reviewed medical research to ring the alarm bell. Right up front in Chapter 1 of their book, they wrote:

> The scientific literature is filled with data that strongly make the case that long-distance runners are much more likely to develop cardiovascular disease, atrial fibrillation, cancer, liver and gallbladder disorders, muscle damage, kidney dysfunction (renal abnormalities), acute microthrombosis in the vascular system, brain damage, spinal degeneration, and germ-cell cancers than are their less active counterparts.[9]

Yikes. That single sentence cited ten different peer-reviewed research papers dealing with each disease it named. Yet when McGuff and Little published these findings in 2009, most of the establishment scoffed or merely ignored their call to arms. Now that the American College of Cardiology's twelve-year mortality study (along with many freshly minted studies I'll cite in *Section I*) have proven them right, I hope you can see why I feel compelled to shout from the rooftops, and I hope you'll join me. If you're still not alarmed, consider this. Between 2009 and 2016 no less than twelve independent medical studies reported a direct correlation between endurance running and other endurance training to: "large-artery wall stiffening and coronary artery calcification;"[10] "increased risk of atrial fibrillation, coronary artery disease, and malignant ventricular arrhythmias;"[11] "localized myocardial edema;"[12] and "myocardial fibrosis."[13] In a landmark 2015 study published in *Trends in Cardiovascular Medicine,* the authors reported:

> Intense exercise is associated with sudden deaths in athletes harboring quiescent yet potentially sinister cardiac diseases. More recently, there have been an emerging number of reports suggesting that intense [endurance] exercise may have an adverse impact on an otherwise normal heart.[14]

Weren't we always told that running was good for our hearts? Double yikes. Please let it register that these warnings should be considered by those of you who perform any type of long-duration endurance exercise, even if it's on a cycle or a cardio machine. Again, it's easy to acknowledge that endurance training has a few benefits, especially if you're a competitive endurance athlete. But there are far safer and far more effective ways to burn fat and strengthen your heart, and *far* more benefits through workouts that follow the 10 Minute BioLogic approach. Much more on that later in the book. If you're asking how all this could be true when the human body is clearly well suited for running, the answer is found in the *survival of the fittest.* Yes, we were born to run, but with bursts of top speed for short-durations over short distances and extremely low-impact stride technique; not at low speeds for long-durations over long distances while incessantly pounding our heels (and our heart).

Our bodies are simply not designed to sustain health and proper healing when continuously subjected to such repetitive, long-duration beatings. In all my years as a sprinter and speed coach to athletes at every level, I never once met a single competitive male or female distance runner who was more physically fit than an equally competitive sprinter. Yet sprinters do a fraction of the work, typically performing short, explosive sets no longer than four hundred meters and often as short as forty meters, with total time sprinting typically under ten minutes per workout. This is an example of interval training, which represents one of the major breakthroughs the fitness industry is finally embracing—albeit slowly—but still their tendency is to push too much of a good thing on their audiences.

As you'll soon learn, short bursts of highly focused stimuli at extraordinarily low volumes are core principles in BioLogic Workout protocols. Compare the above example of a sprinter's workout to that of an endurance runner, which typically consumes two to three hours every day. Which is more appealing to you? Now recall your visual of the three athletes and be reminded which has the ideal body based on our genetic design. Ask yourself which is most prepared to fight in hand to hand combat against an attacker, or flee a fast attacking predator. The answer is obvious.

Fitness Fads to Die For?

To unveil the most troubling hidden truths that the newest tycoons of the fitness world are dumbing down, let's take a look at the most hyperbolic fitness craze of the twenty-first century, the insanely popular *CrossFit*. In just over a decade it's become a four BILLION dollar brand with eleven thousand locations.[15] *CrossFit* consists of very high-impact strength, agility, and endurance training sessions with boot camp (often vomit-inducing) intensity that typically run for an hour or more.

By its founder Greg Glassman's own admission, *CrossFit* involves potentially deadly workouts. As he infamously boasts to the media, "It can kill you." And though many enthusiasts brush this off as a marketing ploy, the statistics prove Mr. *CrossFit* isn't joking. [16] In a recent study published in the *Journal of Strength & Conditioning Research*, 73.5 percent of *CrossFit* enthusiasts report having suffered a *CrossFit* injury; and far more alarming, seven percent required surgery.[17] Surgery for one out of every thirteen people trying to get fit? Unbelievable. Likewise, a professor of exercise science, who was a *CrossFit* enthusiast at the time of his research, found that among 737 *CrossFit* members in his study, fifty-one percent had been injured during a *CrossFit* workout within the previous year, and as many as fifteen percent required a trip to the hospital.[18]

Before you assume *CrossFit* is only dangerous for its high rate of bone, spine, and soft tissue injury (as if that's not enough), consider this. A 2015 *Journal of Special Operations Medicine* report detailed the potential risks of *CrossFit* and similar "extreme conditioning programs" like *Insanity*, *Gym Jones*, and *P90X*. The study documented several cases of *CrossFit* induced cervical carotid artery dissections—a leading cause of stroke—along with several cases of rhabdomyolysis (dangerously rapid breakdown of muscle tissue that can lead to long-term hospitalization and kidney failure), both of which are of course potentially fatal conditions.[19] In *Issue 38* of the *CrossFit Journal Articles,* Glassman used his own pen to report:

> With CrossFit we are dealing with what is known as exertional rhabdomyolysis [rhabdo]. It can disable, maim, and even kill . . . Each case resulted in the hospitalization of the afflicted . . . The rhabdo we've seen has come from sessions of twenty minutes or less, with mild or low temperature and humidity. The victims were not excessively panting, straining, grunting, or otherwise expressing abnormal discomfort from the workouts. The athletes who came down with rhabdo turned in marginal CrossFit performances and showed no signs of discomfort that were out of the ordinary. They left their workouts seemingly no worse off than anyone else.[20]

How comforting. Glassman is so flippant about this threat that his firm developed a comical clown mascot named "Uncle Rhabdo" who is typically shown in a morbidly bloody and beaten state, clearly in need of surgical care. Do an image search on the web if you're curious, but brace yourself if you just had lunch. Sadly, the explosive popularity of *CrossFit* has been greatly accelerated by their highly entertaining *ESPN* obstacle course fitness events. The athletes who can survive the rigors are absolute specimens of power, but no man knows the ultimate price they'll pay for their body-abusing cravings. Back in the nineties I was among a small group of fitness promoters pioneering obstacle course sports as content for *ESPN.* A couple years in, I became so enamored with the production of these glamorous events, that creating one of my own to promote my Charleston, SC health clubs became my full-time obsession. By 1996, *ESPN* and several newsstand magazines began praising our efforts to so quickly evolve the sport,[21] and it was clear to all that obstacle course sports were here to stay. During this phase of my fitness career, the late Robert "Bob" Kennedy (founder of *Oxygen, Clean Eating, MuscleMag*, and other magazines) was a mentor and dear friend. Together we dreamed up a truly inspired vision for the future of televised obstacle course sports, and Bob and I eventually put it all in writing for an article in the new millennium edition of *Oxygen* (January 2000 issue).[22] Though our vision projected the athletes to look far more like sprinters and dancers than the behemoths and the zero-fat crowd we see in the sport today (both male and female), I regret my role in setting the stage for such a dangerous, vanity-driven variation of the sport to emerge.

No matter how entertaining it may be, and no matter how many of the athletes build exceedingly powerful, massively muscular physiques on their way to gaining fame or fortune in these grand *CrossFit* events, is it really worth risking life and limb? Thank goodness there are several other obstacle course events springing up that are much closer to the vision Bob and I shared at the turn of the century. Some are inspiring, and I hope the best of them begin to win the lion's share of the media's attention going forward.

Hidden in Plain Sight

The most encouraging truth that the fitness industry has dumbed-down for the past thirty years has been more a casualty of ignorance than deception. You can hardly walk into a gym without strength training equipment hitting you right between the eyes, which of course makes its minimization all the more bewildering. Many of you already know that strength training (and certainly not endurance training) is far and away the most important form of exercise where long-term physical health is concerned. Even the notoriously slow-moving American Heart Association (AHA) has recently beefed up their recommendations that we all start a strength training regimen for a variety of benefits that go beyond basic fitness, including healing effects that no other form of exercise can provide.[23] Incredibly, most fitness gurus still don't want to give strength training its proper due.

Even when you find a gym or trainer who gives preeminence to strength training, they are often promoting abusive, long-duration programs or high-risk momentum building movements (think *CrossFit*) while undermining the cascade of benefits triggered by the short-duration, high-intensity BioLogic approach. The AHA now recommends strength training for heart health, fat burning, healthy weight management, bone, muscle, tendon, and ligament strengthening, injury prevention, central nervous system health, stroke recovery, and a "better quality of life."[24]

Do you think any reasonable team of doctors or medical organization would make such claims about any of the long-duration, high-impact exercise activities? No, because it wouldn't be true. A wealth of research proves that over-training is destructive no matter what form of exercise you perform.[25]

Though the AHA's list of strength training benefits is impressive, it's merely a sampling of the far more robust list you'll enjoy by taking the BioLogic approach. As you'll see in Chapter 2, the detailed breakdown of scientifically proven benefits from the short-duration, low-impact strength training protocols that comprise BioLogic Workouts is much longer and genuinely amazing. Many of the additional benefits (over those noted by the AHA) can be explained by the fact that the most popular strength workouts go too far, by edging dangerously close to extreme programs like *CrossFit*. Others miss the proper stimuli entirely by training for long-durations with exercises that don't effectively challenge the most critical *fight or flight* muscle fibers that are fundamental to the BioLogic revelation. So why are most strength training gurus still promoting dangerous or counterproductive long-duration workouts with weights? That's where the ignorance comes in. The *no pain, no gain* advocates and the "must get sweaty" crowd will boast of short-term gains, while entirely ignoring the well-documented long-term and short-term dangers.

Maybe by the time you read this book the tide will have already turned among the weightlifting crowd, but I'm not holding my breath. So please take hold of this paradigm shift. Muscles aren't optimally exercised through the quantity of work but the quality and precision of the stimuli. The most important muscle fiber types can only be optimally stimulated for very short-durations before they fall victim to diminishing returns and the high-risks of overtraining—just as is true for Olympic sprinters.

What About Cardio and Aerobic Fitness?

In 2006, the *Journal of Physiology* published the first of a series of groundbreaking studies performed by a highly respected team of scientists and doctors at McMaster University. To the shock of many, their findings revealed that short-duration, high-rest interval training produced the same improvements in actual endurance when compared to traditional long-duration endurance workouts (a.k.a. aerobics and cardio) like cycling and running.[26] Commonly known as the McMaster University studies, these landmark research projects gained zero major media attention, which by now should be no surprise to you.

Body by Science authors McGuff and Little discussed the profound implications of the McMaster studies with one of the lead scientists, Dr. Martin Gibala, and their conclusions are stunning. In a particular two-week study, Gibala's team tested the maximum aerobic capacity (VO_2 max) among two groups of stationary cyclists. One group rode in the traditional endurance fashion for 90 to 120 minutes per workout. The other group performed short, thirty-second high-speed sprints followed by four full minutes of rest, then again and again until they had amassed a total of two to three minutes of sprint cycling. This is, in effect, the BioLogic approach to that particular exercise (minus the full benefits of a similar strength exercise). Though the endurance group invested 97.5 percent more time cycling than those who performed the relatively no-sweat sprint intervals, the two groups improved their VO_2 max *equally.* To that, McGuff and Little wrote:

> The group that exercised 97.5 percent more did not receive an equivalent benefit from having done so. In fact, they received "zero" additional benefit from all the extra time they spent engaged in exercise. Even in terms of endurance benefit, when the researchers performed muscle biopsies and further tests to determine changes in the subjects' fitness levels at the end of the two weeks, these tests showed that the rate at which the subject's muscles were able to absorb oxygen also improved to the same level.[27]

Keep in mind that this study didn't factor the damage caused by endurance training in their analysis, as they were focusing solely on aerobic capacity. In study after study, colleagues like Gibala, McGuff, and Little, along with many others I'll cite throughout this book, consistently come to the same conclusions that I posed to my peers a decade earlier. Less truly is more—once you understand how to best apply the necessary stimuli—even when greater endurance is your goal. But as I'll continue to reveal, endurance should never be your highest goal in fitness training, as your investment into the superior goals of youthful longevity and strength can produce greater endurance as a byproduct.

Likewise, if you've been told that "calorie-burning" endurance, cardio, and aerobics workouts are effective, healthy, or sustainable ways to burn fat, be prepared to learn you've been fed a big fat lie. After completing Chapter 1, refer to the subsection in Chapter 2 titled *Fat Burning, Body Shaping, and Your Metabolism* if you want to get to the bottom of the "calorie-burning" myth before wasting another hour on a hamster wheel. By the time you finish reading this book, you'll fully understand how all of this could possibly be true, and you'll know exactly what to do to get it right.

Less Is More

Not only is our *10 Minute Workout* (also called *The Healer*) extremely efficient and supremely effective, but it finds its greatest success in our ability to embrace *rest* as we take on the far less burdensome BioLogic approach. This opens another set of crucial truths that the fitness industry has long stuffed away in the fine print of their teachings, despite the overwhelming wealth of scientific evidence proving the invaluable nature of resting protocols. Sure, they'll tell you to get proper sleep, and some even teach that recovery has its place. But the majority are so far removed from properly teaching the essential role of rest and recovery *during* your workout and the absolute need for full recuperation between workouts, that their teachings verge on negligence.

In contrast, the latest research proves that the no-sweat qualities of BioLogic Workouts are not merely "sweeteners" but core protocols in the program. Recovery and recuperation (*R&R*) are in fact among the most rewarding disciplines in the BioLogic Method. I'm confident the research will convince you of these much-welcome requirements, and I hope you start getting a taste of the revelation for yourself early on in this book. Once you do, you'll surely want to help tip the scale to reveal this level path to fitness enlightenment.

During the same era that birthed the *CrossFit* craze and the second big running boom, my colleagues around the world who also caught the "less is more" revelation have mostly been ignored by the establishment. Most of these fellow short-duration low-impact advocates also marry biological fact and simple logic to identify the full potential and vulnerabilities of our genetic design. Their clients are among the enlightened few. Though their methods and results may differ, even the most casual among them have proven beneficial and immeasurably safer than the long-duration high-impact approaches the mainstream establishment pushes on their audiences.

We indeed need measured intensity in our exercise, so please don't get the wrong idea. But the bulk of the effort in the BioLogic Method goes to our ability to focus on the proper stimuli, to understand the need for precision protocols, to ensure proper rest and recovery, and to embrace the discipline necessary to stay the course. Once you try it, you'll never turn back from this easily sustainable approach to a stronger, longer life.

Stepping Into the Light

I hope I've provided sufficient evidence of the industry-wide arrogance and ignorance that is pre-aging and literally killing many of the most active enthusiasts while intimidating the masses into settling for dangerously sedentary lives. If by chance you are an endurance runner, a long-duration cardio machine junkie, *CrossFit* fanatic, or practitioner of any other form of long-duration/repetitive strength or endurance exercise on a regular basis, I implore you. At the very least, take a break until you can fully digest and further research the wealth of under-reported revelations my colleagues and I are striving to share. Same goes for those of you who ingest one of the many "miracle" snake-oil supplements on the market. Your heart and body will thank you for it. As the abundance of research has proven, unless you are a rare anomaly (there are always rare exceptions), all of these activities are causing *more harm than good* for even the youngest participants. Knowing the truth could literally save your life—if you take action.

If you can tune out all the mind numbing noise and deceptive visual stimuli and cravings for the endorphin high that these activities are known to trigger, and simply see and hear for yourself with a renewed mind, you should begin to realize how best to care for your body and achieve your highest fitness goals. It simply cannot be overstated. Anything that damages your body will likely lead to irreversible destruction. The risk of permanently damaging (or killing) our bodies should be avoided or minimized in every way possible, no matter how much fun we have, how much euphoria we feel, how much pride we gain, or how much money we make while causing that damage. Unless, of course, you don't mind losing years of youth (and most likely years of life) in exchange for those temporary gains. It doesn't mean you have to totally give up these destructive activities, just as you don't "have to" give up the bad foods identified in *Section III*. But you will need to make significant adjustments if you want to start healing your body rather than destroying it through repeated lengthy beatings or sedentary living.

This exhortation alone should compel you to see the BioLogic revelation as a gift worth unwrapping. Once there, you will find it surprisingly easy to understand the keys to the 10 Minute Workouts and the overwhelming research that proves it to be a true scientific breakthrough. We finally know a level path to total body health and fitness; a liberating truth that—once sown with discipline—can reap sustainable metabolic health, improve physical performance, and defy the aging process. I'm confident that you desire a longer life with more youth, more strength, more beauty, more joy, and more free TIME to do the things that truly matter to you and your loved ones. So let's continue opening these truths and do all we can to spark the revelation in you. Enjoy!

What's Inside the Book

A Note to the Inactive Masses

For those of you who struggle with your weight and health, or don't currently have a consistent health and fitness strategy, be prepared to celebrate—especially if getting started on a path to lasting health is your paramount reason for reading this book. Ten minutes per workout, six sessions every ten to fourteen days, is truly all it takes. You can also gain similar results in a single twenty-minute variation performed once every week or two, or another variation performed just twice per week (variations called *The Once-a-Week'er* and *The Weekender*) if those better fit your schedule. You'll soon see exactly how each variation works, so be prepared for the light bulb to pop on. Even among the most effective fitness programs your friends or family may be enjoying, aside from the very few similar (and virtually unknown) programs developed by my colleagues around the globe, there is nothing else like the BioLogic approach. For most of you, everything you believe about "fitness" is about to change.

I know you have faced many hurdles, and my team and I stand ready to show you the way to overcome each of them. If you stick with the BioLogic program and converse with us in our online forums and social media when needed, you WILL burn unwanted fat and improve your insulin sensitivity. You WILL gain muscle and strength. You WILL improve your health and slow or reverse the aging process. And you WILL feel better in all facets of your being as you enjoy these simple workouts and the freedom they create for the rest of your life. It's a scientific truth that's wired into our DNA, and it is never too late to spark it into action. So forget all the lies. Put aside all the negative thoughts of hopelessness that might attack your peace. And let's get started on your path to a far better life.

What You Will Learn

Before reading the name of this book, did you believe there was even the slightest chance that a 10 minute, no-sweat workout could be scientifically proven to correct your metabolism, shape your body, heal what ails you, and slow the aging process? Whatever your answer, you're reading now, so you obviously want to investigate. Here's what you can expect to learn:

- How the BioLogic Method **burns more fat** and builds more youth sustaining muscle in just ten minutes per no-sweat workout
- How the BioLogic Method enhances **glucose metabolism** to trigger a cascade of benefits across all body systems, including **hormone production** and metabolic processes that slow or halt the aging process while combating disease; including cancer and diabetes
- How our **genetic *fight or flight* design** dictates everything
- The science that explains how most **traditional exercise** and all **endurance exercise** are pre-aging and even killing their enthusiasts before their time
- How ***sustainability*** should direct all your health decisions
- How the ***joy factor*** empowers or undermines all you do
- How the power of ***R&R***—recovery and recuperation—empower the BioLogic Method
- How proper **focus, isolation, and brain power** techniques can change everything
- How BioLogic Workouts can be **tailored to fit any schedule**
- How **proper nutrition that's enjoyable** reigns supreme
- How to establish fun and sustainable **BioLogic active lifestyle strategies**
- How to fully leverage the **power of walking**
- How the **absolute latest scientific research** from the world's most respected scientists, laboratories, and hospitals prove all of the above to be true

I've also developed a new decision-making paradigm to help you identify and accentuate the proper motivating forces you should weigh before partaking in any form of health or aesthetics-enhancing training, treatment, food, drink, or supplement. The paradigm should further prove that BioLogic Workouts are the only workout *everyone* should perform, especially if they continue running or engaging in other high-risk training programs. When properly prioritized, these motivating forces will combine to ensure you reach your long-term fitness, health, and youth-enhancing goals in sustainable, damage-minimizing fashion to reclaim your present ideal.

How to Best Read This Book

The book is divided into four sections. *Section I* deals with the fundamentals and cornerstones of the BioLogic Method. *Section II* breaks down the protocols and techniques of the actual workouts. *Section III* addresses proper BioLogic nutrition and active lifestyle strategies. And the appendix includes two subsections that take unique approaches to exploring the hundreds of peer-reviewed clinical research projects cited in *BioLogic Revelation*. In these subsections you'll find excerpts from many of these published studies and their abstracts. The research represents the work of more than a thousand scientists from around the world, so I encourage you to access these resources if you're inspired to dig deeper into the many scientific topics addressed in this book.

I'm the type of reader who typically flips to the last chapter of a book first, only to read earlier chapters as needed. My appetite for liberating truth is so insatiable that I prefer the bottom line now, free from the hours it takes to sift through the setup chapters that many writers squeeze into their often non-scientific blog-sized topic just to manufacture a book-sized publication. In contrast, the science and recent research studies that support *BioLogic Revelation* would require multiple encyclopedia-sized texts to fully explore, so I hope my atypical approach to delivering the meat of the revelation right up front—free of excessive "geek speak" and complex scientific diagrams—will suit your personal reading style regardless of your background. But again, if you want to conduct your own review of the science and research that explains the effectiveness of the BioLogic Method down to the molecular level, jump to the back of the book.

Conversely, if you want to jump right in to test the BioLogic Workouts, you can skip ahead to *Section II*. If, however, your greatest current need is to develop a healthier lifestyle and a proper nutrition plan, you would benefit from reading *Section III* as soon as possible. But keep in mind that the earlier chapters of *Section I* can prove crucial to truly setting you free from the old lies and to capture the life-changing BioLogic revelation (the "AHA*!*" moment). All that said, I certainly encourage you to read the chapters in sequence if that's your inclination. However you slice it, my goal is to ensure that each topic is delivered in terms that won't require a degree in cellular biology, physiology, nutrition, or sports medicine, while even the most learned among you will still feel challenged and not left wanting for more.

The Hard Part

Even at ten minutes per day (with at least one day of rest per week), there is still a major hurdle in the BioLogic Workout, as is true for everything that matters to life—getting started. And yes, despite its relative ease and emphasis on rest, BioLogic Workouts will still make you sore, especially in your first few weeks; but it will be a deep, isolated soreness you'll learn to crave once you grasp the various metabolic and physiological processes it represents. This precious soreness is the leading indicator that your *10 Minute Workout* hit the mark. If you can simply discipline yourself to stay the course, you will reap a great harvest of healing power and sustainable strength no matter your age. You can do this. Virtually everyone can.

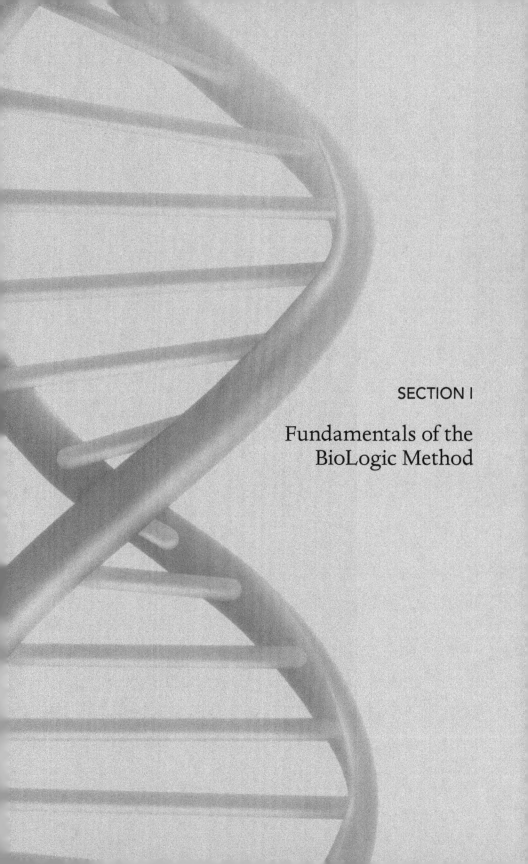

SECTION I

Fundamentals of the BioLogic Method

CHAPTER 1

BioLogic Crash Course: How it Works

> *Therefore, strengthen your feeble arms and weak knees. "Make level paths for your feet," so that the lame may not be disabled, but rather healed.*
>
> — HEBREWS 12:12-13

The Disease of Weakness

In the human body, weakness is the leading symptom of decay and disease. For that, it is also the most common marker of the elderly and the sick. Weakness is, of course, the absence of strength. In its chronic state, it's also the absence of health and youth, which eventually leads to the loss of life itself. Knowing this, we humans would be wise to avoid all things that lead to the weakening of *any* body system, and in turn, develop a realistic plan to counteract all forms of weakness—even more so as we age. It should be simple enough to avoid the easily recognizable weakening of muscle, joints, and bones. But it is far more difficult to diagnose the weakening of your central nervous system, endocrine (hormonal) system, immune system, and body repair mechanisms.

Ignorance of these maladies will unquestionably chip away at your youthfulness and eventually destroy your quality of life and your mental health, typically tearing down your joy and spiritual health along the way. Thus, my repeated warnings against all things that cause *more harm than good*. Protocols that legitimately heal and cure weakness will *never* strengthen one system at the expense (or weakening) of another, and as you learned in the introduction, that sort of weakening is symptomatic of the most popular modes of exercise. In contrast, the BioLogic Method is unique in its ability to stimulate the *BioLogic Cascade* of benefits across all body systems, including those that have been damaged by destructive exercise activities and sedentary lifestyles. For this, the *BioLogic 10 Minute Workout* is also called *The Healer.* Once you give it a try, you'll surely understand why.

A Note to Fitness Enthusiasts

For those of you who are locked into one of the unsustainable *more harm than good* fitness lifestyles detailed in the introduction (and further exposed in the coming chapters), I realize it may be difficult for you to let go. I hope this first chapter will prime your palate for the amazing research I'll share, and maybe you'll be a fast adopter with light bulbs popping on left and right, setting you free from five decades of fitness industry misinformation and vain ignorance. I'm now in my mid-fifties, but when I was in my twenties I was just like you, training hard and looking stronger than most with the endurance to run all day long—but all the while doing *more harm than good.*

I hope the *BioLogic Revelation* will challenge you enthusiasts to begin testing the scientific, time-proven BioLogic Method while weaning off your age-accelerating, destructive training methods before the damage is irreversible. While my primary audience consists of the eighty percent majority who are mostly inactive, I compel enthusiasts like you to read on, as the research shows many of you are in more desperate need of this information than the sedentary majority. Even more, never forget that many of your loved ones, friends, co-workers, church family and others in your community look to you for sound advice—or look at you as a role model. As you have likely realized, most of these folks have concluded they simply cannot or will not ever adhere to your relatively extreme fitness lifestyle. In the end, if you decide the BioLogic approach is not for you, I pray you'll recognize it surely should be for them. Most fitness enthusiasts dismiss the concerns of the majority as the product of laziness, and that's definitely part of the problem. But it may also be that their natural instincts are telling them there is something inherently wrong with the way you exercise and the time you invest into your workouts. For many of the folks I've interviewed, both are true. Whatever the case, I trust you will read on with an open mind, and I hope you join discussion threads in our blog and social media so we can continue this journey of fitness enlightenment together.

What Is the BioLogic Revelation?

The *BioLogic Revelation* is the biologically factual, entirely logical, inspired approach to long-term youth and total body fitness. As detailed in the introduction, the revelation has been proven by thirty years of peer-reviewed research that debunks five decades of fitness expert confusion, body-destroying crazes, gimmicks, gadgets, diet fads, and risky supplements while revealing the simplest, most natural path to holistic wellness. While the revelation first struck me during rehab workouts after one of my many sports injuries, even the most casual reasoning reveals that the metabolic processes responsible for youth and healing have been refined through millennia of adaptations in the human gene pool. One need only consider the *fight or flight* stimuli that shaped modern humankind to understand the broad-ranging implications. For this, BioLogic Workouts are designed to stimulate the muscle fibers most responsible for *fight or flight,* which in the modern era are the very muscle fibers most neglected by couch potatoes or most damaged by the vast majority of training regimens. Applying proper stimuli to these highly specialized muscle fiber types alone can trigger the *BioLogic Cascade* of benefits across each of your body systems, and this profound metabolic cascade reaches well beyond the basic benefits of traditional strength training methods reported by the American Heart Association (as detailed in the introduction).

Once the stimuli are properly applied to these neglected or abused muscle fibers, the *BioLogic Cascade,* in turn, awakens other inter-dependent metabolic processes that in effect have also been stunted, weakened, or damaged. Each life-sustaining process begins to spring back into action, sparking a chain reaction of sorts to perpetuate the cascade through all body systems around the clock—all while burning fat to fuel the healing process—even while you sleep. Many of these neglected metabolic processes are crucial to our ability to sustain youthfulness and to fight diseases like cancer, cardiovascular disease, diabetes, obesity, muscle wasting disease, and the other dreaded disorders that are reaching epidemic levels in our sedentary modern culture.

Every day that passes absent the proper stimuli is another day of potential decay. In addition to the decades of scientific research, the principles that comprise the *BioLogic Revelation* have been well-proven by the lasting results enjoyed by a growing community of doctors, sports medicine professionals, fitness innovators, and their enlightened clients from all demographics. Among these blessed few, the most revealing are the seniors and other folks over fifty (myself included), who after twenty or more years training the BioLogic way, appear and feel ten to twenty years younger than peers who have traveled a different road. But it's never too late to correct your path, no matter your age or current condition. That indeed is very good news.

What Are BioLogic Workouts?

In short, BioLogic Workouts consist of broadly scalable strength building exercises. If you have little to no experience with strength training, many of the following terms might seem like "Greek" to you, but rest assured you'll have a full understanding of these terms before you reach *Section III*. While the exercises and equipment may be common to many of you, the physical and mental protocols that ensure you are effectively stimulating your most neglected muscle fiber types within your largest muscle groups are entirely unique to the BioLogic Method. Even the most avid weightlifters are more than likely neglecting or destroying these fibers. If that's you, don't be fooled by the simplicity of this "short" description. There is far more to this than merely "lifting weights," so please stick with me. The most popular variation of the workout is *The Healer*, and it requires at most four minutes of highly isolated strength exercise spread over each ten-minute session, with resting periods of one to three minutes between each set. This is the variation my wife and I perform most of the year. I know this might sound a bit technical to folks who have never worked out with weights, but I assure you that once you read the book and watch the demonstration videos, it will all seem like child's play. So don't get overwhelmed by any of this "gym talk."

In each *10 Minute Workout* you will typically perform just three sets of a single exercise, using the same weighted resistance for each set. Within each set, you will perform just six to twelve repetitions (reps) per set, and except in rare situations, never more. The weight you use will remain the same for each set and should be approximately seventy-five percent of your single rep maximum for that exercise. This maximum is much simpler to calculate than you may be thinking, so don't get tripped up by the thought of ever having to test this max weight in your workouts. You won't. Each set consists of very simple isolation exercises made effective through the application of four distinct BioLogic Protocols, all of which combine to optimize the stimuli to your *fight or flight* muscle fibers in unprecedented fashion. Though this might sound very "old school" to many weightlifting enthusiasts, there is nothing old about the four protocols. The BioLogic Method simply leverages easily accessible strength exercises to deliver extraordinary stimuli in ways that traditional "old school" protocols can never achieve. The four protocols cover a full spectrum of physical and psychological skills and techniques that you'll seldom if ever see performed in your local gym. And the novices among you will appreciate that the protocols are all so elegant and modest that you'll never have to worry about drawing attention to yourselves.

It's important to know right up front that none of these skills require athletic ability, though it obviously helps speed the learning curve, so please trust that even true beginners can master these protocols after just a handful of workouts. Knowing that the *10 Minute No-Sweat Workout* can actually spark the tremendous cascade of benefits you'll learn in Chapter 2, I hope you can fight the temptation to jump ahead in the book just yet. Even if it's more science than you feel you need, I believe the research will ensure you fully receive the revelation, and thereby commit to this seemingly *too good to be true* workout for the rest of your life.

Fundamentals of the BioLogic Revelation

1. Genetic Design: Enhanced through Fight or Flight

Anthropologists and biologists alike have long recognized that environmental factors, food sources, and other daily survival challenges weeded out the weaklings and promoted the strong in our ancestral gene pool. The human body is wired to survive and thrive when our *fight or flight* muscle fibers are effectively stimulated to fire to their highest potential. So, effectively stimulating (as opposed to abusing) these fibers will trigger the robust health, aesthetic appeal, and youth retention long associated with the most prolific procreators among our ancestors.

The earliest, most fruitful reproducers were the alpha males and females who best survived the trials of life through *survival of the fittest*. They in turn birthed the generations with the fittest genes, thereby establishing our modern gene pool. Fruitful reproduction has always been a primary theme in art and literature, and it also happens to be the very first instruction recorded in Bible. The second instruction is to conquer all the challenges the earth can throw at us, whether environmental or predatorial. It's easy to see that the primary, interconnected purpose of these two missions was well obeyed by our ancient ancestors who survived to reproduce. These alphas had their *fight or flight* muscle fibers stimulated in real hand-to-hand battle or surges of speed to escape attackers and predators—all while engaging in highly physical (and highly intelligent) lifestyles as hunter-gatherers, nomadic shepherds, or farmers. How many of us live up to their lifestyles? Not many.

Even today *survival of the fittest* is a rule of nature, but the path through our ancestors' refining fire hardly exists in our retail, corporate, and industrial wastelands. Thankfully, we no longer have to deal with the daily threats and challenges most of our ancestors faced just a century ago. But our gene pool is still wiring our bodies for *fight or flight* survival, and the metabolic processes that adapted under the same *fight or flight* realities are now dying on the vine, right along with the muscle fiber types that once distinguished the strong from the weak. Absent this *fight or flight* stimuli, we are sending the message to our body systems that we no longer have need for these youth sustaining metabolic processes; so over time they systematically shut down to conserve energy and store more fat. This adaptation to sedentary lifestyles is proving disastrous and helps explain why the average human life expectancy is rising at a snail's pace despite miraculous advancements in medicine and surgery.

We clearly need to identify activities that simulate *fight or flight* stimuli, and as we learned in the introduction, the best ideas cooked up over the past fifty years have proven woefully destructive. Thank God we now know a way to trigger these same alpha responses in our bodies despite lavishing in the comforts of the modern era. That's where the BioLogic revelation comes into play. Just like our alpha ancestors, we also need to apply our intelligence to master our environmental variables and the health of our food supply; but more than ever, we need to avoid sedentary lifestyles if we hope to optimize the *fight or flight* stimuli. You can be sure you'll be fully equipped to tie it all together by the time you finish this book. That said, I strongly encourage you to get started with the actual workouts as soon as possible if you continue with any of the long-duration activities exposed in the introduction. Even professional athletes with rigorous time and energy demands can and should incorporate the BioLogic Method into their training regimen without delay, and many already have—especially those whose professions or sports involve *fight or flight.*

As I continue sharing crucial facts that have been kept from the uninformed masses, I promise to avoid complex geek-speak to ensure you don't get bogged down by continuous complex biology lessons. So please bear with me the few times I use scientific lingo. You most likely already know there are three major types of muscle: cardiac, smooth, and skeletal. But unless you're a true fitness enthusiast you probably don't yet know there are many different skeletal muscle fiber types that bundle together to work as a team, kicking in only when needed for their specialized purposes.

You might recall from high school biology that every muscle fiber is a single muscle cell, so when you see the word "fiber" keep in mind that I'm talking about a single living cell with a highly specialized purpose. While the majority of researchers use scientific terms like type I, type IIa, and type IIx when referencing these skeletal fiber types, most fitness professionals use their common names—*slow twitch, fast twitch, and super fast twitch muscle fibers* respectively. I'll continue to use just these common names throughout the book. Though there is a broad range of fiber types that fit between these three major types to form a broad spectrum from the lowest-order (*slow twitch*) to the highest-order (*super fast twitch*), most researchers group them into three basic fiber categories as *slow twitch, fast twitch,* and *super fast twitch,* and so will I.

2. Super Fast Twitch Muscle Fibers Hold the Keys

Most important to the BioLogic Workouts are the physical and psychological protocols that apply the proper stimuli to your ***fast twitch*** and ***super fast twitch muscle fibers*** (also collectively referred to as *fight or* *flight* muscles throughout the book). These are not the *slow twitch muscle fibers* that power your mundane daily tasks and perform most of the work in endurance running and other forms of long-duration high-stress activities. Due to the principle known as *orderly recruitment,* you cannot fully stimulate your *super fast twitch fibers* until you've already applied more strength or speed stimuli than your *slow twitch* and *fast twitch fibers* can handle.[28] Thus explaining why many fitness enthusiasts can exercise for hours a day yet never effectively train their critically important *fight or flight* muscles—often damaging them beyond repair in the process.[29]

While your *fast twitch fibers* absolutely play a major role in the BioLogic Method, it's important that you focus on stimulating increases in strength and size of the relatively rare, extraordinarily potent *superfast twitch fibers* if you hope to trigger the full *BioLogic Cascade* detailed in Chapter 2. The scientific term for healthy growth of muscle fibers is hypertrophy (the opposite of atrophy), which I'll discuss in detail throughout the book. Before I explain exactly why hypertrophy of these supercells is so crucial to our youthful longevity, let's review why their scarcity should ring an alarm bell.

On average, *slow twitch muscle fibers* make up roughly fifty percent of a healthy human's total muscle mass. The balance consists predominantly of *fast twitch fibers,* while the most important *superfast twitch fibers* round out a relatively small percentage of that balance. As a sedentary couch potato begins to age, their stalwart *slow twitch fibers* hold their ground, but their rare *super fast twitch fibers* atrophy and eventually die—as do their *fast twitch fibers,* albeit at a slower pace. For this, couch potatoes typically suffer with a sixty to seventy percent ratio of *slow twitch* fibers, while the combined number of *fast twitch* and *superfast twitch fibers* take a startling nose dive as they age. This dramatic drop has devastating metabolic consequences. Through continued inactivity, the ratio of *fight or flight* muscle fibers spirals downward over time until these youth-sustaining, disease-fighting fibers comprise just ten to twenty percent (or less) and the lifelong sedentary seniors who suffer this effect tumble toward their premature death. Similarly, those who consistently practice long-duration endurance activities also see their combined *fast twitch* and *superfast twitch fiber* content plummet even before they reach their golden years.

Far more relevant, their invaluable *super fast twitch fibers* all but disappear, while their *fast twitch* partners can dwindle below twenty percent—numbers even lower than those suffered by aging couch potatoes. This startling fact gives a glimpse into the American College of Cardiology's twelve-year mortality study findings (detailed in the introduction) that revealed endurance runners suffer *equal or higher* mortality rates compared to sedentary folks.[30] Conversely, those who have avoided endurance training while applying proper hypertrophy stimuli to their *fight or flight* muscles enjoy the opposite response, often gaining increases in *fast twitch* and invaluable *super fast twitch fibers* to reach as high as seventy-five percent of their total muscle mass.[31]

Fat Burning Warriors: Glycolytic Fibers and the Blood Sugar Burn Factor

While *slow twitch muscle fibers* primarily use oxygen to fuel their comparatively weak contractions, *super fast twitch fibers* stand supreme in their "glycolytic" ability to burn glucose (blood sugar) as fuel, starting with the glucose they uniquely store in relatively high quantities within their cells in the form of glycogen. In comparison, though lower-order *fast twitch fibers* also store and burn varying amounts of glucose as fuel, they're far less efficient than their *super fast twitch* counterparts. *Fast twitch fibers* are blended, as they have both *slow twitch* and *super fast twitch* properties and thereby also use oxygen to fuel their contractions. Knowing that our *fast twitch* and *super fast twitch cells* are major storehouses for excess blood sugar (second only to our liver) should speak loudly to anyone concerned about obesity or diabetes; especially once you consider that *slow twitch cells* are grossly inferior where storing and burning glucose is concerned.

As I'll continue to detail with great emphasis throughout *Section I*, your ability to efficiently burn blood sugar enhances your fat-burning metabolism. It also plays a leading role in catalyzing the amazing *BioLogic Cascade* of vital metabolic processes through all your body systems, including improved resting metabolic rate and proper hormone production and hormonal balance. For this, the BioLogic Method is designed to capitalize on *orderly recruitment* to minimize the work performed by *slow twitch fibers* while optimizing *super fast twitch fiber* stimuli. To put it in the most practical terms, when you're endurance training or performing other long-duration exercise routines, your muscle cells are primarily burning oxygen for fuel. When you're performing BioLogic short-duration workouts, your muscle cells are primarily burning blood sugar for fuel. Yes, both burn recently consumed calories, but as this book exposes in great detail, calorie burn during intense exercise is shockingly low and is in effect a red herring that leads to much of the confusion that keeps enthusiasts overtraining. Ask yourself, would you prefer to invest an hour burning primarily inhaled oxygen during your workout, or would you rather invest just ten minutes while burning stored blood sugar? Once you clear your mind of all the confusion, unless you're a professional athlete, surely you'd choose the latter, and save the high-volume oxygen burning for daily life and recreational activities, yes? If not, read on and I'm sure you'll change your mind.

The Best Kept Secret: How Skeletal Muscles Really Work

If you want to combat aging and premature decay, your total muscle mass should comprise about half of your body weight, yet most adults in their thirties have already fallen far below that mark due to atrophy and cell death from neglect or abuse. Unless you are among the enlightened few, you've suffered more than your share of health-diminishing muscle atrophy in direct correlation to your age and are thereby speeding yourself toward a premature death. You'd think the fact that your heart is made of muscle would be a clue, but alas. For this, I need to hammer home the following process, as it is without question the overarching mechanism that establishes the physical and psychological protocols of the BioLogic Method.

Due to *orderly recruitment,* where actual mechanical work is concerned, your muscle fibers contract in sequence according to the order of their respective roles. These roles range from the low-strength, low-speed, high-endurance *slow twitch fibers* at the bottom of the hierarchy, to the high-strength, high-speed, low-endurance *super fast twitch fibers* at the top. For a more practical perspective, in everything you do, whether rising from your bed in the morning to pushing a broken-down car off the road, these fiber types kick in only when they're needed for their specialized purposes. So your *fast twitch* and *super fast twitch fibers* (your *fight or flight* muscles) will hardly participate unless an activity requires unusually high levels of strength or speed.[32] Sadly, neither of these is a common need for sedentary folks or long-duration endurance trainers.

Now that you have an adequate grasp of the roles of each fiber type, please note that, while the speed names for the various fiber types do in fact indicate the speed of their contractions, it's far more relevant to identify their name with the speed at which they fatigue while being used. *Slow twitch muscle fibers* fatigue much slower than their faster twitching companions. They move you through all of your daily activities—everything from getting out of bed and getting dressed to walking (and sitting) through your day to brushing your teeth at night—all with great endurance even if you never work out. *Slow twitch fibers* alone are designed to resist fatigue (and their own cellular aging) efficiently enough to keep simple activities moving you into your senior years without fail. They're also the skeletal fibers least in danger of premature death from overuse and the least in need of training. Make sure you highlight that fact.

When you exercise for long-durations, *slow twitchers* are performing the majority of the work, but sadly they're far and away the least capable of burning fat or blood sugar. And as previously discussed, they're even less capable of empowering you in a *fight or flight* crisis—even when that fight is against disease or serious injury. Knowing that their primary fuel is oxygen, it should be obvious that *slow twitch muscle fibers* burn calories at a terribly ineffective rate. And far worse, they will eventually turn first to burn muscle as fuel when calories in your blood become scarce—not fat as you've likely been misled to believe. Conversely, your *super fast twitch fibers* have two major jobs. They step up like Superman when great power is needed, and they burn relatively large quantities of blood sugar as fuel. Both of these activities add significantly to your youthfulness and your ability to survive disease and other threats, so it stands to reason that you should optimize their health and development in every way possible. This is why effective hypertrophy of *super fast twitch fibers* is the primary goal of the BioLogic Method, and therefore the primary trigger for the *BioLogic Cascade* of benefits—including fat burning and increased metabolic efficiency around the clock.

As you read on, you'll see that the latest research supporting the *BioLogic Revelation* is exceptionally encouraging. Thanks to the biological process of *orderly recruitment,* ensuring that you maximize the proper stimuli to your *super fast twitch muscle fibers* should be your highest fitness goal, no matter your age, and you don't even need to break a sweat to make it happen. This is the best-kept secret in fitness.

Keeping Superman Alive

While most *old school* approaches to strength training can still preserve and build the middle-of-the-spectrum *fast twitch fibers*, most enthusiasts tend to over-train their most important muscle fibers. So they too are sacrificing their highest-order *super fast twitch fibers* in exchange for more mass in their slower, weaker, far more numerous lower-order muscle fibers. This is yet another fact the fitness industry is tamping down, as most traditional bodybuilders enjoy the extra bulk this sort of over-training triggers in both their *slow twitchers* and their lower-order *fast twitchers*. For this, most are simply unaware of the premature death sentence they're in danger of signing for their super-human, blood-sugar scorching, *super fast twitch fibers*.[33]

Now factor in the unfortunate reality that *super fast twitch fibers* are programmed to progressively die off as we age, especially if we don't use them according to their design. Their wasting directly correlates with our own age-accelerated march toward death, thereby in large part explaining why most folks over sixty have lost any semblance of youthful muscle mass, especially if they spent their lives running or training for excessively long-durations.[34] These facts should greatly motivate endurance enthusiasts to immediately start reversing the destruction. Bodybuilders and *old school* strength trainers are in a *far* better position, but they also need to pause long enough to learn how to maximize their *super fast twitch fibers* in a sustainable fashion before returning to the gym. If that's you, I'll be sharing new research that demonstrates the phenomenal potential for dramatic *super fast twitch fiber* gains (in both strength and size) stored up in your *fast twitch fibers*, so you'll definitely want to stick with me.

Please don't miss the following crucial points, as they're well worth emphasis and review. Our invaluable *fast twitch* and *super fast twitch muscle fibers* can only perform for short bursts before fatiguing and failing due to exhaustion and depletion of their glycogen stores. Once they fail, they are immediately in danger of being burned as fuel and forever destroyed if you continue to burden them, especially your super-human *super fast twitch fibers*. Those of you who are endurance athletes aren't enjoying any of the advantages being gained by bodybuilders, as you are destroying both types of fast-fatiguing fibers to a devastating degree.

If you've been tracking with me since the beginning of this chapter, you surely realize you're losing more than shapeliness and strength; you're also losing the *fight or flight* muscle fibers that are the very tip of the sword in the battle against aging. In 2002, a landmark study published in the *Journal of Medicine & Science in Sports & Exercise* rocked the fitness world, yet the findings have at best been treated as an urban legend by the mainstream fitness media. The study revealed that by the time lifelong strength training enthusiasts reach the age of eighty-five, they are still as powerful as healthy sixty-five-year-olds who don't strength train. The report concluded their findings "would therefore represent an apparent age advantage of approximately twenty years for the weightlifters."[35]

My colleagues and I were preaching this *too good to be true* message a full decade before the report was published, yet in all likelihood, it has never reached your ears. And if it has, someone you trusted probably discounted it for reasons of their own, or else you surely would have taken tangible steps to start cashing in on that extra twenty years by now, yes? We never know when we'll need super-strength or super-speed in *fight or flight* situations, including fights to repel and overcome disease and injury. For this alone we should make every effort to avoid losing our ability to call on our "Superman" muscle fibers to save the day—even at the age of eighty-five.

The Lobby, the Hallway, and the Golden Door

Metaphorically speaking, the effective application of the *super fast twitch* stimuli that activates hypertrophy is similar to opening a golden door at the end of a hallway that is lined with doors to the full spectrum of lower-order *fast twitch fibers*. Very few fitness activities require sufficient time in this hallway, let alone ever reaching the golden door at the end of the hall. In the *BioLogic 10 Minute Workout*, we make a beeline to that door, and along the way we quickly open all the other doors before knocking on the golden *super fast twitch* door at the end of the hall. This is the goal of the BioLogic Method, as your lower-order *fast twitch muscle fibers* receive their proper stimuli along the way to opening that final golden door. Once there, it takes less than ten seconds to apply the proper stimuli, at which time all the "work" in the BioLogic workout for that muscle group is complete.

As you'll soon learn in detail, many strength training enthusiasts spend most of their time over-laboring in this hallway, often kicking down the *super fast twitch* door until it no longer functions as designed. Likewise, the inactive masses and nearly all endurance or aerobics enthusiasts spend most of their lives dawdling in the outer lobby (the *slow twitch fibers* in our metaphor), only occasionally touching the doors in the hallway while never even getting close to the golden door at the end of the hall. For most lobby dwellers, that final door gets smaller and smaller over time, until it eventually disappears. My goal is to get you out of that couch-filled lobby and move you quickly through the hallway to open the door to *super fast twitch* stimuli before you lose another fiber. The lobby, the hallway, and the golden door reveal the pathway that is *orderly recruitment.*[36] If by chance this metaphor confused those of you who are new to fitness, please don't ever forget that this journey takes just ten minutes of no-sweat effort per workout. I promise that by the time you finish reading *Section I* you'll know exactly why every man and woman alive needs to catch this revelation.

As alluded to above, where endurance training and other long-duration activities target your *slow twitch fibers,* they also diminish your critically important *super fast twitch fibers,* thus stunting or damaging many of your youth-sustaining metabolic processes. If you read the introduction, it should be no surprise why the mainstream fitness industry has failed to proliferate these extremely important facts despite the concerted efforts of the scientific community and the world's top fitness researchers. These experts have long touted the youth-preserving potential locked away in these fascinating *super fast twitch* powerhouses, but the average man on the street would never know it.

Consider these profoundly revealing facts. Not only do your *super fast twitch fibers* burn far more glucose per fiber than their lower-order *fast twitch* brethren, but they also deliver two times as much power in strength and speed in their response to *fight or flight* stimuli. Far more extraordinary, your *super fast twitch fibers* deliver a whopping *ten times* more strength and speed than your *slow twitchers*. Surely these superhuman *fight or flight* supercells don't exist just to sit by idly until they/we die. It's high time for you, your friends, and your family to learn about the miraculous potential waiting to burst forth from your *super fast twitch muscle cells,* as many of my colleagues and our students already have. If you've ever seen a senior citizen with the strength, vigor, and body of a person far younger than their years, they are surely practicing many of the protocols you will learn in this book. The more you read, the more clearly you'll see how every man and woman alive should immediately start practicing *BioLogic 10 Minute Workouts*.

When combined with a more active lifestyle (especially less sitting and more walking!) and proper nutrition (add the good, eliminate the bad), the BioLogic approach will prove fruitful no matter where you stand today. These active lifestyle and proper nutrition components of the BioLogic approach are common to nearly all fitness programs, so I'm confident you're aware of their overarching necessity. For that, I'll refer to this necessity as *The Great Requirement* going forward. As I proceed with this crash course, let's uncover the most valuable research that the establishment has been keeping hidden away.

Atrophy Versus Hypertrophy

To put it bluntly, if you lack healthy *fast twitch* and *super fast twitch muscle fibers* that enjoy a purpose filled life of flexing, glucose burning, healing, and growing stronger (hypertrophy, which by now you know is necessary for optimal longevity) you are in effect aging at an accelerated rate as your muscles atrophy and die day after day. And as logic would dictate, this sort of premature aging can and likely will lead to your premature demise. Please don't ignore that fact, and ask yourself why you don't hear it more often. The healthiest among us trigger the metabolic process of muscle hypertrophy on their *fast twitch* and *super fast twitch muscle fibers,* which is the enhancement of muscle composition, strength, and health. As previously noted, muscle hypertrophy is the opposite of muscle atrophy, and I'm sure most of you already know that atrophy is the leading symptom of muscle decay and death.

When you see a picture of an anorexic person or the tragic photos of starved Holocaust victims clinging to life, you are seeing palpable evidence. As we proceed, you are going to hear a lot about hypertrophy of your *fast twitch* and *super fast twitch muscle fibers*. Though I'm committed to speaking in simple terms throughout the book, hypertrophy is probably the most important scientific term for you to retain. After all, you probably already knew the definition of the negative term "atrophy," so isn't it revealing that most of you have never been taught its positive antonym? Let's change that trend. Muscle hypertrophy in your most important fibers is marked by increases in two characteristics. First is the increase in actual fiber size, which is possible for all fiber types. Second is the increase in glucose (blood sugar) storage in the form of glycogen, which is virtually impossible for *slow twitch fibers*. Glucose storage occurs in progressively larger quantities across the fiber type spectrum until we reach the *super fast twitch fibers* that can store the greatest quantities. As you'll soon learn in detail, this sort of glycogen storage provides the primary fuel for the BioLogic Method, thereby establishing *super fast twitch muscle fiber* hypertrophy as the key that turns on the amazing *BioLogic Cascade* of health benefits.

Metabolic Fat-Burning Catalysts

I know many of you are reading this book with high hopes that *BioLogic 10 Minute Workouts* might finally help you burn away your excess fat and speed up your metabolism without having to sweat through hours of pain and drudgery every week, so fear not. Your hopes have brought you to the right place. The fast fatiguing, *fast twitch* and *super fast twitch muscle fibers* are without a doubt your highly specialized fat-burning catalysts. In fact, properly stimulating these *fight or flight* muscle fibers is the most effective physical activity for ramping up much-needed insulin sensitivity in the fight against obesity and diabetes. With 10% of Americans suffering from the debilitating age accelerator that is diabetes, this alone should close any doubts you may have about getting started today. For that, these most basic effects of *fast twitch* and *super fast twitch muscle* training go well beyond the desirous aesthetic benefits (less fat, more lean muscle mass).

In 2011, award-winning research scientist Dr. Nathan LeBrasseur and his team at the Mayo Clinic found that the crucial link between glycolytic muscle fibers and insulin sensitivity proved that muscle hypertrophy is a key trigger *"in the powerful and complex cross-talk between metabolically active tissues."* This speaks directly to the scientific bases of the logical processes that drive the full *BioLogic Cascade* of benefits detailed in Chapter 2. In Dr. LeBrasseur's findings published in the *American Journal of Physiology, Endocrinology and Metabolism*, he wrote:

> Collectively, these data suggest that even modest increases in skeletal muscle mass, the growth of [fast and super fast twitch] glycolytic fibers and modest changes in glycolytic capacity can have remarkable effects on metabolic homeostasis. They also suggest that interventions targeting skeletal muscle may directly or indirectly alter the metabolic profile of other organs affected by insulin resistance and [type 2 diabetes]. It is now evident that skeletal muscle is a key node in the powerful and complex cross-talk between metabolically active tissues . . . In view of the coordinated responses of muscle, liver, adipose tissue [body fat], and the vasculature highlighted in these models, it is likely that 1) increasing skeletal muscle mass will have favorable effects on affected tissues of [type 2 diabetes] and cardiovascular disease; and 2) a network of hormonal communication exists between muscle and other metabolically important organs . . . Although a growing body of experimental evidence suggests that resistance training improves metabolic homeostasis in a manner distinct from endurance training, our understanding of how this precisely occurs is rudimentary.[37]

Let's make sure we don't gloss over the revelatory points of these groundbreaking findings, as they point directly to the table-flipping truths the fitness industry has long ignored. Even modest increases in your *fast* and *super fast twitch muscle fibers* will spark positive changes in your glycolytic capacity. This, in turn, delivers remarkably favorable changes in your metabolism while combating diabetes and obesity. It is now evident that your fastest twitching fibers are a key node in the powerful and complex cross-talk that prompts favorable effects on every metabolically active system in your body, including your endocrine system (your hormones). Be reminded that just a few minutes of proper training can trigger far more than modest increases in your glycolytic muscle fibers, using no-sweat methods that are free of all the life-threatening risks exposed in the introduction. Knowing this, can you see why "the powers that be" are working so hard to hide this revelation from the masses?

When I first read Dr. LeBrasseur's research, I thanked God for such a succinct scientific explanation of what I call the BioLogic Method and the resulting physiological processes that trigger the *BioLogic Cascade*. We now know that *super fast twitch muscle fiber* hypertrophy should be the preeminent goal of all exercise, thanks to the unrivaled glycolytic (blood sugar burning) capacity of these fibers, as this burn factor is a *key node* in the chain reaction of metabolic processes found at the very top of this amazing cascade. Once you consider the reality that both *fast twitch* and *super fast twitch fibers* progressively die off as we age—especially if we ignore or abuse them—you should feel a sense of urgency to start applying the proper life-sustaining stimuli as soon as possible. The wasting of these precious glycolytic muscle fibers directly correlates with our age-accelerated march toward death, so please make sure you're catching the implications of Dr. LeBrasseur's findings. The dramatic decay of invaluable glycolytic muscle fibers reveals why most folks over sixty have lost any semblance of youthful muscle mass and are especially vulnerable to the dreaded diseases noted above, and further identified throughout the first two chapters of this book.

While Dr. LeBrasseur has revealed much about the metabolic benefits of *fast* and *super fast twitch* strength training (hypertrophy), don't let it escape you that his Mayo Clinic team's findings indicate that these hypertrophy protocols should be prescribed to all who suffer from cardiovascular disease as well. Conversely, the study ensures that readers realize the same cannot be said of endurance training. With heart health being the primary reason most people engage in running and other endurance activities, that's quite an indictment. But as you'll soon see, the good doctor was being very conservative. Over the next half decade, the scientific community stepped up to substantiate his conclusions in overwhelming fashion, with not a single dissenting opinion to be found. You can refer to the research in the Appendix for a wealth of evidence, but I'll be sure to highlight the most compelling research as we continue.

Through this crash course, I hope you are beginning to see that the proper stimulation of your powerhouse *super fast twitch fibers* is not merely an easy alternative approach to aesthetic fitness, but is in fact the primary physical catalyst for a profound cascade of metabolic and hormonal enhancements. As the research reveals, these boosts in turn can heal and restore youth to all of our vital body systems through stimuli that take mere seconds to apply. Talk about a revelation! These are just a few of the truths that the mainstream fitness industry is either too busy to see, or simply doesn't want you to know. Let's hope this book opens their eyes, and their mouths.

We All Have a Gland Problem

While some of us suffer from endocrine system disorders for various genetic and environmental reasons, our hormone-producing glands generally get a bad rap as the culprit behind every fitness and weight management failure known to man. Many fitness professionals are quick to claim that their favored type of exercise will help counter some of these shortcomings, and a small percentage of them are right. Unfortunately, the majority reserve their discussions of hormone levels to serve as the primary excuse to explain why all the hours, weeks, and months of long-duration training failed to help their clients lose weight or gain muscle at a rate commensurate with the time invested. But as we've already discussed, their training protocols are among the primary culprits.

Aside from the *Great Requirement* of proper nutrition and a more active lifestyle (which includes effective management of environmental variables, see *Section III*), nothing naturally empowers you to overcome critical hormone deficiencies and correct hormone imbalances better than *fast twitch* and *super fast twitch fiber* hypertrophy.[38] This is especially true when following the short-duration, high focus protocols you'll perform in BioLogic Workouts. While the earliest research scientists were all over the map concerning exercise-induced natural hormone optimization, as demonstrated by Dr. Nathan LeBrasseur's Mayo Clinic study (noted above), the preponderance of new research reveals an undeniable correlation between proper hormone production and *fast twitch* and *super fast twitch muscle* hypertrophy. Now we know the same stimuli that give life to our *fight or flight* muscles also burns the most blood sugar (and fat) to increase insulin sensitivity. Likewise, these same stimuli also trigger proper production of the hormones that regulate your resting metabolism, tissue function, sexual function, sleep, mood, speed of healing, immune system, and the all-important youth-sustaining hormone commonly called HGH (human growth hormone, or somatotropin); just as logic would dictate.

Though I could dive deep into the cause and effect for all the hormones enhanced through proper stimuli, I'll center on HGH as a case in point. Being one of the master hormones, HGH typically garners the most attention for its popular use (or abuse) by celebrities, top athletes, and anyone in the social elite who can afford synthetic replacement therapy. Much like your muscle mass, your natural production (bioactive production) of HGH begins to drop dramatically after the age of thirty; and most people over forty can readily attest that this drop-off coincides with the onset of a wide range of aging symptoms, both aesthetic and health-related.

While this unfortunate effect of the aging process has become common knowledge, the discovery that effective stimulation of *fast twitch* and *super fast twitch muscle fibers* boosts natural HGH production to more youthful levels (minus the potentially life-threatening side effects associated with synthetic injection therapies) has been widely ignored by all but a small minority of my peers. Though a gradual reduction in HGH production is normal, as previously noted, most people stop producing HGH to a detrimental degree once they enter their mid-thirties. This is due in large part to the neglect of glycolytic muscle fibers, and the combined effect greatly accelerates aging (decay) of all vital body systems.

To put it all in the simplest terms, if you're not sending the necessary stimuli to your body in accordance with your *fight or flight* design, by default you're telling your body that anti-aging and longevity are not real needs, so your body responds accordingly. For further evidence that our bodies cannot sustain substantive benefits from endurance exercise or aerobics training, consider this. In 2014 a team of scientists representing three American universities published a study in the *Official Journal of the Growth Hormone Research Society* that concluded not only that resistance training enhanced HGH bioactivity, but also that aerobic exercise inhibited HGH bioactivity.[39] If these findings don't immediately unnerve those of you who are endurance and aerobics enthusiasts, I believe that by the time you finish reading *Section I*, the alarm bell will ring loudly.

If you're over sixty but never developed a consistent strength training regimen, please don't despair. While there is much evidence to prove that those of us who began strength training earlier in life have long enjoyed enhanced HGH levels, in 2015 the *Journal of Aging and Physical Activity* published a study that revealed hypertrophic resistance training can stimulate growth hormone increases regardless of age.[40] And if by chance you've been told that endurance workouts can accomplish these same hormonal improvements, don't believe it. If all the negatives of endurance training exposed thus far haven't proven enough to make you pause, then consider this. A 2010 study published in the *Journal of the Growth Hormone Research Society* concurred that HGH and related hormone concentrations are significantly increased by short-duration hypertrophic muscle training, while no such increases can be associated with high-volume endurance training.[41] But even if the research wasn't so compelling and bountiful, doesn't simple observation prove their findings to be exceedingly obvious? It does for any honest fitness professional. I hope you're starting to see why the *BioLogic 10 Minute Workouts* are far more than an easy way around long, sweaty workouts. Less truly is more, once you understand human design and how all the systems in our bodies are in fact interdependent.

The Muscle Stem Cell Phenomenon

Now that you likely have a fair grasp of the fundamentals of *BioLogic Revelation*, let's take a look at an especially important biological fact that many of you will be learning for the first time. Most fitness professionals (and medical doctors for that matter) don't even know how to properly discuss this topic, let alone teach it with a legitimate understanding of its urgent health and anti-aging implications. Of all the truths I've revealed so far, I hope you've locked in on the fact that the most important actionable component of the BioLogic revelation is our need to activate and extend the lives of our highly vulnerable, limited-lifespan *super fast twitch muscle fiber cells*. If so, you should also have recognized that reducing the volume of work heaped upon their highly durable, longer lifespan *slow twitch* counterparts is integral to that mission. Please lock in on those facts as you read on.[42]

You've likely heard about the prodigious capabilities of embryonic stem cells and their highly controversial use. It's less likely that you know about the extraordinary adult stem cells that are found dormant throughout the body, including our muscles, where they are also called satellite cells or myosatellites. They're also referred to as myonuclei once they enter an existing fiber or generate a muscle fiber of their own. These quiescent satellite cells act as an incredibly dynamic talent pool of sorts, as they literally hang around in our muscle bundles waiting for a reason to spring to life, and—even more fascinating—for their specific assignment within their host muscle fibers *if* ever called upon.

It is that "if" that creates the urgency to get started with BioLogic Workouts as soon as possible, for these invaluable stem cells become more difficult to activate with age,[43] and will eventually die if they're ignored. While research into the harvesting of adult stem cells for a variety of cures is non-controversial and well under way, I find it shocking that the fitness industry finds no reason (or courage?) to discuss the extraordinary capabilities of our invaluable muscle stem cells. I'm even more disturbed that most fail to discuss the destructive effects that over-training and endurance exercise has on these precious pearls. After all, we're talking about stem cells . . . in our muscles . . . waiting to be harvested or "assigned" to perform a life-extending role that they alone can serve.

Muscle stem cell harvesting is a major facet of the BioLogic revelation, so please pay special attention whenever they're mentioned throughout the book. Though they were first discovered in 1961,[44] only recently have scientists begun to publish clinical studies touting their miraculous healing abilities. As you might imagine, now that the previously noted studies are reaching the scientific community at large, new research confirming the virtually supernatural behavior of these myosatellites is finally trickling in. In January of 2016, the *Journal of Experimental Biology* published what I consider to be a definitive review of the muscle stem cell phenomenon. In the publication, the respected research biologist Dr. Kristian Gundersen recommended that every adult should begin strength training early in life to ensure maximum myosatellite harvesting, and suggested that the critical importance of these cells should be widely discussed as "matter of public health."[45] Such a call to public arms is the mark of a true scientific breakthrough, yet have you received this "public health advice" from your government or the major media? Your doctor or personal trainer? I'll bet not a word.

Your satellite cells cling to your muscle fibers in great numbers, and are hanging around for three basic reasons. First, they repair muscle damage. Second, they will replace muscle fibers lost due to severe injuries. Third, they enhance the role (power and activity) of muscle fibers that are subjected to consistent hypertrophy. From our perspective, these satellite cells are standing ready to supercharge the strength and speed of the muscle cells responsible for *fight or flight* survival—our *fast twitch and super fast twitch fibers.* But if their host fibers are neglected, these myosatellites will atrophy or downgrade for mundane *slow twitch fiber* support. If this neglect continues they'll eventually die, never to fulfill the highest purpose of their amazing design. So unless you train your muscles through protocols that effectively stimulate your *fast* and *super fast twitch fibers,* you are wasting (or killing) the super-human stem cells that would otherwise sustain and optimize your *fight or flight* capacities and trigger the *BioLogic Cascade* of benefits well into your senior years.

This, to me, is one of the greatest biological discoveries of the modern era; yet only a handful of scientists and writers are celebrating this "super" human potential. When properly stimulated, these satellite cells repair and rejuvenate our muscle fibers. Upon receiving proper stimuli they will move like an army to infuse themselves into the individual muscle fibers that they have clung to in large pools for the entirety of their dormant lives. Consider that for a second. You probably didn't realize a single muscle cell could contain many nuclei. But once you spark hypertrophy through consistent low-volume, highly-focused stimuli (the BioLogic Method), you can activate these satellite cells to fuse into their host fiber cell as a response to meet and exceed the increased demands. To revisit the metaphor of *the lobby, the hallway, and the golden door,* this is the highest achievement upon entering the golden room behind that final door. The more myosatellites that are recruited into each *super fast twitch fiber,* the more powerful and invulnerable that fiber becomes, as these additional myonuclei team up to exponentially empower each and every fiber involved. Amazing.

Even more awe-inspiring, research has shown that once recruited, these myonuclei will maintain their role within their host fiber for fifteen years or more—possibly even on a permanent basis—even if the fiber is never again stimulated.[46] This is the actual, biological explanation of "muscle memory," a phenomenon that most folks consider to be a pie-in-the-sky myth. Among fitness experts who teach muscle memory, you'll hear most talk about it in metaphorical terms. You'll hear that it's merely a mental placebo effect enjoyed by those who brainwash themselves into accelerating their strength gains through a purely psychological event; as if harkening to earlier days of hard training gives us the mental capacity to regain strength and muscle hypertrophy earned and lost years earlier. Others teach that muscle memory is the result of neural adaptations and motor skill learning, driven primarily by our brains. While both theories have merit in discussions about our ability to adapt to various physical skills more quickly after long layoffs, neither reveals the science of muscle memory as it occurs in our muscle fibers. Only satellite cell activation can explain that effect, as every myosatellite you recruit today is an investment in your fiber strength (and muscle memory) in the future.

To underscore the importance of this phenomenon, please note that satellite cells typically die when their host muscle fibers die.[47] So just like the *fast* and *super fast twitch fibers* to which they cling, if you don't use them you lose them, forever. But as noted above, once you properly stimulate these *fight or flight* muscle fibers to activate and recruit their respective pools of satellite cells, they will remain alive in that fiber indefinitely (even if you never strength train again). Also, they will work together to extend the life of that fiber, ready and waiting to spring back into action when *fight or flight* stimuli are again applied.[48] If you consider all this phenomenon implies, you should quickly catch the revelation. The sooner you recruit these myosatellites through proper and consistent hypertrophy of your *fast twitch* and *super fast twitch muscle fibers,* the more of these satellite stem cells you'll retain well into your senior years, and the longer your *fight or flight* muscles will live on to trigger the full *BioLogic Cascade*—even if you stop training for years at a time. Amazing! See Figure 1 for Dr. Gundersen's simple model that shows how the invaluable muscle stem cell harvesting works.

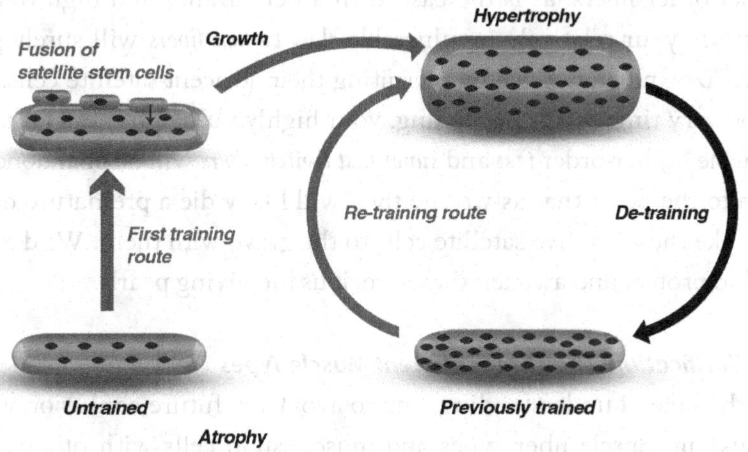

Figure 1: Gundersen's satellite stem cell fusion and muscle memory diagram (reproduction)

I personally take a week or two off every season, but I don't recommend you taking month-long breaks unless necessary, especially if you're over forty or fighting obesity or some other disease. So please don't miss the greater point. The sooner you start training with BioLogic Workouts, the more of these precious pearls you'll activate and retain to extend or regain your youthful health well into your golden years, and the more equipped you'll be to battle major injuries or diseases that might require prolonged bed rest or inactivity. So even if you continue with your body-abusing lifestyle (I hope I'm only speaking to professional athletes who have no choice), taking ten minutes per day to apply the proper stimuli will counter some of your ongoing damage while also "banking" on a more youthful future once your body-beating days are over.

You'll soon learn more about how these satellite cell pools are in fact a literal fountain of youth for your *fast twitch* and *super fast twitch fibers*. You will also learn that the same effect occurs when you stimulate your lower-order fibers, though in their case (absent effective hypertrophy stimuli to their faster twitching counterparts) virtually none of the cascade benefits detailed in Chapter 2 will be triggered.[49] But hypertrophy of your lower-order fibers *will* give you a more muscular waistline and thicker ankles, if that's your thing.

When you over-train your *slow twitch muscles* and neglect your higher-order fibers (as is the case with all endurance and high-volume exercise), your relatively invulnerable *slow twitch fibers* will surely gain some size and endurance by recruiting their adjacent satellite cells. But at the very time this is happening, your highly vulnerable and far more valuable higher-order *fast* and *super fast twitch fibers* will be abandoned—even to the point that as we age they will likely die a premature death and take their inactive satellite cells to the grave with them. We'd all do well to protect and awaken these precious life-giving pearls.

For Clarification: The Three Different Muscle Types

For the sake of understanding, and to avoid any future confusion when discussing muscle fiber types and muscle stem cells with others, let's take a quick look at the three very different muscle types that exist in the human body.

1. **Involuntary smooth muscle:** Found in our organ walls, these muscles run on autopilot (aren't controlled by your conscious mind) to keep our organ systems operating around the clock.
2. **Involuntary cardiac muscle:** Similar to smooth muscle, this most-specialized muscle type of all powers the non-stop beating of our hearts.
3. **Voluntary skeletal muscle:** These most common muscles are the object of our discussions concerning muscles and muscle stem cells. These muscles power our physical movements and determine our physical strength and speed. They are comprised of the *slow twitch*, *fast twitch*, and *super fast twitch fibers* that are the primary "clay" of the BioLogic Method.

Be reminded that every muscle fiber is an individual muscle cell, so you will see the terms "fiber" and "cell" used interchangeably throughout the book. While skeletal muscle stem cells (myosatellites) have been known as the source of emergency muscle repair and optimal fiber hypertrophy for more than half a century, evidence of cardiac stem cells (resident in the heart) wasn't proposed until 2003.[50] Research into these highly specialized stem cells (along with their smooth muscle counterparts) is robust, and though this research is all over the map and still considered controversial, no such doubts exist concerning our prodigious skeletal muscle stem cells.[51] While discussions of the various adult stem cells is without question a compelling and important effort, it's beyond the scope of this book; but we'll be sure to spark discussions about these non-skeletal pearls in future texts and online discussion threads as continued research warrants. For a deeper study of satellite muscle stem cells, be sure to review the wealth of published, peer-reviewed research I've outlined in the categorized research section of the Appendix, but let's continue discussing these pearls in straight language.

CHAPTER 2

The BioLogic Cascade of Benefits

The Waterfall of Cascades

Once you learn how to properly and consistently stimulate your *fast twitch* and *super fast twitch muscle fibers* absent destructive forces, you will begin the amazing *BioLogic Cascade* of benefits across all your body systems—corrections that will trigger positive changes in your body composition and produce new found youthful vigor. As you've likely surmised, the BioLogic Method actually triggers many interdependent cascades with their own sub-cascades. Most are metabolic enhancements that take place the moment the stimuli spark your *super fast twitch fibers* to burn the glucose stored in their cells. Others are secondary cascades that stem from the actual physical effect the workout has on cell health within your major structural systems.

Each of these is a basic metabolic process our bodies are genetically designed to perform for survival, and most people are neglecting each to dangerous degrees. Such negligence stunts the activity of your endocrine system and thwarts the release of crucial youth-sustaining hormones. This "master breakdown" plays a major role in the subsequent collapse or pre-aging of your fat-burning metabolism, and nearly all other metabolic processes that are genetically predisposed to perpetually replenish, heal, and fuel the full waterfall of cascades had the chain reaction of stimuli been put into proper motion. Since greater strength and a better body are the most obvious benefits of BioLogic Workouts, I'll save those discussions for later chapters and get on with the benefits that fight disease and systemic breakdown to extend your life. For summary purposes, the top level cascades can be grouped into the following five categories. Each represents several lower-order cascades that I'll further detail in this chapter and throughout the book:

- Immediate strengthening of our muscular, skeletal, and central nervous systems
- Immediate enhanced activity in our blood sugar (glucose) metabolism
- Optimal production of crucial youth-sustaining hormones
- Enhanced fat-burning metabolism and reduced fat storage
- Optimal health of our cardiovascular system

Many fitness gurus claim to target *fast twitch muscle fibers* within portions of their workout program and thereby claim many of these same benefits. However, the BioLogic Method is unique in its development of highly engaging, energizing, and logical isolation techniques and recuperation protocols that greatly enhance the key *super fast twitch* stimuli and the subsequent harvesting of their satellite muscle stem cells. In contrast to other short-duration no-sweat fitness programs on the market, the BioLogic Method is not merely a "better than nothing" approach to fitness, but instead has been proven to be more effective in delivering its promises than anything else being taught, especially for the masses who simply don't enjoy working out.

Let's take a survey of the unrivaled benefits of the *BioLogic Cascade* and debunk a few myths along the way. Please don't just skim over these benefits. I'll start out with the benefits that you're most likely hoping for, and I'll wrap up with a few that should blow you away. You will be hard pressed to find a single alternative approach that can legitimately claim even half of these scientifically proven life-extending benefits. Several are so amazing that you'll wonder how on earth you're just now learning of them. Enjoy!

Fat Burning, Body Shaping, and Your Metabolism

In short, the more *fast twitch* and *super fast twitch muscle fibers* you have, the better your body composition, the higher your resting metabolic rate, and the more stored fat you burn twenty-four hours per day, seven days per week, even while you sleep. These are typically the initial concerns for most people seeking an effective workout. Once a BioLogic 10 Minute workout is complete and our hearts are still racing, our blood-sugar metabolism is immediately put into action as the glycolytic fibers strive to replace their burned glucose stores and begin the healing process. This of course immediately improves insulin sensitivity and the overall hormonal response. This instant response is a highly taxing event on calories in the blood stream (what we call "afterburn"), and—far more important—sustained practice will spark a marked increase in our fat-burning metabolism to fuel this cascading effect around the clock. Over time, through hypertrophy, muscles grow according to their genetic design, and (if you've corrected your food intake) excess fat stores are reduced to a degree that the major muscles begin to dictate the visible shape of your body. Revisit your visual of the sprinter/dancer to be reminded where you'll be headed.

On the other hand, long-duration, high-volume exercise primarily targets *slow twitch fibers* and other lower order fibers that store little-to-no glucose and primarily burn oxygen to fuel their contractions. So, though these long-duration workouts indeed get your heart pumping (to what many researchers have determined a dangerous degree) and burn recently consumed calories, once the activity ends there isn't a whole lot of metabolic activity required to wind down. *Slow twitch fibers* are genetically predisposed to handle prolonged workloads with very low energy requirements, and the burned oxygen is easily replaced once we inhale it back into the bloodstream, so you'll be hard-pressed to find any "afterburn" here. Likewise, relatively few favorable metabolic processes have been triggered, and as you now well know, our bodies and critical life systems are often left worse for wear.[52]

Before moving on to my overview of what I consider the more amazing benefits of the *BioLogic Cascade,* we need to clear up a couple of especially destructive myths concerning calorie-burning and it's role (or lack thereof) in fat-burning. Similar to running and other forms of endurance exercise—though they have their uses—treadmills, steppers, stationary bikes, and other "cardio" equipment do not burn fat or calories the way most of you have been told. The same goes for the plethora of sweaty, long-duration "aerobics" workouts. Unless they're employed for short-duration interval training (see HIIT in Chapter 1), they simply cause *more harm than good* to your invaluable *fight or flight* muscles and other body systems. Though cardio machines can play a minor role in your effort to achieve a more active lifestyle (see *Section III*), they're far removed from their mythical fat-burning and calorie-burning claims. For clarification, in reference to the aforementioned *Great Requirement* of proper nutrition and a more active lifestyle, it is "proper nutrition" that plays the lead role in the reduction of stored fat, not the "more active lifestyle" component. Increased activity is far more important to our efforts to counter structural decay and the diseases detailed in the Introduction (see *Speaking of Emperors: Get off Your Throne*), not the modest increases daily calorie-burning as you may have assumed. All we need is to apply some basic logic and simple math to see why this is true. As we proceed, don't be ashamed if you've been duped into believing that cardio or aerobic training burns enough calories to effectively or efficiently burn stored fat during your workout in a sustainable, beneficial fashion.[52] It simply isn't true.

Myth: A good measure of an effective and sustainable fat-burning fitness program is the number of "calories burned" during each workout.
Truth: The number of calories you burn during a workout is virtually meaningless.

Those of us involved in fitness research groan every time we hear that medieval calorie-burning distortion of fact being further perpetuated. So if you do nothing else, please refrain from being misled into that hamster wheel ever again. In reality, most calorie-burning cardio or aerobic workouts performed in effort to burn stored fat do exactly the opposite over time, as they neglect your blood-sugar burning *fight or flight* fibers, and—as detailed above—almost exclusively employ your oxygen-burning *slow twitch muscle fibers* to perform the work. For that, as discussed in Chapter 1, these long-duration workouts lead to atrophy and eventual death of your invaluable *fast twitch* and *super fast twitch muscle fibers*—the obesity-fighting fibers that are most responsible for increasing your resting metabolic rate (and, more important, your insulin sensitivity), 24/7. Never forget that we can't effectively train our *fast twitch* and *super fast twitch muscle fibers* during a long duration cardio or aerobic workout. And when you don't ever use them, you most definitely lose them. Don't let anyone tell you otherwise.

If someone you know swears that consistent cardio training has helped them lose significant fat stores, odds are that the real reason for the weight loss or size reduction was a dramatic correction in their diet and (or) a tragic loss in muscle mass. Similarly, many of the folks I've met who believe cardio or other endurance training played a major role in their weight or size loss had not only corrected their eating habits, but had also begun strength training. Those combined lifestyle changes get the credit for any sustainable improvements, not their cardio work.[53] This psychological switcheroo is similar to the response you'll hear from folks who get duped into buying one of the many miracle snake oil supplements on the market. They've been convinced that the supplements were the reason for their improved health when it was actually the dramatic changes they made to their diet and lifestyle that were the true heroes. Yet even those improvements can be lost if they fail to properly train their highest order muscle fibers or ever revert back to old habits.

It's very important to realize that the calories you burn during a workout come primarily from the food you most recently consumed. If those fresh calories are fully burned away, only then will your body begin any form of extra-calorie burning, and sadly, our genetic design dictates that we consume unused muscle mass before consuming fat stores. Be reminded that food abundance is a modern day phenomenon, and our often-starving ancestors (who developed our gene pool over the millennia) needed stored fat to survive frequent food shortages and outright famine. And since sedentary muscle is metabolically expensive to carry, our genetics are programmed to burn it up well before dipping into our famine-fighting fat stores. For this, our bodies are wired to stockpile much more fat than muscle. Look around for mounting proof.

Let's consider a practical application of this reality. Consider a man who consumes 3500 calories per day and a woman who consumes about 2500 calories per day. Many consume well beyond those numbers, even in a single meal, but let's do the math with those numbers to keep it simple. Please remember that everything you do, including sitting on a couch all day or running on a treadmill for an hour, will require calorie burn. Hypothetically speaking, if the man and woman in our application burn seventy-five percent of their freshly consumed calories by living an average life, that would leave a daily surplus of 875 calories for the man and 625 calories for the woman. Most of these surplus calories will be stored as fat if not somehow burned as fuel. If they choose to use cardio machines, running, or walking as their primary means to burn this surplus, they'll most likely fall short in their effort to burn these newly consumed calories, let alone ever burn any stored fat. A full hour of these activities performed at an average rate will burn somewhere between 200 and 500 calories. Every remaining calorie will be stored as fat, so please do the math. Sure, they could stay at it for another hour or two in effort to burn even more of their daily surplus calories. But don't forget that once they burn the calories readily available in the bloodstream, their bodies will tend to protect their fat stores and look elsewhere for fuel.

Even if they could somehow trick their bodies to first go after the stored fat during that extended workout, consider that just one pound of fat consists of a whopping 3500 calories. If they're burning a relatively high 500 calories per hour, once they finally burn their calorie surplus, it would take them an additional seven hours of exercise in that single workout to burn just one pound of fat.[54] But again, that's NOT how a healthy body burns stored fat. Yet that's exactly what many of the folks who pound down the streets for miles every day have been led to believe. It's insane. Any "certified" weight loss expert who teaches otherwise is still living in the eighties. For those of us involved with real research, this particular form of fitness industry misinformation is unconscionable. Sadly, despite all the time lost and damage done, when a runner or cardio junkie loses one or two pounds after a workout, it's mostly water loss that they'll regain as soon as they rehydrate.

All that said, there is in fact a type of person that can actually enter the "fat burning zone" during an extended cardio, aerobic, or other type of high-volume endurance workout: those who have so restricted their caloric intake and stayed on this destructive cardio path for so long that they've burned up all their *fight or flight* muscle mass, along with all other tissues that their bodies deemed expendable. So, once they burn through their minor calorie surplus, they start burning stored fat right there in the moment as they crank along. And though they will typically enjoy a season or two where they truly "look" fit in the mirror, these folks have in effect headed down a path to anorexia nervosa. Many in fact would already be diagnosed with the disorder if they were to visit a physician, even while looking fairly healthy, but these folks seldom seek wise counsel. In my days as a health club owner back in the nineties, my staffs and I had to conduct more interventions to save the lives of these types of individuals than I want to remember. Think about that. I've actually had to trick members of my "health" clubs into joining me in my office where one of my fitness directors and a friend or family member (if we could locate one) were laying in wait to plead with them to seek professional help and end their "cardio" obsession before it literally killed them. Even today when I walk into a large gym loaded with cardio machines, I often see many headed down that horrifying path. Most are women. If you know someone who fits this description, please intervene. Or at very least alert their loved ones before it's too late.

Again, remember your visual of the gaunt marathon runner discussed in the introduction. Do you see any quantities of youth-sustaining muscle on their frail physiques? Not much. The high-calorie demand of their extreme training tricks their body systems into feeling starved, which in effect puts their body into famine survival mode where their combined metabolic processes desperately attempt to conserve fat at all cost, not to burn it. That's a truly sad irony. This is the same phenomenon that occurs when you starve your body through crash diets. You might temporarily lose a few pounds, but you are programming your body to store even more fat as soon as the "crash famine" is over. Are you starting to see the futility in using cardio or aerobic exercise as your primary fat burning activity? All you're doing is encouraging greater fat storage while destroying the muscle fibers most responsible for curbing excessive fat. For this, many of you would be better off taking a one hour nap than running on a treadmill for that hour, especially if you're performing *BioLogic 10 Minute No-Sweat Workouts*.

Myth: Exercise in itself burns significant amounts of fat as fuel for that exercise.
Truth: Fat is effectively burned only through sustained metabolic processes.

As I wrap up this very important subject, it's essential to realize you should never exercise with the mindset that your primary goal is to burn calories or fat, but rather to train in a way that converts your body into a 24/7 fat-burning machine. Since this can only be sustained through effective hypertrophic strength training (following the principles that comprise the BioLogic Method), it's equally important to realize most strength training programs are nearly as ineffective and unsustainable as endurance programs. So don't let anyone convince you that all weight lifting is the same. Consider our *CrossFit* discussion in the introduction for the most revealing evidence. More on this topic later.

Beware of the "No Pain, No Gain" Lie

This topic is both a benefit and a myth-buster that leverages a lot of the same science and logic detailed above. To ensure that you didn't miss the health components built into this time-redeeming benefit, let's take a more scientific look. If your main goal is to burn fat, then you must train your metabolism-enhancing muscles in a very specific, sustainable fashion. As previously discussed, the problem with most of the hyped-up strength training regimens being peddled today is their tendency to over-train muscles to the point they stunt your metabolism boosting cascade rather than enhance it, while often producing *"a similar physiological stress response to [an endurance running program]."*[55] This is true even if we begin to look more muscular and lean over the short term. So if that's you, please realize you're burning your fat in a far less efficient fashion and enjoying aesthetic gains that are far less sustainable than you think, and the potentially irreversible damage you're risking goes far beyond your body composition.[56] Most strength training enthusiasts have twisted the truth within the "no pain, no gain" concept and have over-blown it into an especially dangerous untruth. Yes, pain can fill a positive role, but this is not one of those cases. For many bodybuilders and body shaping enthusiasts, their painful overuse abuse can completely destroy their *super fast twitch muscle fibers* in exchange for hypertrophy in their far more numerous, far less efficient *slow twitch fibers* and other lower-order counterparts.[57] Please be reminded that your calorie consuming, blood sugar burning, *super fast twitch muscle fibers* are TEN TIMES more powerful than your *slow twitch fibers* that primarily use zero-calorie oxygen to fuel their contractions.

Knowing this, you've got to wonder how so many people are being duped into training their low power, low burn, *pedestrian* muscles in a way that destroys their high burn *super-human* muscles. Craziness.

Even worse, research has shown that these long-duration strength programs can damage your heart and other vital body systems to the same devastating degree suffered by endurance runners. In fact, the *American Journal of Hypertension* published a University of Texas study that showed these workouts increase arterial stiffness and aortic wave reflection in young healthy women, and cited a wealth of research that proves the same destructive effect is true for young men.[58] If overtraining with weights can stiffen your aorta just as it does for endurance runners, what else is being damaged? Only time and more research will tell. But all indicators reveal that too much of any form of activity causes *more harm than good* for all systems in your body.

The truth is, many long-duration strength training enthusiasts could have achieved sustainable results and a lasting boost to their resting metabolic rate, had they simply known when to cut their workout short and start allowing their muscles to recover before burning them up. Talk about diminishing returns! During my decade as a competitive sprinter, football player, and "no pain, no gain" weightlifting junkie, I was among the misinformed masses. So I empathize with those of you who are still living that life, and I have the memories from those glory days and the irreversible joint damage to prove it. If you're still a competitive athlete, I've developed reductionist protocols that will help you continue incorporating these high-risk activities in a way that both minimizes the damage and improves your performance, despite cutting back on the abuse. It's just another extraordinary example of the healing power of the BioLogic approach.

Optimal Hormone Stimulation

Though I briefly covered this topic in Chapter 1, this subject holds such a high degree of preeminence that I need to share a bit more research to ensure it doesn't fall victim to the establishment's efforts to silence the alarm bells. If there's anything about the BioLogic revelation that I fear you'll fail to properly retain, it's this awesome all-encompassing benefit. You probably already know that hormones regulate virtually every biological process in your body. Yes, that includes your metabolism, your stress levels, your brain activity, the rate at which you age, your sex drive, etc., etc.—everything. Aside from strict control of our diet and our environment, how do you think we can best maintain proper hormone balance? We do this through effective short-duration hypertrophy strength training and sufficient rest before, during, and after each workout, all while avoiding high-volume, high-stress exercise. Yes, the BioLogic Method.

In a key study conducted in 2009 by a team of scientists at the Neuromuscular Laboratory at Appalachian State University, researchers compared alternate long-duration training methods to short-duration BioLogic-style hypertrophy resistance training protocols. In their study, the "hypertrophy" test involved just four short weight lifting sets with ninety seconds of rest between each set, using seventy-five percent of their maximum weight (which likely took about twelve minutes to perform). Then the scientists compared the hormonal response to that of two other long-duration (high-volume), more highly intense tests. No surprise to me and my colleagues, the researchers' conclusions read like a physiological definition of the BioLogic Method:

> These data indicate that significant acute increases in hormone concentrations are limited to hypertrophy type protocols independent of the volume of work completed. In addition, it appears the hypertrophy protocol also elicits a unique pattern of muscle activity as well. Resistance exercise protocols of varying intensity and rest periods elicit strikingly different acute neuroendocrine responses which indicate a unique physiological stimulus.[59]

Put in simpler terms, the Neuromuscular Laboratory team's findings demonstrate that the hypertrophy protocols of the BioLogic Method are unique in their ability to stimulate "acute increases in hormone concentrations," and that quantity of work (time investment) is virtually irrelevant. BioLogic Workouts are designed specifically to spark this "unique physiological stimulus" through the most efficient and sustainable hypertrophy protocols possible. This unique stimulus sparks remarkable neuroendocrine responses across every system in our bodies, and is therefore a major facet of the BioLogic revelation.

If you didn't catch this in Chapter 1, BioLogic Workouts produce this stimulus by following very specific protocols and techniques across just three sets, consisting of six to twelve repetitions, using about seventy-five percent of your maximum strength for that exercise. Each set also requires one to three minutes of rest before moving on to the next. Through sheer coincidence, the researchers tested the *BioLogic 10 Minute Workout*, albeit with an extraneous fourth set, which they concluded was unnecessary due to the virtual irrelevance of volume of work. Please trust this Appalachian State University study was conducted entirely independent of any influence from my colleagues or me.

As we proceed, it's important to note that not all research is equally reliable. There are companies that pay millions for studies like the one cited above, and many pressure the researchers to emphasize the bits of their findings that support their product or cause. In contrast, I go to great lengths to cite only independent research projects, and will spend far more time in this book detailing clinically controlled peer-reviewed findings over my two decades of real-world observations, especially when dealing with all-important hormone issues. This sort of vetting has become easier every year, as a wealth of new research has shown that of all the varied approaches to strength and speed training, those that follow the hypertrophy protocols inherent to the BioLogic Method best trigger the optimal balance of your most important hormones. This includes adrenaline (for *fight or flight*) and Human Growth Hormone (HGH, which you should recall is in effect human "youth" hormone), as well as testosterone in men, and a full "cocktail" of crucial hormones[59] that together ensure greater health and longevity for women and men of all ages.

Even more, when properly performed, the BioLogic exercises that target your *super fast twitch muscle fibers* reign supreme in their ability to *increase the production* of the master hormones, especially HGH, well after most people have lost their mojo. As mentioned in Chapter 1, please be aware that most adults stop producing HGH in quantities sufficient to prolong youthfulness somewhere between the ages of twenty-five and thirty-five (roughly a fifteen percent reduction in HGH). Far more alarming, by the age of fifty-five, HGH production drops to a scary twenty percent of youthful levels (an eighty percent reduction).

Logic would say that HGH deficiency is a precursor to death, and the scientific community is in full agreement, as ever-increasing volumes of research from around the globe have been proving this tragic reality for more than a decade. One such study used unambiguous language to ensure that the gravity of this epidemic could not be missed, though the establishment and major media have continued to ignore the alarm bells. In a 2013 study published in the journal *Frontiers in Endocrinology*, a team of scientists representing major universities in Washington, Florida, Massachusetts, California, Virginia and Japan together concluded:

> Deficiency of growth hormone in adults results in a syndrome characterized by decreased muscle mass and exercise capacity, increased visceral fat, impaired quality of life, unfavorable alterations in lipid profile and markers of cardiovascular risk, decrease in bone mass and integrity, and **increased mortality.**[61]

Notice the direct link between "decreased muscle mass and exercise capacity" and "increased visceral fat" with the host of life-threatening symptoms brought on by HGH deficiency. This is a classic example of the bio-loop that exists between hypertrophic strength training and proper hormone production. If you're not stimulating the cascade to fight aging, your neglect of this critically important loop is speeding you to a premature demise. Take a long look at most seniors and you'll see more than enough evidence. Is hypertrophic training of your *fight or flight* muscle fibers the proverbial fountain of youth? The evidence leaves little room for doubt.

Insulin Sensitivity and the Fight Against Diabetes

While I've already discussed the "top of the cascade" importance of blood sugar burning and the resulting increases in insulin sensitivity enjoyed by those who practice the BioLogic Method, I want to ensure the reduced risk of type 2 diabetes is not lost among the more glamorous benefits of fat-burning and body shaping. If by chance you skipped over Chapter 1, this would be a good time to go back and read the section on Dr. Nathan LeBrasseur's landmark research published with his team at the

Mayo Clinic. Those of you who suffer or have a family member who suffers from diabetes or morbid obesity already know the crucial role of *insulin sensitivity* in muscles and the critical importance of flushing excess glucose and insulin out of your bloodstream.

With one in ten of us likely to be struck by this debilitating disease at some point in our lives, it's worth repeating the glucose/insulin relationship for proper emphasis. Please recall that your *fast twitch* and *super fast twitch muscles* are second only to your liver as primary storehouses for glucose, as it is stored in these highest order muscle cells (in the form of glycogen) to serve as instant fuel when called upon for *fight or flight* situations. This is where the BioLogic approach triggers one of the most beautiful harmonies between our body systems. Not only does BioLogic training burn those glucose stores for fuel in an extraordinarily efficient manner, but, as previously noted, it also triggers the release of a full cocktail of youth-preserving hormones. This elusive bio-loop (which is entirely neglected by most adults) exponentially increases our power and speed and draws very large amounts of glycogen out of the muscle cells, regardless of your age.[62]

This amazing enhancement of your *glucose metabolism,* in turn, clears the way for blood sugar to be filtered out of your bloodstream to replenish even larger stores in your *fast twitch cells* and far more so in your *super fast twitch cells.* This is a cycle that enhances insulin sensitivity and corrects insulin production to optimal levels while eliminating or greatly reducing the extreme fat storage that occurs absent this cycle. When you have low insulin sensitivity, as is nearly inevitable if you fail to properly train your glucose burning (glycolytic) *fight or flight muscle fibers,* you put your glucose metabolism in danger. The increased insulin in your blood stream literally blocks the proper release of the all-important anti-aging hormones, HGH included.

Your doctor may tell you that the effort to increase your insulin sensitivity is one of the primary reasons you need to exercise, but have they ever told you that this goal can only be optimally achieved through effective hypertrophy training of your *fast* and *super fast twitch muscle fibers*? Or have they told you that endurance training and most other forms of exercise can eventually block or stunt this cycle? Probably not, as the pharmaceutical industry has kept most doctors too busy pushing their pills to find the time to keep up with the latest anti-drug research. If you are ever in doubt, be sure to survey the categorized research section in the Appendix for a wealth of concurring evidence from the world's most respected medical research experts. Diabetes and obesity are becoming global pandemics, and we should all do everything in our power to ensure the truth finally reaches the front lines of the battle.

Glucose Metabolism and the Fight Against Cancer

You should already know that every man, woman, and child alive should cut ALL non-naturally occurring sugar from our diets; but it appears that Americans are more consumed by consumption than we are concerned about self-inflicted disease. As we'll discuss in *Section III*, while the human body without question needs naturally occurring sugar, the quantities most Americans consume and push on their children is unconscionable.[63] Though the diabetes and obesity epidemics have failed to snap most of us out of our illicit love affair with sugar and simple carbohydrates, maybe "the C word" will do their bidding.

In my family, we call the "white stuff" poison, and with every passing year, new research proves that's not hyperbole. As we learned from the Mayo Clinic study cited above, our glucose metabolism (blood sugar burning metabolism) affects the health of virtually every cell in our bodies. Scientists around the globe have been sounding the alarm concerning the likely connection between sugar and cancer for many years. But in the absence of definitive research at the highest level indicating a direct link between dietary sugar and the most deadly cancers, the media and their high-sugar advertising partners have tiptoed around the subject. Then came 2016, when three independent studies by three of the most reputable cancer research teams ever assembled identified those direct links, and the major media response was nearly nonexistent.

Most recently, the *Journal of the National Cancer Institute* published a study by a team from Harvard University led by Dr. Susanna Larsson of the University of Cambridge (and the Institute of Environmental Medicine in Stockholm, Sweden) that identified a direct link between sweetened beverages and gallbladder cancer.[64] Just weeks earlier, a team of six scientists from the highly respected M. D. Anderson Cancer Center at the University of Texas identified a direct link between high glucose levels and lung cancer.[65] But most alarming of all was the freshly inked landmark study published in the journal of *Cancer Research*. Conducted by a team of eight scientists also at M. D. Anderson, the study noted that a number of preceding *"Epidemiologic studies have shown that dietary sugar intake has a significant impact on the development of breast cancer,"* while concluding that *"dietary sugar [increases the] risks of breast cancer development and metastasis."*[66]

It's clearly time we stop waiting for the media and the government to wake us up to the facts about the sugar plague. Rather than destroying or deactivating the very muscle fibers designed to maintain a healthy glucose metabolism, we should be strengthening and developing them to fight disease, yes? As one who has lost several beloved family and friends to this dreaded disease, including my mother-in-law at far too young an age (while writing this book), I had to pause to dry my eyes while typing this section. If you find yourself wondering why I'm so emotionally driven to share the BioLogic revelation, please reflect on this chapter in its entirety, but especially this section. If we can turn from our ways to see with our eyes and hear with our ears, we can be healed.

Heart Health and the Cardiovascular Effect

When I touched on this topic in the introduction, I could hear some of you saying, "Okay, that's all fine and dandy, but can a *10 Minute No-Sweat Workout* really train my heart?" or simply, "What about 'cardiovascular' fitness?" I'm glad you asked. First, let's agree that heart health is best defined by a heart that can perform with strength well into your senior years. Any other definition is skewed or short-sighted. Your heart's primary job is to keep you alive as long as possible.

From my perspective, cardiovascular endurance is best measured by maximum aerobic capacity, also called VO2max. Believe it or not, that's a metabolic strength issue, not an endurance issue. *Fast twitch* and *super fast twitch* muscle hypertrophy can significantly enhance endurance and stimulate our lower-order (*slow twitch*) muscles to greater health. But endurance training can never stimulate the highest order (*super fast twitch*) muscles, so they cannot trigger hypertrophy in these muscles nor enhance their glycolytic and *fight or flight* capabilities. While this refocusing on the actual results of endurance vs. strength should have revealed that hypertrophy strength training is superior to endurance training in nearly every way, please note that the latest research reveals a parallel phenomenon is true of our heart health as well. There has been a lot of confusion and misinformation put out there by so-called "aerobics" gurus, running enthusiasts, cardiovascular machine manufacturers, and the health clubs that invest tens of thousands on profitable treadmills and steppers, so we'll be sure to help you separate the fiction from the little fact that remains. The truth is, you're always training your cardiovascular (heart/lung) system 24/7, so there is no need to focus on your heart's endurance (which does nothing to significantly enhance its strength).

Heart strength is trained with far better effect—especially where the health of other body systems and longevity is concerned— through short-duration, highly-focused, relatively intense training, as compared to any of the hamster wheel methods that the *old school* gurus have touted for far too long.[67] There has been a virtual tidal wave of new research this decade that should prove beyond any reasonable doubt that the traditional methods of stimulating heart health are both dangerous (as already well documented) and vastly inferior to short-duration, rest-infused interval training programs like BioLogic Workouts. Again, refer to the categorized research in the Appendix for a wealth of clinical studies, including excerpts from their respective peer-reviewed conclusions.

A Quick Look at HIIT

There are several popular short-duration "speed" interval training methods that also target *fast twitch fibers,* and they're generally categorized as *high-intensity interval training* (HIIT or HIT) programs. Together, the various HIIT programs have produced tens of thousands of success stories, and my colleagues and I applaud them. Though few involve strength exercises similar to BioLogic's, the goals are mostly the same, but the differences are significant. Where BioLogic Workouts involve sets of isolated muscle strength bursts in non-variable exercises, most HIIT workouts involve intervals of total body speed bursts using highly variable exercises. Likewise, where BioLogic Workouts are sweat-free by design, most HIIT workouts are developed with sweat in mind. It's important to remember that our *super fast twitch muscle fibers* have two mechanical purposes, to generate short bursts of maximum strength, and to generate short bursts of maximum speed. That's why I refer to them as our *fight or flight* muscles. If you can truly generate a maximum speed stimuli (your personal maximum, not the max speed of others), you can also spark hypertrophy in your speedy fibers (recall our visual of the sprinter).

In that most important respect, HIIT practitioners are our like-minded peers. At the same time, multiple studies have recently shown HIIT enthusiasts would benefit from adding BioLogic styled strength exercises to their regimen.[68] Some are calling this merger high-intensity *interval resistance training*, or HIIRT.[69] Not a great marketing acronym, but it works. When I add track sprints to my workout, I basically practice HIIRT in reverse. All that said, HIIT enthusiasts might understand why the vast majority of adults I've surveyed find it far easier to attempt bursts of maximum strength than bursts of maximum speed, so prolonged sustainability is another challenge for many HIIT exercises.

I still enjoy sweat-inducing speed intervals in various exercises, (not the sweat, just the exercise), but my early sports injuries bar me from practicing each of them more than once per week, at best. Even if you don't deal with injury limitations, maximum speed stimuli are far more difficult to apply than maximum strength stimuli. And measuring quantifiable performance gains (the capstone protocol in the BioLogic Method) is often impossible with HIIT exercises.

In my personal observations across 30 years as a fitness professional, I've found that folks who solely practice speed intervals appear to fall short of their goals where muscle hypertrophy is concerned, but more studies are needed before I would draw any conclusions. The track sprinting routine I've developed teaches how to sprint according to our design (most of my students are competitive athletes), and it's an especially effective hypertrophy workout that can be classified as HIIT. But there are several added risks to running sprint intervals and other HIIT speed workouts, so we have to take great care when rapidly propelling ourselves (and our joints and spine) to the edge of our limitations. Ultimately, most of you HIIT enthusiasts already strength train as a supplement, so I hope you'll be fast adopters of the BioLogic "high-intensity interval" workouts.

To continue with the subject of heart health, in a landmark research paper published in the February 2016 *Journal of Heart, Lung, and Circulation,* a team of scientists conducted ten independent studies at six different hospitals involving 472 coronary artery disease patients. Their findings were indisputable. In their conclusion, the authors revealed that short-duration, high-intensity interval training improves peak aerobic capacity in patients with coronary artery disease more effectively than long-duration, steady-state training.[70] Don't let that escape you. If this paradigm shift is true for heart disease patients, how much truer is it for those of us who are hoping to avoid that dreaded disease? Amazing.

For me, even if the study showed short-duration training *equal* to long-duration training, I'd obviously choose the shorter program. My time is invaluable, as I assume is yours. But when proper short-duration exercise is found to be *more* beneficial to your heart health than traditional hamster wheel training, that's something to celebrate. Once again, less is more. For those who might be thinking speed training intervals on cardio equipment should be more beneficial to heart health than strength training intervals with weights, not so. In their book *Body by Science,* McGuff and Little explain in the simplest terms how this mini-paradox is true.

> Your heart and lungs cannot tell whether you're working your muscles intensely for thirty seconds on a stationary bike or working them intensely on a leg press. The heart and lungs know only about energy requirements, which they dutifully attempt to meet. Four thirty-second intervals of high-intensity muscular exertion is four thirty-second intervals of high-intensity muscular exertion, whether that takes place exclusively in the lower body, as in stationary cycling, or in both the upper and lower body, as in resistance exercise. In either scenario, it is mechanical work by muscles that is the passkey to the aerobic and other metabolic machinery within the body's cells.[71]

Nearly every promise of greater health and body shaping the fitness industry touted during the eighties to promote the supremacy of "aerobics" and other long-duration "cardio" training has been proven dead wrong in the twenty-first century, and it shouldn't take a physiology degree to understand why. As I'll continue to underscore, traditional sweat-inducing, long-duration cardio training has its benefits. But now that you see that the scientific community is trending toward discounting the best of these benefits—due in large part to the potentially devastating harms already detailed—I find it very difficult to edify anything about endurance training, except for competitive endurance athletes, that is.

I personally have never run a mile in my adult life, nor have I ever participated in any form of so-called aerobic or long-duration cardiovascular training program of any sort, yet my resting heart rate hovers around fifty beats per minute and my blood pressure has been approximately 110/70 for more than fifteen years. I can walk or hike or cycle for hours without tiring, and I'm seldom quick to lose my breath when playing tennis or other high-intensity sports, all thanks to my consistent use of the BioLogic Method.

If for competition reasons you're looking to improve your endurance in a particular sport, I recommend *BioLogic Interval Training* workouts that incorporate sprinting or sprint cycling (see Chapter 6). These will get you where you want to go without all the excessive damage. Many scientists and health professionals believe that the human heart can only sustain so many beats in a lifetime. While there is empirical evidence to support this theory, basic logic also plays a role. I take great care to avoid burning up the only "candle" I have, and so should you. Yes, if you've been sitting on a couch all your life you can in fact increase many aspects of your current heart health through steady-state endurance training. But as you'll continue to see throughout the book, the risks that these *more harm than good* methods bring to your heart—even more so over the long run—can be life threatening. Be assured no such risks exist with BioLogic-styled strength workouts. Refer to the categorized research in The Appendix for more than thirty sources and excerpts supporting these conclusions.

Significant Reduction in Blood Pressure

In 2015 the American Heart Association (AHA) presented their strongest-ever plea that every person begin a strength training program as soon as possible. In their article, titled "Can Strength Training Help with Blood Pressure?" the AHA wrote:

> Studies have reported several benefits of resistance training—or weight training—including strengthening of bones, muscles and connective tissues (tendons and ligaments). Additionally, weight training may lower your risk of injury. And increased muscle mass may make it easier for you to burn calories and maintain a healthy weight. You'll feel better and stronger and want to do more . . . Researchers reported that only four weeks of [strength training] exercises resulted in a 10 percent drop in both blood pressure measures. Aerobic exercise, however, has shown [at best a 5% reduction in both measures]. [72]

That's a strong, overarching exhortation for an article about blood pressure. We are simply designed to grow stronger, not weaker, and that can only be accomplished through hypertrophy strength training. Speaking of common measures of heart health, I could easily add another full section on the cholesterol reducing effects of strength training. By now that benefit is well known, so I won't belabor that point here. The media and medical community have done a (rare) fair job of publicizing that nearly all forms of exercise to reduce cholesterol levels, though few can do it to a greater degree than a proper hypertrophic strength training program like BioLogic.

Optimal Harvesting of Muscle Stem Cells

As you'll recall from Chapter 1, when it comes to increasing the overall percentage of our *super fast twitch muscle cells* in a sustainable fashion, only our satellite muscle stem cells can deliver. Of course the *Great Requirement* of proper nutrition and a more active lifestyle must have its due, but it can be argued that the harvesting of these invaluable pearls is the single most important benefit of the *BioLogic Cascade.* Two of the leading experts on the subject, Dr. J. L. Andersen and Dr. P. Aagaard of the Institute of Sports Medicine at the University of Copenhagen, were among the first to publish this now widely accepted revelation. In their 2010 landmark study published in the *Scandinavian Journal of Medicine & Science in Sports*, the team concluded that the two primary processes leading to hypertrophy are, *"(1) increase in muscle protein synthesis and (2) [muscle] satellite cell proliferation.*"[73] So for those of you who might still be struggling with the logic behind claims of greater muscle hypertrophy through less work, this should be your tipping point. You've been led to believe strength and muscle gains (hypertrophy) are caused by increased protein synthesis and high-volume, high-pain exercise. But as you're surely starting to see, you've been fed a half-truth to support a massive lie. Protein is absolutely needed to grow your muscles. As you know, that's *mostly* what they're made of. But what have you been told about the crucial role of muscle stem cell harvesting to extend the life of those muscles? Virtually nothing, I'm sure.

While serious muscle trauma (loss of muscle from external injuries or prolonged illness) will instantly call these stem cells (myosatellites) in to repair and replacement mode, the harvesting of large numbers of these super-charging myonuclei into a single *super fast twitch muscle cell* can only be accomplished through optimal *fight or flight* hypertrophy training followed by prolonged recovery and recuperation.[74] The more *super fast twitch fibers* you supercharge through this type of hypertrophy harvesting, the more age-defying, youth-sustaining, fat-burning, blood sugar scorching power you'll sustain well into your senior years. Study after study continues to prove these super-charged supercells take on an indestructible nature.[75] It's this nature that ensures the *BioLogic Cascade* continues well into your golden years, *if* you can sustain your *10 Minute Workouts* without giving in to the temptation to over-train. And yes, you'll also build stronger, more shapely muscles along the way despite all the extra rest.

Harvesting these precious pearls reminds me of the not-so-old riddle that asks, "if you had just one wish, what would it be?" The answer of course should be "more wishes—many more wishes." If *super fast twitch muscle fibers* hold the keys to the cascade, and only the activation of their attached stem cells can keep these youth sustaining cells alive indefinitely (and vice versa), the resulting bio-loop reveals a perpetual motion machine of sorts. This self-regenerating lifecycle of your highest order of *fight or flight muscle fibers* is beyond invaluable if healing and anti-aging are important to you. Pay special note to the next benefit for proof, and refer to the notes and research in the appendix for a wealth of supporting evidence.

Miraculous Stroke Recovery and Prevention

By now I hope you would already guess that strength training might also be able to prevent stroke and heal significant neurological damage, and you'd be right. In another commendable public enlightenment effort by the AHA, their continued documentation of the healings of special needs fitness trainer Tom Wisenbaker is both inspiring and inspired. For fifteen years, Wisenbaker has broken decades of medical conventions to pioneer the exclusive use of strength training to bring miraculous healings to stroke victims that mainline physicians had all but abandoned. In the 2013 AHA/American Stroke Association article "Weight Training After Stroke," Wisenbaker delivered a compelling testimony:

> I get people after everyone else has given up on them, and they've been going downhill a long time. So many doctors and therapists who assess stroke survivors give only a few tests to decide if someone has plateaued. What we have found is that plateauing in one area doesn't mean they've plateaued in every area. We have not seen someone who doesn't continue to improve. We had a lady from Denmark who was more than 20 years post-stroke, and she got her gait back after limping for all those years. People actually develop new muscle on their affected side. The experts didn't think that was possible, but we clearly see it. One of my clients was talking to his neurologist, who was impressed with how much improvement he had made. He asked the patient if we had planned that improvement because he didn't believe that you could target areas and have them improve. The big thing I've learned is how amazingly adaptable and capable we are. The medical community is so external and passive and unwilling for us to look inside. When are they going to realize that the head is part of the body, that the brain cells are attached to the body, so our thoughts and desires are part of our body? It's amazing what we can accomplish when we stop focusing on our limitations.[76]

How can you read that and not be inspired to add at least a little bit of strength training to your life? Maybe you can fit ten minutes into your day? If you're wondering where all that healthy nerve-infused muscle is coming from, we can thank the divine design of satellite muscle stem cells for that (Chapter 1). All we have to do is stimulate them into action, and they'll work medical miracles.

Spine, Bone, Joint, and Central Nervous System Health

Unless you've been avoiding fitness related information for the past twenty years, you already know that proper strength training is your number one physical defense against osteoporosis and other bone mineral deficiencies. Likewise, if there is a risk factor that should slam the door on all the high-impact, high-stress endurance training and long-duration gym training methods (as well as most sports as forms of exercise), their abuse of your skeletal and central nervous systems is it. If you read the introduction, you're already well informed on how dangerous these forms of exercise are to our long-term health and youthfulness. Why anyone would choose a form of exercise that damages the spine, bones, joints, and thereby the central nervous system—which of course is the primary life-sustaining body system—is beyond comprehension.

If you're a professional athlete or fitness model that needs an extreme pseudo-fitness body type, then you have a "reasonably" good excuse. Trading longevity for wealth or some other personal gain is as old as time. NFL football players are the prime example in the modern era. God bless those guys. And then there are those who can't let go of the endorphin high they get from their favorite body-beating activities. And I guess it can be argued that the *joy factor* is sometimes more important than sustainability or longevity, but I don't see it. Ask any NFL veteran in his sixties who played "for the love of the game," or any professional marathon runner nearing seventy (if you can find one), and the vast majority will tell you they wish they could undo most or all of it. Just one look at their pre-aged, often crippled bodies should serve as a wakeup call for all of us.

Those of you who are into abusive activities simply for good times or temporary vanity (both of which suffer greatly diminishing returns) should be considering an about-face right about now. It only takes a little bit of vision to see where it will lead you if you stay the course with your body-beating fitness lifestyle. The medical community may be a decade away from truly effective artificial joints, but is that your retirement plan? And there will likely never be such a thing as a full spinal column or cranial replacement, so please start listening to your body and respond accordingly.

Along with increases in bone density, the BioLogic approach also promotes lubrication, stability, and healing in joints. Most popular strength programs and nearly all endurance exercises do the opposite over time. So all who suffer from joint injuries (like me) have that benefit to look forward to as well. Joint injuries might not be a major concern of yours, but to me and millions of others, it's huge. We'll address these topics in greater detail later in the book, so until you get there please take heed. You only get one lifetime in that skeleton you have, so for God's sake please try to make it last.

Greater Strength and Capacity to Survive

Okay, this benefit is the poster child of *obvious*, but the depth of the cascade that spring from this *fight or flight* empowerment cannot be overstated. Where other programs list strength among several other goals, few focus on strength gains like the BioLogic Method. Strength has always been the primary reason we survive as a species in a hostile world, and it's no less important today. A strong person can survive illnesses or severe injuries that would kill a weaker neighbor. A strong person can evade or repel a predator that would overtake most others. A strong person can participate in physical activities and play heartily with their children and grandchildren. And where the weak project weakness and laziness, a strong person inspires discipline and leadership. These are a few of the markers of the alphas of most animal species.

Improved Mental Health, Cognitive Activity, and Anxiety Management

While all forms of exercise are known to improve mental health, most research during the twentieth century measured only the effects of endurance activities. Over the past decade, prompted in part by the AHA's shift in their recommendations, the medical community has finally begun cracking into these benefits as they result from strength training. In a 2010 landmark study published in the *American Journal of Lifestyle Medicine* titled "Mental Health Benefits of Strength Training in Adults," a team of scientists from the University of Georgia conducted seven different randomized controlled studies, and just as you should expect, their research findings were no less than astounding.[77] So much so that the authors recommended resistance training for:

- Profound and marked improvements in **memory and memory-related tasks**, most notably in "executive function," which is the "command and control" conductor of cognitive skills.
- Extraordinary **reductions in chronic fatigue** for as many as ninety-four percent of test subjects, producing success beyond any pharmaceutical or cognitive-behavioral interventions previously researched.
- **Intervention for sufferers of anxiety**, even those suffering from prolonged or heightened symptoms.
- **Improved self-esteem** for all, regardless of health or age, including sufferers of cancer, cardiovascular disease, and depression.
- **Healthier sleep patterns** and lower risks of sleep apnea, including a thirty percent improvement in sleep for those suffering from depression.
- **Marked increases in central nervous system health and function**.

If you read the section on Stroke Recovery above, you probably already assumed most if not all of these unprecedented neurological benefits, as the American Heart Association's case studies of Tom Wisenbaker's groundbreaking work surely proves their validity in the real world. This University of Georgia study has become the launching pad for almost forty additional studies and peer review articles, and I have found nearly complete agreement across the board. In one such article, a team from the University of New Mexico (UNM) added that the cognitive improvements were likely due to multi-factorial adaptations involving new nerve cell generation in the brain, increased neurotransmitters, and the formation of new brain blood vessels. In their final thoughts, the UNM team concluded:

> The evidence is quite impressive how resistance training can improve several major mental health issues. In addition, the research is convincing that resistance training can appreciably improve cognitive function. An exercise professional's bottom line message to clients is clear. For a mental lift, you should weight lift.[78]

Honestly, you've got to be asking yourself right now why these findings haven't been trumpeted by the fitness establishment and major media with great excitement. There's just not a whole lot of money to be made selling ten-minute strength building workouts. But selling running shoes and elaborate long-duration training regimens? Billions every year. If you have a family member suffering from any sort of cognitive or mental disorder, please get this book in their hands as soon as possible, or teach them the BioLogic Method once you have it well in hand.

Pain Management

Nearly all consistent workout programs can release naturally occurring pain and stress fighting endorphins from various body systems. But sadly, most fitness enthusiasts are causing so much pain from exercise-related damage that they totally miss out on the soothing effect these natural pain killing chemicals can have on pre-existing pain or chronic pain disorders attacking their bodies. In contrast, the damage free BioLogic approach isolates soreness to just a single muscle group per workout, thereby optimizing the endorphins' benefits. Before receiving the BioLogic revelation I suffered more irreversible sports injuries than most professional athletes, so I occasionally battle chronic pain as a result. When I perform my *10 Minute Workouts*, nearly all pain in my body subsides. That alone is miraculous to me. There is nothing I can do that better removes my pain and stress than a BioLogic Workout, so I have no need or desire for over-the-counter or prescription painkillers. Nothing can even come close to delivering the energy, vigor, and outright euphoria I often feel while walking out of the gym after my *10 Minute Workouts*. Give it a try, and you'll see soon enough.

Sweat: The Stinky, Drippy Truth

Over my past forty years as a year-round athlete and fitness professional, I've studied many thousands of people of all ages before, during, and after their sweat-inducing activities. In the informal studies I conducted at the seven health clubs I owned during the eighties and nineties, those who sweat profusely during their workouts were easily the least healthy looking folks, and those who sweat lightly enough to avoid requiring a post-workout shower were typically the healthiest. Though sweat has its essential purposes (body cooling being primary among them), soaking your skin, hair, and clothing in salty, toxic perspiration offer no benefits at all. It can even turn the cooling process into a negative when the exercise stops and the air conditioner kicks on or the outdoor temperature drops considerably. After a long workout, have you ever been soaking wet with sweat in an air conditioned room, or outdoors when the temperature drops below fifty degrees? If so, you surely realized it wasn't a healthy experience. While I hope you've been drawn to BioLogic Workouts for their ten-minute no-sweat protocols, I'm confident by now that you realize the program's no-sweat design is not an attempt to pander to the lazy among us (though lazy folks will surely love it). Instead, like everything else I've proposed in this book, it's rooted in clinical research and decades of observations in real world venues.

The minimization of sweat and stress are fundamental (physiologically and psychologically speaking) to what makes BioLogic Workouts so exceedingly effective, sustainable, and enjoyable. While I personally promote naturally occurring perspiration's potential detox benefits as a secondary purpose, many of my colleagues are beginning to flip tables on the pro-sweat crowd much more aggressively than I have. In a recent *New York Times* article titled "Is It Good to Sweat?" Dr. Oliver Jay, a professor of exercise physiology and director of the Thermal Ergonomics Laboratory at the University of Ottawa in Canada, threw a massive wrench into the fitness establishment's pro-sweat propaganda machine. Jay insists that exercise-induced sweat is futile at best, as aside from cooling the body it adds no additional benefits while exacerbating the very real risk of dehydration and leaving you a sweaty wet mess. *"There's this entrenched idea that it's good to 'sweat things out,'* said Jay, but *"sweating, per se, provides no health benefits."*[79]

Myth: Long sweaty workouts are beneficial for good health and longevity.
Truth: Long sweaty workouts do *more harm than good* and are unsustainable over time.

From a BioLogic Workout perspective, perspiration is a lot like *slow twitch muscle* activity. If we're eating well and living a relatively active lifestyle (see *Section III*), sweating is a normal process that never needs to be forced into prolonged and profuse volume. Unless you have a rare condition that hinders proper sweat gland activity, you are sweating for physiological reasons all day long, but it's hardly noticeable unless some environmental, physical, physiological or psychological stimuli causes you to sweat enough for it to bead up before it can evaporate. As Jay insists, each of these instances is designed primarily to cool your body temperature when it begins overheating.

Additionally, Dr. Joseph Mercola suggests several other benefits, including its potential to more quickly expel toxins that may collect in your skin and to more effectively eject bacteria and blockages from your pores.[80] But again, none of this condones the extreme practice of exercise-induced profuse sweating. Unless you've been told by a medical professional or have legitimate reasons to believe you are carrying high quantities of toxins or harmful metals in your skin (which is unlikely if you're healthy and eat well), the preponderance of research shows there is zero benefit from exercise-induced *profuse* sweating. Even then, barring a rare health condition that may block proper sweat production, our bodies will automatically perspire heavily to expel excessive toxins and bacteria or to fight viruses whenever they become a threat. You've more than likely experienced this process through occasional inexplicable sweating, or feverish sweats, or a rare bed-soaking night sweat. A healthy body has all of this well under control. Sweaty exercise enthusiasts need to stop buying into and perpetuating archaic lies, and start shifting their focus onto scientific truth.

If by chance you have grown psychologically addicted to heavy sweating or are genuinely concerned about the effectiveness of your automatic perspiration, I suggest you fill your perceived need for profuse sweat by allowing heat to do the work for you. Take more frequent, longer-lasting hot showers or baths (yes some of our best sweating happens while washing ourselves in hot water), spend regular sessions in a sauna or steam bath, or partake in playful activities or physical chores in hotter environments (my personal favorites). I haven't broken into a drippy, disgusting body-soaking sweat in a health club for more than twenty years, and in all humility, I'm in better condition than all but a tiny percentage of folks from my generation. When I feel the need for a great sweat while at the gym, I sit in a sauna until I'm drenched, then shower it off well before it starts to attack my skin and hair. Otherwise, I know my body will sweat whenever it needs to, on auto-pilot so to speak.

Goodbye Fad Diets and Crash Dieting

Two of my personal favorite benefits of the BioLogic approach are 1) my optimized metabolism and insulin sensitivity allow me to eat more of the foods I love without fear of storing excess fat, and 2) the workouts have a way of naturally reducing my appetite, especially for late night snacking. While you likely know that proper nutrition is eighty to ninety percent of the battle, partial starvation or expensive (mostly useless) supplementation is NOT part of the BioLogic program. In *Section III* I'll ask you to start cutting out the foods that are poisoning or aging you, and I'll also make a few recommendations of proven whole food supplements. I'll also offer healthy and delicious alternatives while teaching you approaches to curb your chemically stimulated hyper-appetite back to the levels of your genetic design. This is the appetite you would have had if not for the cultural brainwashing and resulting chemical addictions that tripped you down a path to inactivity or obesity. That, of course, is a subject worthy of its own book; so until we get there, you'll find a great starter plan for BioLogic nutrition in *Section III.*

Healing Power and Anti-Aging

In addition to a profound reduction in injuries and chronic joint or spine problems, thanks to the *BioLogic Cascade* and the resulting increase in natural HGH and other age-defying hormones, this workout enhances and speeds healing in all our body systems, just as it can for stroke victims. Have you ever wondered how an NFL running back like Adrian Peterson can take a beating on the field that would kill an average man, then engage in six days of "rehab training" before heading back to the field for another beating (rinse, repeat)? Be encouraged to know that the core principles that speed healing for professional athletes in sports medicine rooms gave rise to the BioLogic Method.

This approach has healed dozens of my own sports injuries and further ensured I'm not a virtual cripple now that I'm in my mid-fifties, and I thank God for it every day. Even more, I also suffer from a relatively rare but often debilitating thyroid condition (Graves Disease) that hit me twenty years ago, just before receiving the BioLogic revelation. I believe that my adherence to BioLogic principles all these years has played a key role in my ability to recalibrate my glands and get my thyroid disorder firmly under control with far greater speed and more lasting success than the typical patient following conventional prescriptions—and my personal physician agrees. In fact, not only is my HGH production far greater than most people my age, but all of my hormones (including testosterone) consistently test out at optimal levels.

Today I'm seldom, if ever, ill and I tend to bounce back from injuries and viruses faster than others much younger than me; yet the opposite is usually the case for sufferers of thyroid disorders like mine. As I review my research notes, I see many benefits that clearly fall under the umbrella of the cascade of benefits noted above. So please be assured that BioLogic strength training workouts can more than likely help, heal or improve whatever ails you, whether it be gastrointestinal transit issues, arthritis, lower back pain, or most other ailments. I'll spend more time discussing how and why this is true in the coming chapters, so until then, may the healing begin!

Reversing Age at the Genetic Level

Speaking of anti-aging, please be assured that each of the benefits detailed in this chapter also applies to senior citizens, often to an even higher degree. Far more compelling to me and my peers have been the revolutionary implications of the new research into the effects of strength training on atrophy, functional impairment (sarcopenia), and related cellular dysfunction in the skeletal muscle of aging adults. While numerous research projects blazed the trail ahead of them, in 2007 the medical journal of the *Public Library of Science* published the six-month research study conducted by a team of scientists from the Buck Institute for Age Research (California).

This startling study revealed that strength training not only significantly increased the youthful strength and muscle hypertrophy in their senior test subjects, but it literally transformed the genes of these seniors to more closely resemble the genes of much younger trainees.[81] Never before has science shown that we could reverse human aging at the genetic or molecular level. To me, this is truly earth shaking news. Some readers would say I'm guilty of "burying the lead," for surely this extraordinary biological discovery can logically explain the molecular science behind every benefit under the *BioLogic Cascade*. Maybe that's true, but I find it far more important to speak directly to the masses that need the proper motivation to start working out rather than geek-speak my target audience out of the discussion.

When you start talking about something as revelatory as our newly found ability to reverse the aging of our genes, it becomes far too easy to lose sight of the forest for the trees. That said, I can't offer that same defense to the news media, the fitness establishment, or the medical community at large. Each has mostly sidestepped the implications of this astonishing discovery, despite more than fifty peer-reviewed articles and additional studies adding validity over the past decade. If you're still wondering why I have spent so much time railing against the establishment and their motives for hiding new research while perpetuating profitable old myths, I hope by now you understand what we're up against. In their book *Body by Science,* concerning the Buck Institute's breakthrough, Dr. Doug McGuff and fitness journalist John Little were so inspired by the implications and so shocked by the absence of a commensurate response from the establishment that they used the final paragraphs in their eleven chapter entirely scientific text to close out their book:

> When the drug Resveratrol was shown to produce some reversal of aging in mice and worms, it flew off the shelves as an age-reversal agent—without any proof that it had a similar effect in humans. Now here, after millennia of searching for the "fountain of youth" . . . a clinical study has essentially said, "Look, here it is—an actual functional reversal of aging at the molecular level!" . . . But it's not surprising to us, nor to anyone who performs the type of training that we advocate . . . Having said this, the most amazing thing that happened after this study came out in 2007 was—nothing. That news of this magnitude should come out during our lifetimes and not be on the front page of every newspaper and on every evening news program was inexplicable to us. Perhaps it failed to garner much attention because people are more than willing to take a pill, thinking it's going to reverse their aging, and it's only the exceptional individual who would hear such news and say, "I can do something for myself, by the

> sweat of my brow; by applying my own effort and my own work ethic, I can achieve this for myself!" Perhaps. [82]

Strength training your *super fast twitch muscles fibers* is a potential fountain of youth. Skim back over this chapter right now, or at least read just the headings, and you tell me, can any of the popular fitness activities honestly make such claims and back them up with independent scientific research? The answer is no. Isn't it scientifically clear and exceedingly obvious that only low-volume, high-rest hypertrophy training of your *fight or flight* muscle fibers can reverse or at least slow the aging process? What now will you do with that revelation?

The Great Benefit: Greater Freedom and More Time

Before 1998, my workout schedule was a primary factor in how I mapped out my week. Now it's virtually an afterthought as I step into the gym (at home or right around the corner, whichever is most convenient that day) for a quick *10 Minute Workout*, and my family, my ministries, and other service projects have gained back all the hours I once burned up while over-training. Likewise, as you'll learn in greater detail in this book, once you've set a strong base through six months or more of training, the BioLogic Method also benefits from occasional long breaks of four weeks or more. For this, BioLogic Workouts have also freed me up to go on long term mission trips and take prolonged family vacations without missing a beat.

After fifteen years raising my daughter as a single dad, I finally remarried in 2014. I'm exceedingly grateful that I had the freedom to pursue my bride and to build a strong family with our three kids without a time-consuming workout program getting in the way. Even more, my wife has fully caught the revelation, and with just over two years of BioLogic Workouts the results show in every way imaginable. Most important of all, we no longer have to choose between optimizing our health or freely living our lives to the fullest, and we sincerely want the same to be true for you.

CHAPTER 3

Fitness Defined

The Eye Test

Look at the people around you. Do they appear to be growing stronger or weaker? Younger or older? Among those you consider to be fitness enthusiasts, which look like they're on a sustainable path to true fitness even into their senior years? Everyone involved in high impact joint-endangering workouts is instantly disqualified. Please consider that to be an undeniable fact, as it's a pivotal truth that will open your mind to greater understanding of the *BioLogic Revelation*. You cannot judge a workout program by its apparent short-term results, yet that's exactly what the fitness fad fanatics and snake oil hucksters do.

The only true measures of success are the long-term results a person can sustain into their senior years. Good luck finding a marathon runner or high-volume high-impact gym enthusiast who looks younger than their age and still moves like an athlete well into their seventies. There are always exceptions and enigmas, but I've yet to meet one. If you have, please ask them to contact met. I'd like to know their secret!

In contrast, when you see an exceptionally fit man or woman in their senior years sporting an athletic build and gate and looking ten to twenty years younger than their age, you can be sure they're doing things the right way. Invariably, they long ago abandoned high-volume high-impact workouts. I know many folks who sat on the couch for a decade or two, never participating in any sort of fitness program, until they finally tested BioLogic styled workouts and nutrition/lifestyle guidelines. The speed of their transformations has amazed me every time. We should marvel at these folks, find inspiration in them, and follow their lead. Even the most beaten down and sedentary among you can do this workout. You just have to understand your genetic design—as proven by the very real science revealed throughout this book. Your body, without question, yearns to retain youthfulness and strength through the *fight or flight* stimuli delivered through the very simple BioLogic protocols detailed in *Section II.* If you catch this revelation, I can promise you, you'll never turn back.

Defining Fitness

If you make the mistake of listening to those who earn their living selling extreme approaches to fitness, you'll find yourself buying into a counterproductive or destructive definition of the term that has been tailored to fit what they're selling. Before we can fully define true fitness, let's first round out a logical survey of what true fitness is not. True fitness is not defined by your ability to run a marathon every year or a treadmill for hours at a time no matter how thin you get or how strong you *think* your heart is becoming.

If you've read every preceding word in this book, you likely already know this. But if you disagree, I believe you'll change your mind before the end of this chapter. To continue, true fitness is not defined by a six pack of abs or muscles so large they don't fit into clothes bought off the rack. True fitness is not defined by your ability to perform extreme physical acts that would cripple most people. And true fitness is definitely not defined by *skinny-fat* people who look trim in clothes but (due to their very low muscle to fat ratio) are no more fit than their obese friends. Most waifish super models suffer from this *skinny-fat* disorder, and they are often in far worse health than the couch potatoes. Their starvation diets and overall poor lifestyle is destroying their *super fast twitch muscles* and damaging each and every one of their vital life systems. In a time of famine, a thin frail woman will die of starvation long before her obese neighbor. So which of the two is most fit? While that's obviously a dramatic hypothetical, I need to underscore the point. It's not that the obese person is doing anything right, but that her waifish neighbor is doing everything very wrong.

While these and other examples of pseudo-fitness types each have sincere motivations for what they do, and often look fit for a decade or two, each are training and shaping their bodies in extreme ways that do far more long-term damage to their bodies than the temporary results could ever justify. Each of these extreme pseudo-fitness types is simply causing *more harm than good* to their bodies, regardless of how fit they look or feel through a relatively small window of time. Short-term fitness is simply not true fitness, as true fitness is best identified by its ability to enhance sustainable "whole body" health. We'll be repeating that overarching truth as the *Sustainability Axiom* continuously throughout this book (especially in Chapter 3), and you can't deny its veracity. So if you fit one of the groups identified above, don't despair. The BioLogic Method can and should help you minimize (and often reverse) the damage you've done while still upping your game. Keep an open mind and you'll soon see how this is true.

Myth: Short-term results are leading indicators of a beneficial/sustainable workout.
Truth: Short-term results are often misleading and are typically unsustainable.

Pseudo-Fitness Extremists

Many fitness extremists are rebelling against healthy logic or are simply unaware of the long-term consequences of their favorite exercise pastimes. Free will is for everyone, so if that's you, please trust I'm not judging your intelligence or your heart, just your decision making paradigms. If you currently work out on a regular basis, then you most likely fall into one of the many pseudo-fitness types without even realizing it. Maybe you're a "gym rat" (that was me back in the day), or a gimmick workout believer, or a *CrossFit* warrior, or an avid runner or cyclist, or an aerobics enthusiast, or a cardio machine fanatic. If so, as detailed in the introduction and previous chapters, you're more than likely over-training your joints and invaluable *super fast twitch muscle fibers*, and thereby causing *more harm than good*.

I know this can all sound downright insulting to some of you, particularly if you teach one of these extreme methods, in which case it's probably fitness blasphemy to your ears. But please hang in there with me. If you're not quite ready to consider alternative paths, the research in this book will help you adjust your training regimen in ways that will reverse or greatly reduce the damage while also conditioning your body to better excel at your favorite activities. I know you may have some sincere objections. Everyone does until they accept the overwhelming scientific truth and logic found in the volumes of research I present in this book. I also realize many of you will go to the grave defending your favorite regimen. I remember when I would have done the same for my own pseudo-fitness addictions—the very activities that have left me with severe joint scarring and much regret. Extreme body types have long been idealized in the media as specimens of fitness despite the relatively short number of years they can maintain their pseudo-fitness glory before breaking down. I have to admit I took that bait and swallowed that hook back in the days of my youth. For this, I hope you'll start reconsidering your path sooner than later . . . especially if you're already on the downslide with your best years behind you. Whatever the case, let's dispel another fitness myth once and for all.

Myth: Fitness extremists make great fitness teachers and role models.
Truth: Extreme fitness methods typically damage various body systems, and should only be practiced by those who are willing and able to accept such damage to attain a short-term goal.

If you've avoided a consistent fitness plan most of your life, you obviously don't fit any of these pseudo-fitness types and are among the majority who never set any sort of extreme fitness goals. But you also may be among the thirty-five percent (in America) whom the government labels as clinically obese.[83] For most people in this group, simply losing twenty-five pounds of fat or gaining ten pounds of *fight or flight* muscle would be a wonderful accomplishment. BioLogic Workouts will empower you to set far more ambitious fitness goals regardless of your current state—even many of the goals set by the extremists—without all the wasted time and body abuse that has been pre-aging the extremists, and without all the negatives that have derailed so many of you all your fitness lives.

The Candle Metaphor

As you continue coming to terms with these paradigm shifts, I suggest you start recognizing that, metaphorically speaking, our bodies are a lot like a burning candle. We only have so much wick to sustain our lives before there is no more candle to burn. We have just a few prime decades in our lifetimes to get our candle to a sustainable state before all our wick is gone. You may have enjoyed how your candle looked at times during your life, especially if you burned away all the excess pounds that made you feel unattractive or overweight. But in your zeal to burn fat, you have more than likely been burning away your life-sustaining wick when you could have been conserving it and adding to it through more efficient and effective means using focused protocols that burn away excessive wax without destroying the candle.

This is a metaphorical goal of the BioLogic Method. It builds, strengthens, and restores your wick while burning away only the unwanted wax, even while your candle *isn't* burning. All it takes are very simple movements that wake up the wick (your critically important *super fast twitch muscle fiber* percentage) and build it up for greater strength and longevity.

From Marathon to Fixx: Historically True Parables

Many of you already know that the term "marathon" in a sporting sense was born from the exploits of the historic Grecian courier Pheidippides (Fy-dip-id-ees), who after running approximately twenty-six miles from the city of Marathon to Athens to announce victory in battle over Persia, uttered the word "Joy" and dropped dead on the spot. That's about as loaded a factoid as you'll find in history. For the sake of full disclosure, most historians also believe that Pheidippides had previously run 150 miles as a messenger during the days leading up to the final victory, so he was surely in a weakened state before his final epic run. This of course serves well to underscore my point. Had he been a man who trained to fight and sprint according to genetic design rather than run cross-country with little to no sustenance, he may or may not have reached his destinations as quickly, but he surely would have had the strength and body composition to survive the journey.

Even more, Pheidippides could have enjoyed the "Joy" of his message at the victory feast that followed his historic announcement. I have A LOT of friends who are avid runners. Your accomplishments have been very impressive. I've congratulated you upon every victory and personal best, and my kudos to you have always been sincere. After seeing the joy and vigor and spiritual clarity your runs brought you, I can see why Pheidippides was joyful even in death. But I desperately hope for a better end to your final run.

As I'll continue to admit, there is high value in the *joy factor.* From a scientific standpoint, it is greatly magnified by a cocktail of released endorphins and other hormones along with numerous psychological rewards. I'm not saying you should entirely give up the spiritual high you gain from your endurance activities. But there is clearly a better way to accomplish your personal goals and get that joy rolling without all the debilitating damage you risk with each additional long run. And for anyone who thinks the Pheidippides reference is a bit dated or historically questionable, please look up "Jim Fixx."

Jim is widely known as the father of the modern running craze; a phenomenon that gave birth to the fitness explosion of the eighties. His seminal work, *The Complete Book of Running,* was the *New York Times* #1 Bestseller for more than two months after its release in 1977. Just seven years later, during a normal run, Fixx tragically died of a heart attack. At the time of his death, Jim was just fifty-two, which happens to be younger than my age while writing this book. I have complete respect and gratitude for Jim's role in history and his positive impact on my life and career path. Rest in peace, Jim Fixx. But I hope that mentioning his premature demise helps to ensure he did not die in vain. I pray the truth saves many lives as I fight the "the powers that be" to get this message out to the masses. If you haven't already, please read the research on endurance running detailed in the introduction, as the scientific community is working tirelessly to reveal that Jim's endurance running tragedy was by no means an anomaly.

Most recently, in a review published in the April 2016 issue of *Sports Medicine,* a team of award winning cardiologists and scientists representing six research institutions in three nations (most notably the Mayo Clinic in the US), used the most conservative language possible to report:

> Although low- to moderate-intensity exercise has well-known cardiovascular benefits, it has been increasingly suggested that prolonged strenuous endurance exercise (SEE) could have potential deleterious cardiac effects. In effect, the term "cardiac overuse injury" (or "over-exercise") has been recently reported to group all the possible deleterious cardiac consequences of repeated exposure to SEE or "over-exercise".[84]

It's hard not to read the warnings implied between those lines. Have you ever heard of the medical terms "cardiac overuse injury," or the acronym "SEE" as real threats to the average endurance enthusiast? Have you ever heard that it was even possible to "overuse" your heart during exercise? Probably not, as they've been freshly coined for use in this growing field of cardiac overuse research. Now reconsider my Candle Metaphor.

In addition to the growing number of "deleterious cardiac consequences" known to be caused by strenuous endurance exercise, it does in fact appear that the human heart can be "beat" to death simply through "overuse." Many of you know someone—possibly someone very dear to you—who has suffered from the plague of "SEE," though the clear and present dangers have clearly been hidden in plain sight. I can only pray that you have eyes to see and ears to hear that the minor benefits of "SEE" are simply not worth the potentially deadly costs. For more eye-opening research on the subject of heart health, please review the many research studies and excerpts I cite in the Appendix. If by chance you're thinking that only marathon runners are at risk, please be sure to dig deep into the *Journal of the American College of Cardiology's* twelve-year mortality study discussed in the introduction.

Eye Witness Fitness Parables

Before proceeding, I want to share two case studies from my days in the health club business that detail the learning curves of five very different people across several decades. As you'll soon see, their stories are loaded with life lessons and honest perspectives. Once considered in full, these eye witness accounts should help harmonize everything I've shared about the *BioLogic Revelation* up to this point, but in far more practical terms. Since their workout programs varied greatly, the five principle characters in these two stories represent the majority of folks who exercise, through both their motivations and results. If you don't relate to any of the first four enthusiasts, you'll probably see yourself in the fifth and final character introduced, a normal middle-aged man named John. As you read, be reminded that the *BioLogic 10 Minute* workout involves stimulating specific muscle fibers using safe strength exercises in controlled settings—not any of the high stress types of exercises the four lead characters practiced most of their lives.

Though sprinting (which is a primary activity in the first case study) is one of the most effective exercises when targeting *fast twitch muscle fibers*, we only recommend it as a form of exercise to competitive athletes or lifelong sprinters. The risks involved when running at one-hundred percent of your maximum speed, which is necessary if you're trying to apply the optimal stimuli to your *super fast twitch fibers* through speed alone, are simply too high for most. Most of you will never incorporate sprinting into your program, but there's a lot to learn from a lifelong sprinter like Jen, below. As you read these stories, see if you can glean a few key facts that could help you or your friends make BioLogic changes in your lifestyle sooner than later. And don't worry, none of these stories end with someone dying, as there's far more to learn than how to avoid premature death from "cardiac overuse injury."

The Story of the Runner and the Sprinter

Jen and Lori were on the same high school track team, and they loved to run. Both were champions in their events, but only Jen continued as a college track athlete. No longer having the opportunity to run organized sprint races like her teammate, Lori began running a mile or two at least four days per week for health, fitness, and the joy of running. The two women remained friends, and both looked great well into their twenties. As a collegiate sprinter, Jen looked every bit the athlete, sporting low body fat and feminine muscle mass across her entire physique, including her arms. In contrast, Lori became exceptionally lean, just as she had hoped. Despite developing far less muscle mass and looking a bit soft when standing side-by-side with Jen, the majority of their friends felt Lori had the more enviable body. Most (like the masses of women they represented) preferred the petite body Lori was sculpting through her endurance running, and some feared Jen may eventually start to look too muscular over time if she continued training as she did. For that, their friends were far more inclined to adopt Lori's approach over Jen's.

Once Jen ended her track career, she had no interest in switching over to distance running as Lori did. So Jen adapted her college training regimen to a much reduced, once or twice per week sprint regimen that seldom took more than 30 minutes, and she stayed this course into her late thirties. Both women were maintaining similar healthy diets, and both women still gained great pleasure from their workouts; often referencing the mental and spiritual high they would feel after each outing. While Jen was surprised how easily she maintained her muscular build—albeit a bit less extreme due to the greatly reduced workouts—Lori was looking more like an endurance athlete every year, and she loved the results she was seeing, so she began to gradually increase the frequency and duration of her runs. Lori felt great pride when people asked her if she was a competitive runner, and the fact that she could fit into the smallest sizes on the rack drew great praise from her friends. She was now running five to ten miles per day at least three days per week, and began entering 10K and marathon races at an increasing rate. As Lori trained for these challenging competitions, inclement weather would often force her into the gym where she would spend hours on a treadmill. Maybe you know someone like Lori.

The Relentless Impact of Time

By the time the two friends were in their mid-forties, Lori had been investing as many as ten hours per week into her passion for running. Jen had also ramped it up a bit, as she began sprinting in Masters Class track meets and was now investing more than two hours per week to train and compete. Jen also began adding strength training sessions into her schedule, as that's what many of the top masters class sprinters were doing. At forty-plus, Jen still looked like a competitive sprinter, and hardly a soul believed she was a day over thirty. But Lori, despite her many road racing medals and her enviable "zero" dress size, was looking tired and aged no matter how much makeup she applied.

Even compared to her inactive friends, Lori's face was looking bit old for her age, as her skin was showing wear and tear from all the years of profuse sweating, excessive sun exposure, and forces of gravity (compounded by the excessive pounding against the pavement). Lori was also dealing with unwanted "peach fuzz" hair all over her face, but she didn't seem to let it bother her too much. Her friends, however, were noticing that she had lost her curves and was now built like a pre-teen boy, nearly void of shapely muscle.

By the time Jen and Lori were in their fifties, Lori had begun experiencing a host of joint, bone, spine, and muscle injuries. Her race performance was dropping at a steady rate, and she was starting to admit her immune system was also taking a beating, as illness and chronic fatigue became harder to shake off with every passing year. As a notable sidebar, over the decades, Lori also experienced several scares involving motor vehicles, stray dogs, and an occasional nearby lightening strike, so she began training more frequently on treadmills.

As she approached sixty, Lori knew that, "at her age," the runner's lifestyle was no longer sustainable. She knew it was time to cut back on her running, but it had become a physical, mental, and spiritual addiction for her, so Lori found the transition to low impact exercises more than just a bit disheartening.

Also approaching sixty, Jen the sprinter likewise began dealing with frequent aches and pains. She also suffered occasional muscle injuries (though nothing of the severity Jen was enduring), so she too hung up her competitive track shoes. In contrast however, Jen easily transitioned to two or three workouts per week in the gym, performing the type of strength exercises she had begun employing in her early fifties—exercises that had the similar effect on her body as sprinting. For this, the transition was especially easy and rewarding for Jen. She continued sprinting three or four times per month whenever she needed that mental and spiritual high, and began feeling even greater strength and energy as the aches and pains decreased over time. Jen was now looking as strong and fit as she did in her forties, while Lori looked every bit of sixty, and then some. Across the forty years of this case study, Lori trained approximately twenty-thousand hours in total. In stark contrast, over the same time frame, Jen logged just under four-thousand hours. That's a sixteen-thousand hour difference. Consider their respective costs compared to their end results. Shocking, yes?

The Story of the Bodybuilder and the Rehabber

Kevin and Glenn grew up in the seventies and both were greatly inspired by Arnold Schwarzenegger's advice in the landmark book *Pumping Iron*. Both were highly motivated and dedicated to build muscle and to get "yoked," as we called it in those days. Arnold's way was the roadmap to all (like me in my teens) who were his admirers and considered him their top role model. If you've ever seen pictures of Arnold from his days as a young bodybuilder, you know why the boys of my generation were motivated to get start hammering the weights as early as possible.

As Kevin and Glenn progressed through the years, Glenn decided to become a competitive bodybuilder like his hero Arnold. He spent two to three hours per day, five to six days per week, lifting weights, performing hardcore muscle building exercises, and pounding the calories like a glutton. Meanwhile, Kevin continued with similar bodybuilding exercises to build more muscle (to a lesser degree), as sports like basketball and touch football were the interests that consumed most of his free time. Kevin's typical day consisted of an hour in the weight room to build muscle, followed by two to three hours playing his favorite sports.

Over the next decade Glenn became a behemoth of a man. Thanks to rollercoaster crash diets and calorie-burning endurance training sessions lasting hours at a time, his body fat would often dip below eight percent leading up to competitions. He was looking like a true specimen of muscularity, and his skin would often appear nearly transparent. During off-seasons, Glenn would return to eating incessantly, and avoided calorie-burning endurance exercise like the plague. Talk about yo-yo dieting. So Glenn got "big as a house" between competitions, and his gut would eventually bulge like a gorilla's. He looked freakish to some and inspiring to others, but he was a spectacle of inhuman muscular potential to all.

In contrast, despite being plagued with many sports related injuries during the same time frame, Kevin had developed above average muscle mass and an athlete's body fat ratio, yet he still looked almost scrawny standing next to his bodybuilder friend. Then, while simply jumping one day, Kevin blew out the major ligaments in his right knee in the worst possible way. Two years of considerable rehab later he attempted a return to his pre-injury lifestyle and soon blew out his left knee. Over the course of a single decade, Kevin suffered too many major injuries to count. Surprisingly, not one of these injuries was the result of contact with another athlete, as the impact and high speed movements of competitive sports alone were gradually breaking him down—especially in the extreme way he played. By the time both were in their mid-thirties, Glenn the bodybuilder had suffered just a few minor injuries and was more Arnold-like than ever. Kevin, on the other hand, had given up most high-impact sports altogether, and had begun a strength training regimen that adapted the rehab strategies he learned from his sports medicine therapists. Glenn felt like a champion, and Kevin was filled with regrets.

We speed ahead two decades and both men are now in their mid-fifties. The often injured Kevin has given up nearly all high impact sports activities and reduced his gym workouts to thirty minutes per session, as that seemed to be all it took to maintain his muscle mass. He hadn't suffered any new injuries to his joints and had surprisingly maintained the physique he enjoyed in his late thirties. In stark contrast, though Glenn never lost his love for massive muscles, his fast-aging body could no longer keep up his former pace. It simply was no longer sustainable. He tried a variety of potent performance supplements and even experimented with performance enhancing drugs, but all proved to have little sustainable effect. Far worse, Glenn began suffering from a variety of health issues, including organ damage likely caused by his radical body fat swings and chemical use. Likewise, his joints and even his spine began breaking down under all the years of high-impact load-bearing wear and tear. He was still much more muscular than Kevin, but was actually a fraction of his former hulk-ish self. Glenn's highly stressed skin, his hunched posture, and his utter lack of youthful movement made him look many years older than his age.

Enter John Stage Right

One day, the two men were talking at the gym when John, a common friend from their college years, stopped to chat. After beating around the bush, John eventually asked the two "experts" for some tips on how to start showing muscle tone and shape through his formerly flabby physique. John was never an athlete, nor did he even start working out until his forties. But he had recently been diagnosed as morbidly obese by his family doctor, which alarmed him enough to clean up his diet and start working out as time allowed. Proper eating alone got him out of the "morbid" category, but he had yet to figure out how to effectively build muscle in a way that he could sustain. John never experienced the joy of competitive bodybuilding like Glenn, nor the athletic "glory days" success like Kevin the jock. However, at the age of fifty, John also never suffered a serious joint injury, and looked a heck of a lot younger than Glenn the bodybuilder—especially in his skin and hair.

Both Glenn and Kevin were envious to learn that John was playing a lot of tennis and golf and didn't hesitate to join in a game of pickup basketball or football with his kids—activities Kevin and Glenn would seldom risk for fear of injury. Like Lori in the previous story, up to that point in time Glenn had logged more than twenty-thousand hours beating his body. And though Kevin tracked right along with Glenn for his first decade, ironically, his many sports injuries kept him from logging more than nine-thousand hours in total.

What about John? Having neglected his body up to the age of forty, John had invested just over two-thousand hours to date, and all things considered, is actually in a better overall state of health than his two old friends—proving injuries and overtraining should be avoided at all cost. It's worth noting that in the case of an emergency, if "*fight or flight*" was ever required, John would be the man among these three who would be most capable of answering the call with his full physical faculties ready to respond at one-hundred percent of their genetic design. I'm sure you can glean a lot from the health mistakes all three of these friends made, but which would you say is the healthiest among them? Who among them has the brightest potential outlook where health and fitness are concerned? Clearly it is John, the former couch potato.

Learning from the Mistakes of Others

As a sprinter, my personal fitness path had a lot of similarities with Jen's; but if you haven't already figured it out, I'm the real life Kevin in the second story. I of course changed the names for the privacy of the other four, but I'd venture to say hundreds of my past clients would believe I'm talking about them. That's how common these stories are in the fitness world.

In retrospect, I gladly would have given up my extremist lifestyle had I known then what I know now. No amount of fleeting glory justifies the damage I've done to my joints. Likewise, there is little doubt that John wishes he had begun correcting his nutrition and lifestyle while he was still in his twenties, as only time will tell how much he pre-aged his vital life systems during all those years of toxic eating on the couch. Though we can't change the past, we can definitely reverse some, if not most of the damage. I'm living proof. For that, my goal is to help every type of person—from the Jens to the Johns—to eliminate or correct all the stumbling blocks and immediately jump over to the ultra-low-risk, uniquely potent, entirely sustainable BioLogic Workouts as soon as possible.

The Motivational Paradigm: The Four Cornerstones

What Proves a Beneficial Workout?

There are dozens of workout programs that produce some sort of results. As you've likely noticed, the workout programs I most strongly criticize in this book often produce short-term results that can appear quite impressive, for a while. Even more, I hope you realize that the people who are pitching most of these workouts (or magic elixirs) typically looked great well before they began practicing or consuming what they're selling (if in fact they ever truly did either). In all likelihood they've changed their regimen many times over, often over-training in spurts to produce abnormally statuesque physiques that can only be sustained for a few weeks at a time.

Most fitness models and bodybuilders have mastered this practice, and there are many books and published articles that teach it. Of the most legitimate programs being pitched on the web or in health clubs, several will indeed reduce your weight and shape your body—for a while anyway. And then of course there are the yo-yo's—folks who look great for a couple of months, then look sloppy, then great, then sloppy… rinse, repeat. Most of us fully realize this is an especially dangerous lifestyle. Although competitive bodybuilders have a reasonable justification for taking this unsustainable yo-yo approach, most others have no pure motivation for this counterproductive practice. So before you get started with any new program, make sure your motivations are in order, and you will better ensure your efforts are not done in vain.

The Four Cornerstones of Motivation

While the previous chapters detailed the science behind the revelation, the purpose of this chapter is to take a deeper dive into its logic. If you're currently choosing your first real workout program, or if you're searching for a brand new approach to reverse past damage and reboot your machine, let's first get your priorities in order. There are four obvious motivational forces that should determine all of your health and fitness decisions. These four cornerstones drive all of us to choose our workouts and virtually all other activities. For that, identifying their combined intersection is the purest decision making paradigm where your health and longevity are concerned. Understanding each motivation, and the unique physical and psychological benefits that result when they all overlap, will establish a firm foundation on which to build a fitness lifestyle that can stand the test of time.

Once you're fully motivated, you will without question stick with it and reach your goals. So although you may be tempted to skip ahead to study the actual workouts, If you realize that staying the course will remain your biggest challenge, then please digest the remainder of this chapter before getting started with the workouts. As you consider the four cornerstones, ask yourself if your current or past workout activities were truly driven by all four of these motivational forces in unison.

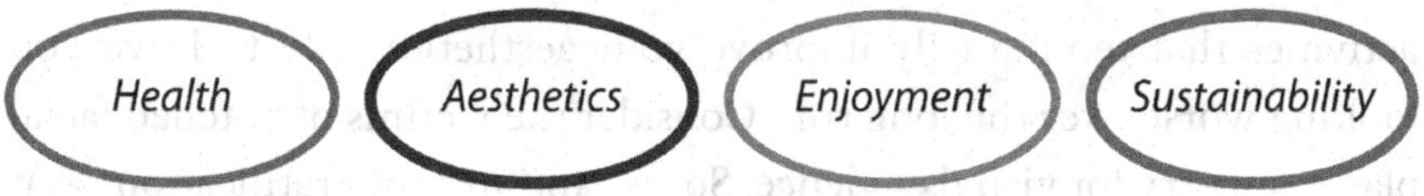

Cornerstone 1: True Health

Health—this most obvious of motivators is at the root of true fitness. To satisfy this cornerstone you must identify programs that strengthen and benefit ALL your body systems, not just your current favorites (see the outline review at the end of this chapter). It's imperative that you come to terms with the fact that any program that damages your joints or any of your body systems cannot produce sustainable good health. If it causes permanent damage, it simply does not satisfy the health cornerstone, no matter how impressive the short-term results may be. You will continue to hear me echo this principle over and over (and over) again. If it does *more harm than good*—if the net effect is damage or pre-aging of any of your body systems (no matter how strong or healthy you feel over the short run)— then the activity does not satisfy this primary motivational cornerstone. As you now know, that axiom eliminates nearly all of the most popular "fitness" programs out there today, and all forms of sedentary living as well. If you can't face that fact, you're bound to continue on a destructive path.

Cornerstone 2: Aesthetics Matter

Aesthetics—for many of you, the way you look in the mirror is your top motivator among the four. As I address the motivational force of aesthetics throughout the book, it will always be viewed from the perspective of fulfilling our genetic design, not for the fulfillment of our ego or vanity—though taking *healthy* pride in your improving aesthetics is indeed fruitful, both emotionally and spiritually. Few people are happy when they look fat or frail or both; and there's absolutely nothing vain about wanting to look strong and healthy, but many in the health industry have perverted this otherwise sincere concern. And many of those have exploited it to an unethical degree.

As is true with all matters dealing with your health, there are many activities that temporarily improve your aesthetics only to leave you looking worse over the long run. Consider the victims of botched facial plastic surgery for visual evidence. So, as "anti-instant gratification" as it may be, the only honest measure of aesthetic gains produced by a fitness program is found by asking this question: "How will that program affect my youthfulness many years from now?" Not, "How will it make me look next week?" Knowing that the most popular fitness activities actually pre-age their enthusiasts dismisses any claims that they can satisfy the aesthetics cornerstone, no matter how well your abs show today.

Cornerstone 3: Enjoyment Is Imperative

Enjoyment—I'll often call this motivator the *joy factor,* or simply "Joy." What good is a workout that you don't enjoy? If there's anything that I learned about the fitness industry early on that is still absolutely true, it's this simple fact: no one sticks with a program they dread. Year in and year out, 99% of the people who try to turn their fitness lives around jump into programs that bring them little to no joy, only to jump back off the ship once the drudgery (or injury and weakness) kicks in. Even when they see results, most inevitably realize the ends will not justify the means when there's no joy in the process. Conversely, no amount of joy justifies a workout program if it damages your joints or other body systems; thus the need to find the overlap in all four cornerstones before considering a new program. This clear logic should be a final wake-up call to endurance runners, *CrossFit* members, and other high-impact long-duration fitness enthusiasts. I know that's an overwhelming challenge for extremists, so I'll keep hammering that point until you get it written on your heart. Your beloved program might light up your joy in ways too profound for words, but if that's the only cornerstone it's hitting, you're probably killing yourself. So, at the very least, come to terms with the fact that you accept the damage and pre-aging as costs you're willing to pay to get the temporary results and momentary joy-filled "high." Once you do that simple math, maybe the truth will finally push you to make substantive changes.

Additionally, time consumption is a major component of enjoyment, so I hope that once you reach the end of this book, you'll start giving even greater value (and joy) to your free time. Life is a series of decisions, and few decisions are more important than determining how much time to invest into yourself versus how much time you invest in your loved ones and others. At the end of our lives, we won't be begging for another workout, but the vast majority of us will without question be praying for more time, as nothing this side of heaven can be enjoyed without it. Take that to heart as soon as possible, and you'll increase your chances of gaining more joy, even today.

Cornerstone 4: The Sustainability Axiom Trumps All

Sustainability—sustainable activities strengthen, heal, and protect ALL body systems while never posing a high-risk of damage. By definition, sustainable workouts remove or greatly minimize the risks to any system in your body, especially to your joints, spine, metabolism, and hormonal balance. Going forward I'll refer to the preeminence of sustainability as the *Sustainability Axiom*. As you may have surmised while reviewing the other three cornerstones, sustainability truly does trump all—though it too must pay homage to the others. There are highly sustainable activities (kicking back on a couch all day, for instance) that do not enhance your health, or your aesthetics, or your continued enjoyment of that activity. The four cornerstones of the Motivational Paradigm overlap to form a Venn diagram that reveals a central window. This window helps to identify which activities you should engage in your lifestyle and which should be forever deleted—or at least greatly reduced to help curb the damage they cause. Just as is true with the *joy factor*, time investment is a major concern when testing the sustainability cornerstone.

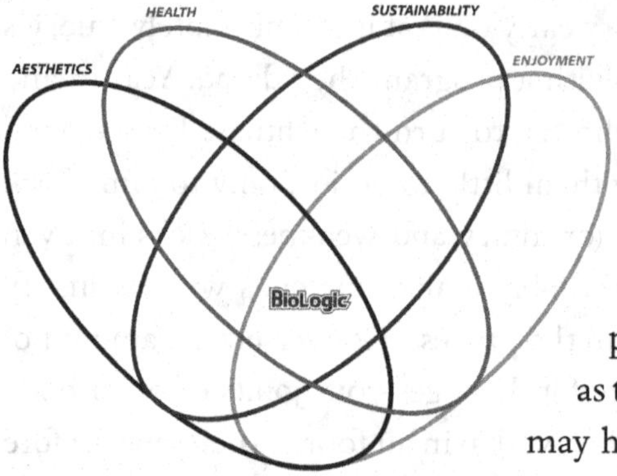

Even the most hard-core fitness enthusiasts inevitably reach a point where they dream of a way to sustain their physique in less than the hour or more per day that most invest into their already unsustainable regimen. For them, we have a thirty to forty minute version of the BioLogic Workout that can produce extreme results with far greater sustainability. As you will soon see, only BioLogic Workouts and others built on the same sustainable principles can satisfy all four cornerstones and hit the sweet spot of the Motivational Paradigm. No amount of gain from one cornerstone should ever justify setbacks in the others. Please take that as an absolute truth. If you don't agree with that, I hope you're either a professional athlete or a soldier who realizes and accepts the sacrifices, and the greater risks. Otherwise, it's a good time to talk through your decision-making paradigms with a trusted advisor.

The Tragedy of NFL Great Terry Long

If you've seen the film *Concussion* starring Will Smith, you know that it details the Chronic Traumatic Encephalopathy (CTE) crisis that is killing so many retired NFL football players. You were also introduced to the story of Terry Long, who was the third Pittsburg Steeler driven to self-inflicted death (at least in part) by the brain destroying disorder. He was in effect the man who provided the tipping point for the doctors trying to prove the crisis was real. I've known Terry since I was a teenager, and his training methods deeply impacted my own approach. My brother Rally was his teammate and one of his closest friends while playing football at East Carolina University, so he was much more than a casual acquaintance. Through my brother I knew things about Terry that only his closest teammates knew.

Terry was a U.S. Army Special Forces soldier assigned to the 82nd Airborne before playing college football. He was fearless. Even before he earned his way into the NFL, he was already an inspiration for his service to our country, his tireless work ethic while transitioning into major college football, and his unmatched determination to become the strongest football player ever—no matter the cost. Terry was also a heavy steroid user, as the combination of his fearless Special Forces mentality and his "joyful" desire to play in the NFL was so powerful that he refused to consider the long-term damage to his health. Terry was willing to risk *all* to make his dreams come true. He was a truly great athlete, and according to my brother, he was an even better friend and teammate. Everyone loved the gentle giant. He was, by all accounts, a sweetheart of a guy who truly loved life. Terry eventually achieved all of his highest fitness goals, including gaining notoriety as the strongest football player ever on record. But after eight successful seasons with the Steelers, he was left brain-damaged and broken down—a mere shadow of his former self. Soon thereafter, at the far-too-young age of forty-five, Terry ended his own life. Had he known that he would one day be driven mad by his lifestyle decisions, I believe it's safe to say he would have chosen a different path, and would likely still be alive today.

If you're not building your fitness lifestyle on the fundamentals and motivational cornerstones I've shared so far, you're setting up your body to break down well before it's time. You're most likely far from the extremes pursued by Terry, but don't let that numb you to the long-term cost of the risks you are taking. As a recovered muscle junkie, I'll readily admit I was part of the problem back in the eighties. Due to my years in the same football culture that led to Terry Long's demise, I had traded my proper focus—the cornerstones of the Motivational Paradigm—in exchange for unsustainable macho ego boosts and aesthetic vanity. But when the blinders finally fell from my eyes, the "AHA!" light bulb popped on. I refocused on the truths of this decision making paradigm even before I had received the BioLogic revelation in a teachable form, and I chose more life over vanity. Once in the right state of mind, I was in effect born anew as one who would no longer act out in the gym with vain pride as my motivation. And I began teaching the truths I had long known but failed to obey during my years as a wannabe professional athlete.

I've paid a heavy price with my many joint injuries and bone breaks suffered across many weeks and months that I wish I could have back. Nonetheless, my regrets are wiped away by my gratitude. I'm alive. Had my brother Rally or I have had Terry's extreme opportunities and drive to play at the highest level, we might have stumbled down a similar path. Thank God we were spared. Before proceeding, I want to offer a simple disclaimer for parents out there whose sons dream of playing full contact football at any level. The sport has come a *long* way since the CTE crisis was brought to light, as the training methods, the rules, and the code of ethics among the players of the game have changed dramatically. So Terry and Mike Webster and Junior Seau and Dave Duerson and the many other victims of CTE did not die in vain. No contact sport is risk-free. And for the sake of proper perspective, the Centers for Disease Control and

Prevention report that most youth head injuries are suffered from everyday falls from bikes or skateboards or playground equipment or from simple stumbles while playing hard.[85] With any sport, if you ensure your children are well coached and well equipped, I firmly believe your best course is to honestly weigh the Motivational Paradigm, let your kids be kids, and cover them with *confident* prayer.

True Fitness is Holistic Fitness

As we head into *Section II* to begin discussing the techniques and protocols of *BioLogic 10 Minute Workouts,* never lose sight of the fundamentals and motivational cornerstones detailed in *Section I.* If necessary, review chapters one and two until it gets you so excited that you joyfully embrace your next session. As you begin to make all of your health and fitness decisions based on these principles, don't ever forget that an effective *10 Minute Workout* is worth far more than gold or fame, as the return on investment is "more life." I can always find ten minutes. So can you. With consistent application of the ten-minute stimuli fully explored in *Section II*, you will without question trigger the much needed hypertrophy (growth and strength increases) in your most valuable muscle fibers. By doing so, you'll harvest satellite muscle stem cell nuclei into those muscle fibers, and you'll fire up your fat burning metabolism in accordance with your genetic *fight or flight* design. And, as you'll recall from Chapter 1, that's just the tip of the sword.

Never forget that *super fast twitch muscle fiber* hypertrophy is the key that cranks up the full *BioLogic Cascade* of health benefits, which in turn triggers a chain reaction of youth-sustaining metabolic processes with unrivaled efficiency. That's positive motivation, I know, but don't miss the what that actually implies. In contrast to the pseudo-fitness motivations detailed earlier in this chapter, BioLogic Workouts bring about sustainable "whole body" holistic fitness. As we explored in Chapter 2, all life systems in the human body are vitalized, finely tuned, and greatly empowered by every successful ten-minute session. Let's pause for a minute to reflect on the full cascade of benefits across all the vital life systems of the human body, as listed below. As you review this list, ask yourself exactly what you currently do to ensure the health and youth of each system, and question what exactly your current activities (or lack thereof) is doing for each.

- Nervous: Brain, spine, and nerves
- Endocrine: Glands and hormones
- Digestive: Nutrient absorption, stomach, intestines, and colon
- Skeletal: Bones, cartilage, and joints
- Excretory: Skin, kidneys, liver, and urinary system
- Reproductive: Sex organs and sex drive
- Immune: Disease defense systems
- Respiratory: Lungs and oxygenation
- Circulatory: Heart and vessels
- Muscular: Cardiac, smooth, and skeletal muscles

As Dr. LeBrasseur's Mayo Clinic study (discussed in Chapter 1) clearly demonstrates, our highly glycolytic *super fast twitch muscle fibers* are master catalysts in the bio-machine that is the divinely engineered human body. The longevity and proper function of our body systems depends on the "cross talk" these cells spark between each of our metabolic processes, so the earlier you start stimulating that BioLogic conversation the better. Remember, it takes very little time investment to effectively stimulate your *super fast twitch muscles* to trigger greater health in all the systems listed above—for a longer, stronger life, no matter your age. That, to me, is a true miracle. Please don't let it go to waste.

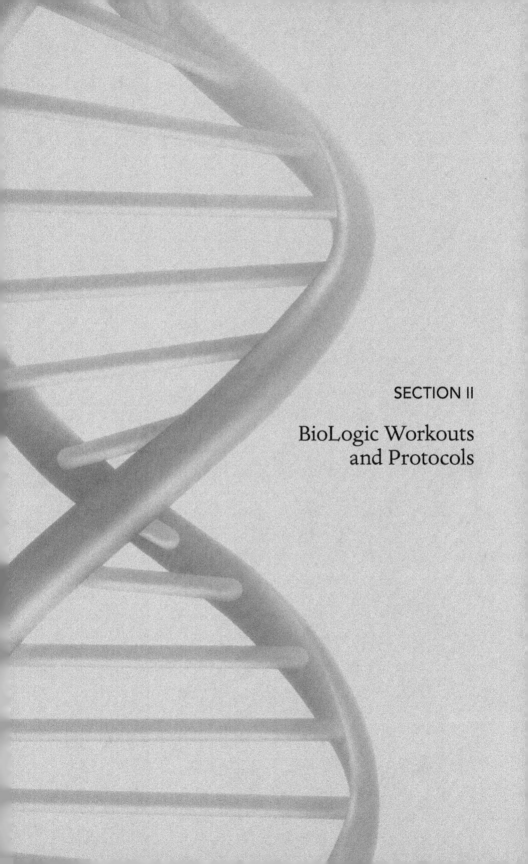

SECTION II

BioLogic Workouts and Protocols

CHAPTER 4

BioLogic Workout Protocols 1 & 2

Building on a Firm Foundation

If by reading the previous chapters you've retained nothing but the fact your *super fast twitch muscle cells* are proverbial seeds packed with youth-sustaining potential, then you've captured more than enough to learn how to sow these seeds. In earlier sections, we discussed how our ancestors conditioned these *super fast twitchers* through real world *fight or flight* survival according to our original design. Thank goodness we now know how to rev-up these super-cells through smooth, stable movements and greater mental engagement in controlled settings—far removed from the mortal threats that triggered these stimuli in the past. As I begin to share the four protocols that make the *BioLogic 10 Minute No-Sweat Workout* a functional revelation, let's be reminded of the fundamentals and motivational cornerstones that form the foundation for these protocols.

Fundamentals

1. Genetic Design: Strength for Fight or Flight
2. Super Fast Twitch Muscle Fibers Hold the Keys

Motivational Cornerstones

1. True Health
2. Aesthetics Matter
3. Enjoyment Is Imperative
4. The Sustainability Axiom Trumps All

These six concepts deal with the logical, scientific building blocks that should be firmly understood and sincerely embraced before proceeding. The four protocols you're about to learn deliver the physical, psychological, and intellectual techniques that empower the actual BioLogic Workouts. These protocols are the steps that stimulate and condition your *fast twitch* and *super fast twitch muscle fibers* to meet their optimal sustainable design in the least amount of time. Your adherence to the fundamentals and cornerstones while challenging your current state is—to borrow a term used in human behavioral psychology—"operant conditioning" in action. The balance between positive and negative feedback from each protocol work together in a highly complex, fast track manner to stimulate the ideal response in your muscles. But don't let that confuse you. If all you do is follow the four well-defined protocols, the re-conditioning of your body and metabolism will soon be child's play.

BioLogic Method Taboos

As we prepare to take our first deep study of the four protocols, let's first identify the three major technique taboos. Sadly, these taboos are fundamental to nearly all other workout programs but are seldom, if ever, found in BioLogic exercises due to their unsustainable, counterproductive nature.

1. High-impact, asymmetrical, uncontrolled activities that engage your entire body
2. Overtraining—too much of a good thing (or a bad thing) is a very bad thing
3. Stationary compound repetitions that employ momentum or variable movements

As you might surmise based on the *Sustainability Axiom* (detailed in Chapter 3), among these three taboos, only number 3 is somewhat negotiable. In fact, many of the strength exercises that fit that description can be adapted for BioLogic Workouts if they are modified using the low-stress isolation and time-minimization techniques detailed below. These *old school* exercises do in fact stimulate *fast twitch muscle cells* even when performed in an *old school* way but at a very high cost. See the story of Glenn the bodybuilder in Chapter 3 for a refresher. These traditional approaches to strength training exercises are generally risky and unsustainable. Unless you're a competitive bodybuilder, these approaches not only consume more time than anyone should ever invest into muscle building, but they can also burn up or stunt the powerhouse *super fast twitch cells* in exchange for bulkier *slow twitch* and lower-order *fast twitch fibers*.

In 2008, a clinical study published in the *European Journal of Applied Physiology* found *super fast twitch fibers* to be "completely absent" in their test group of bodybuilders, while the lower-order *fast twitch fibers* showed up in much higher numbers in this test group compared to the control group of physical education students.[86] By now you know that's not a favorable trade-off. Bodybuilding approaches to popular exercises are mainstays that most gym rats (like me) performed through the seventies and eighties. Even today, most people you see in a weight room are still performing these exercises using dangerous and counterproductive protocols and techniques. But don't be mistaken. If I had to pick a team to fight off a massive predator or rescue a child to the safety of high ground, I'd take the gym rats over the marathon runners any day and I'm confident you'd do the same. So if you're an avid weight lifter and are ready to switch to the BioLogic Method, you're going to be amazed how fast your *super fast twitch fiber* percentage can bounce back even after decades of neglect,[87] especially if you've avoided significant damage to your joints and spine.

If you can forget most everything you ever learned about how and why and when to perform the most popular weightlifting exercises, you're just a month away from seeing and feeling real results and healing as the *BioLogic Cascade* kicks in. Enthusiasts and beginners alike will appreciate the elegance of the no-damage, low-stress protocols we've developed for these popular exercises. Even a basic dumbbell press is an entirely different, exceedingly efficient, far more effective *super fast twitch* exercise when performed the BioLogic way.

Quick Word on Scheduling

As I'll soon detail, there are six basic variations of the BioLogic Workout. Each has been fine-tuned to meet the unique demands of your schedule or your advanced goals. While all six variations will satisfy the BioLogic fundamentals and cornerstones, most of you will prefer the *10 Minute Workout* for its unique efficiency and high *joy factor.* It's the variation I perform most of the year, and for me, it's easily the most sustainable. There's nothing like being able to jump in and out the gym and still grab a bite to eat or knock out a couple errands, all in thirty minutes or less, without ever breaking a sweat. This is ideal for those of you who will work out before going to the office, during your lunch break, or on your way to a dinner date, but it's even more convenient for those who will be training at home. In the basic *10 Minute Workout*, you will train (condition/stimulate) just one muscle group per day, once every seven to fourteen days. Much more on scheduling variations in Chapter 6.

How We Stimulate Super Fast Twitch Muscle

As you've surely noticed, all the exercise programs I've criticized place stress on many of your skeletal muscles and joints in sequence during a single exercise, either through full engagement of your core and all four limbs or through standing or seated exercises that involve compound movements (involving several joints) with a high degree of variability across the range of motion. While your *slow twitch* and *fast twitch muscles* are working hard throughout these exercises, the *super fast twitchers* won't even check in unless there is a genuine need for greater strength (or greater speed) than the less powerful *fast twitch muscles* can provide.

Here's the key. Once you learn to flex the core of a specific muscle group to the extent of its current maximum ability—devoting all your effort and mental focus to flexing that single bundle of muscle fibers—you'll be reactivating (or possibly activating for the first time) your *super fast twitch fibers.* For this, you'll also awaken the satellite stem cell myonuclei you may have harvested into those fibers earlier in life while triggering greater harvesting as hypertrophy begins to kick in. Never forget it's not a matter of the quantity or volume of your work (multiple exercises with multiple sets with dozens of repetitions), but the quality of the stimuli in very short order that sparks your *super fast twitch muscle fibers* to start burning their stored glycogen.

In stark contrast to *old school* approaches, the physical component of the stimuli isn't like the constant pounding of a jackhammer or the incessant spinning of a hamster wheel (*slow twitch fiber* activities) that primarily burn oxygen as fuel. Instead, it's the focused burn of a broad-point laser that torches the blood sugar stored in glycolytic *super fast twitch fibers* over a matter of seconds. Learning to focus one-hundred percent of your effort into the target muscle group is where it all begins. Protocol 1 will detail the specific mental and mechanical techniques that form this high-speed laser, and I'm confident you'll find it all to be as logical as it is easy. While actual hypertrophy conditioning occurs over several successive workouts, with your very first workout, you will have started the *BioLogic Cascade.*

Since most of you have been missing out on these benefits your entire life, this instant positive response in your critical *super fast twitch muscle fibers* should get you more excited than anyone, especially considering the extraordinarily low time demands and no-sweat ease. If you're a well-trained enthusiast you can probably skip ahead to Protocol 1, but the majority of you will definitely want to stick with me as I discuss the science behind *orderly recruitment* and how it leads to the *golden door* of *super fast twitch* hypertrophy. I'll put it all in very simple terms, so don't shy away. I'm confident it will help you fully understand the vital importance of all four protocols.

The Science of Orderly Recruitment

Nearly everything we do during a typical vigorous workout makes use of all the different types of skeletal muscles being worked, but seldom in the fashion or to the degree necessary to generate effective stimuli for *fast twitch fibers* and even less for *super fast twitch fibers.* Refer to my metaphor of *The Lobby, the Hallway, and the Golden Door* in Chapter 1 for a basic understanding of *orderly recruitment*, as I'll continue to reference the metaphor as we proceed. In short, the lobby represents your *slow twitch fibers*, the hallway represents your various types of lower-order *fast twitch fibers*, and the golden door at the end of the hall represents your *super fast twitch fibers.*

Keep in mind that skeletal muscle cells are so elongated that under a microscope they look more like snips of yarn glued into bundles than the semi-spherical discs we typically see characterizing most types of human cells. So when I speak of a "muscle" or "muscle bundle," I'm actually referring to many micro-bundles within each larger bundle, with all three basic fiber types intertwined in fairly arbitrary patterns. To help visualize the actual structures involved, study the cross-sectional graphic that represents a microscopic slice of a skeletal muscle bundle (see figure 2).

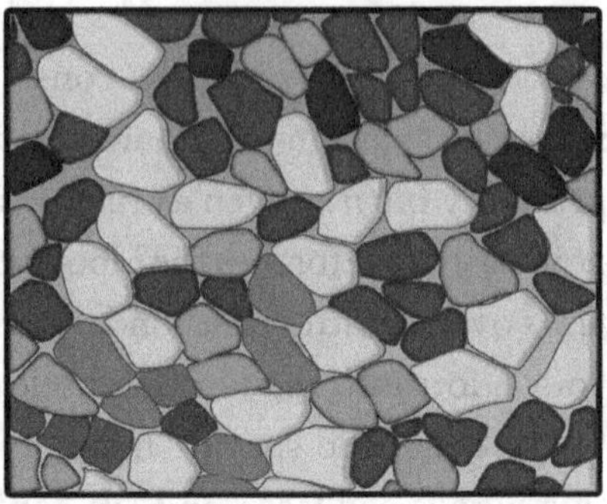

Figure 2: Illustration of a muscle cross-section, if viewed under a microscope

To continue with the yarn metaphor, imagine cutting a hypothetical multi-colored inter-woven bundle of yarn in half, and then studying the cross-cut. As you would see, the fiber types are not grouped together in each bundle according to their type (or shade of red, pink, or white), but instead are intermingled throughout the bundle in random groupings, so a cross-sectional cut reveals a mosaic pattern. Due to their low-power and high-oxygen (oxidative) nature, *slow twitch fibers* are the reddest skeletal muscle fibers in an animal. Likewise, due to their non-oxidative glycolytic properties, *super fast twitch fibers* are the whitest muscle fibers. And since there is a full spectrum of lower-order *fast twitch fibers* that are both oxidative and glycolytic to escalating degrees, these will appear in highly variable shades of pink, with the higher-order (faster twitching) fibers appearing progressively lighter in color. The full spectrum of muscle fiber types exists together like this in all skeletal muscle bundles. The trained condition of each bundle will produce either a reddish shade from high-volume low-power endurance activity or a whiter shade from low-volume high-power hypertrophy.

The most easily observed example of this contrast can be found in raw chicken meat, where the legs and thighs are the dark red meat, and the breasts clearly present as white meat. Being walking birds, chickens seldom take flight, so their legs and thighs carry most of their slow moving workload and thereby contain a majority of red *slow twitch muscle fibers*. Likewise, chickens seldom use their breasts (which propel their wings), and they're only fully flexed during *fight or flight* situations. Keep in mind that even the white breasts of a chicken are still infused with red *slow twitch fibers*, just as the red meat thighs and legs are infused with pink *fast twitch fibers*, but at much lower percentages respectively.

It's even more important to recognize that the *fast twitch* and *super fast twitch fibers* in a well- trained muscle are much thicker than the spindly *slow twitch fibers*. This is evidence of both their greater hypertrophy and their greater glucose storing capacity. As a very relevant side note, don't forget that dark (red) chicken meat has a higher fat content than the "healthier" white meat. This fact should spark a bit of revelation in you, as the same is true in humans. It seems paradoxical that the least used, most powerful muscles are the leanest in a chicken, but I hope you're starting to see why that's true. Notice how the whiter cells in the cross-section (Figure 2) are generally the largest (thickest), while the dark red cells are generally the smallest (narrowest). As you now know, our goal is to increase the number and size (hypertrophy) of the rare and vulnerable *super fast twitch fibers* in all of our muscle groups before they atrophy and die. To do this, it's important to understand the role of *orderly recruitment*, so keep this intermingling of fiber types in mind as we make sense of the protocols needed to reach that goal in a sustainable fashion.

Your Role in Commanding Orderly Recruitment

As discussed in Chapter 1, *orderly recruitment* is a natural and logical progressive handoff of fiber flexing that occurs when a specific muscle group is called into action. To explain our conscious control over this process it helps to use a bit of personification terminology in reference to the three major fiber types. The *slow twitch fibers* in a muscle bundle will fire until they're not strong enough for the activity, at which time they *acquiesce* and the *fast twitch fibers* take over the bulk of the work. Once the load becomes too much for these higher-order fibers to bear, they in turn hand it off to the *super fast twitch fibers*—the Superman of muscle cells—to save the day. Once these highest order fibers have generated their relatively brief burst to accomplish the goal, like a chicken taking flight just long enough to jump a fence while escaping a predator, these Superman fibers quickly fail upon burning all their glucose stores. This happens in the mere matter of seconds[88] (a critical timing issue you must never forget), and immediately shut down to pass the load back to the weaker *fast twitch fibers* that will also eventually fail.

At this point, the load is passed back to the far weaker *slow twitch fibers* that in turn put on the brakes. This is how our skeletal muscles are designed to work. If, however, you refuse to gear down and attempt to strive through the pain and *super fast twitch* failure over and over (as do *CrossFit* and most bodybuilding enthusiasts), you risk destroying or beating these vital glycolytic *fight or flight* fibers into an indefinite comatose state. This taboo severely stunts the glycolytic capacity of the lower-order *fast twitch fibers* as well.[89] The ultimate result will be a net loss in strength, speed, and glucose burning capacity, and you'll risk missing the *BioLogic Cascade* of benefits altogether. You will have left your *fight or flight* muscles so beaten that only your *slow twitch fibers* are left to fight battles for which they were not designed.

Over the course of a few short minutes, the BioLogic Method takes a single muscle group through this fascinating relay of *slow twitch muscle* overloading to *super fast twitch muscle* recruitment and failure to trigger hypertrophy and supercharge your glucose metabolism without causing potentially irreparable damage to any of your fibers. Once you learn the mental and physical techniques that effectively move your muscles through *orderly recruitment* with optimal effect, you'll begin the cellular transformation that sparks the *super fast twitch* hypertrophy and triggers the full *BioLogic Cascade.* When you truly grasp this revelation, you'll without question appreciate its purity and the immediate, recognizable rewards of the *10 Minute Workouts*.

In essence, in order to stimulate hypertrophy and avoid atrophy, *super fast twitch fibers* need to be 1) isolated, 2) fully flexed for relatively short-durations, 3) commanded to reach their flexing threshold to optimize blood sugar burn, 4) challenged to the point of failure (but no further), and then 5) rested until they're completely recovered, healed, and conditioned to make another run at exceeding that threshold.[90]

As you'll soon see, the BioLogic Method gives you a simple mental framework of techniques to ensure you flex and safely "max out" as many *super fast twitch fiber cells* in a specific muscle group as possible. For this, I've found that conditioning individual muscle groups (chest, glutes, shoulders, etc., see Chapter 7), at the rate of just one group per day, allows us to give each group the full mental and metabolic attention to accomplish the proper stimuli in very short order. Thus the *10 Minute Workout*.

BioLogic Protocol 1: Isolation and Focus - Brain Power

It's easy to forget that we are an amazingly complex set of biomechanical systems that each have their own unique intelligent design, all consciously or unconsciously controlled through the neurological activity of our brain and central nervous system (CNS). Within each of these systems, there are even more complex sub-systems comprised of trillions of cells, all miraculously working in concert at the constant command of our CNS.

Likewise, it's important to remember that every single one of your cells is not just part of a larger community of cells, but it is also its own intelligently ordered community of sorts. Each "member" within the cell answers to commands received from their nuclei as they work as a singular body to fulfill their purpose among the team of cells with which they're bundled—all, in turn, answering to *you* through your CNS. We seldom give this wondrous design a single thought, and there's no better time than the present to start recognizing the untapped power within the relationship between your conscious mind and your skeletal muscles.

As discussed in Chapter 2, over the past two decades the research community has proven that hypertrophic strength training can spark neural adaptations that give even greater power to neural capabilities, thus revealing a remarkable bio-loop where mind and body can perpetually rejuvenate the other.[91] That is some elegant design. Through the BioLogic Method, we take full advantage of the simplest approaches to fully empower this mind-body connection. As you'll soon learn (and gain first-hand proof after a few short months of training the BioLogic way), it is all so entirely logical that even an octogenarian with zero experience can kick-start this bio-loop into action—especially if they can take "every thought into captivity" during each exercise.

The Six Techniques of Isolation and Focus

While the most important muscular processes run on autopilot—either through involuntary functions or subconscious activation of learned motor skills (like walking)—the voluntary actions of skeletal muscle should remain under our intentional, well-focused conscious control during exercise.[92] If not, you will never optimize hypertrophy or minimize damage. Conscious control is essential to the BioLogic Method, as it's the primary reason we can apply the proper stimuli in ten minutes or less.

The demonstration videos will indeed show how the actual mechanics are very easy to perform, but demonstrations aren't needed to learn how to take every thought captive during your workouts. Developing the ability to tune your mind to the frequency (the specific mind-body connection) that sends the proper message to an isolated group of *super fast twitch muscle cells* is the holy grail of BioLogic Workouts.[93]

In the seventies, Arnold Schwarzenegger famously stated that "the body is very important, but the mind is MORE important than the body," [94] and in doing so he helped many enthusiasts like me to learn how to bridge the mind-body gap. While I believe Arnold did more to exacerbate the fitness industry's obsession with over-training on weights than anyone else in the modern era, his promotion of this simple truth was, in my opinion, his towering contribution to fitness. While still a pre-teen, that revelation alone set my fitness trajectory. Thank you, Arnold. Four decades later, the scientific community has proven that the mind has the power to trigger motor learning and strength increases in our skeletal muscles, even when we're not using them.[95]

Likewise, professional athletes have long known (and the scientific literature leaves no doubt) that visualization techniques, mental rehearsal (motor imagery),[96] and other mental isolation and focusing techniques can apply hypertrophy stimuli and motor learning to your muscle fibers even before you begin to flex them.[97] Imagine how much more stimuli you can apply when your full focus is aimed at your target muscles during the actual repetitions of your workout. Through the BioLogic Method, due to the preeminent role of mental engagement, I will often remind you to avoid letting your mind focus on the effort of "lifting weights" or pushing/pulling a bar (or your body weight). In fact, you'll want to perfect your ability to tune-out all peripheral elements of the exercise you're performing, as those draw your conscious thoughts onto external things and obstacles. Instead, you should concentrate solely on flexing the isolated target muscle group, and the following six techniques of Protocol 1 will teach you how to accomplish optimal isolation and focus in a simple step by step process. Focus on flexing muscle, not on moving parts.

Once you have a good grasp on these six techniques, your focused flexing will in turn move your body and the source of the resistance through a safe, controlled, consistent range of motion; without distracting you from the only thing that matters—maximum flexing of the target muscle to ensure you reach the golden door of *super fast twitch fiber* stimuli through *orderly recruitment*. In doing so, you'll ensure your head wags your tail, not vice versa. Don't let that revelation escape you. The vast majority of people I've observed performing a strength exercise are focusing on the wrong thing, and by doing so they basically skip right over the mental bridge they need to cross if they want to fully recruit their *super fast twitch muscle fibers* and optimize the hypertrophy stimuli.

As you'll see below, each specific technique in the BioLogic Method ensures proper isolation of the target muscle group while also eliminating the herky-jerky, teeter-totter, spine-stressing, joint-wrecking movements performed by most gym enthusiasts and taught by most of the *old school* trainers (and all *CrossFit* type trainers I've ever observed). Once you begin to properly isolate and flex the target muscle group and maintain a smooth consistently controlled timing cadence through the full rep, you'll find that these techniques make it impossible to create counterproductive momentum. I really need to hammer that home, as the use of momentum is the most common error in most strength training programs and is therefore a major taboo in the BioLogic Method.[98] As you will see in the demonstration videos, if you are properly isolating the target muscle group, you will automatically eliminate momentum while minimizing movement and effort in all other muscle groups outside of the target muscle group.

Here are the six techniques of isolation and focus that comprise Protocol 1.

1. **Proper Posture**: Establish correct, *fixed*, and balanced posture for each exercise, and whenever possible watch yourself in full-length mirrors to ensure you're maintaining this correct posture.

2. **Peripheral Relaxation**: Identify the proper anchor points for each exercise (hands, feet, elbows, knees, backside, etc.) and lock them into fixed positions with as little associated muscle tension as possible. This technique ensures you maintain *peripheral relaxation*, which enhances your ability to maximize proper leverage to focus all of your effort on the flexing of the target muscle group. So no more squirming around or stressing your face and neck by grimacing or clenching during each rep. Not only does this sort of peripheral movement hinder your focus, but over time it also cuts deep wrinkles into your face. All vanity aside, wrinkles serve no purpose, and neither does peripheral stress.

3. **Focused Flexing:** Truly connect your mind with the core of the target muscle group, and mentally command the target muscle group to flex rather than thinking about moving or gripping the weight/resistance. If your surroundings become a distraction, you may want to close your eyes to help focus on the muscle group, but it's generally best to visually monitor your posture, balance, and other techniques in a mirror if at all possible. Limit all other thoughts except what is required to maintain focus on these isolation mechanics, so you need to avoid taking the focus of your mind, eyes, and ears off the task at hand.

4. **Zero Momentum:** When flexing the muscle, your movements should feel explosive while never generating momentum. This can be accomplished by flexing to move the resistance at relatively slow speeds (two to three seconds) through the full range of motion, both during the contraction movement and the release (aka the "negative" of the rep).[99] Again, the demonstration videos will clearly show the finer points of these techniques in

great detail. Once you see and feel the difference, it will all make perfect sense.

5. **Fixed Range of Continuous Motion:** To put it most simply, every rep should move the weight or your body in a consistent maximum range of motion without ever pausing between repetitions. The range may be shortened greatly in the first set to help warm up the muscle group and the active joints, but the track of movement should be identical for every rep even if the range of motion is just a few inches during the initial set. Once warmed up and fully lubricated, maintaining a fixed range of motion requires the preceding four techniques to work in unison.[100] Continuous motion is necessary to ensure you never disengage your target muscles or allow them to rest at any point during a set—not even at turning points of a rep—as any pause or rest will call lower-order fibers back into the effort and hinder orderly recruitment.[101] The demonstration videos will help you make child's play of this technique within a matter of weeks.

6. **Consistent Breathing Cadence:** This is about as *old school* as it gets, but I'm still amazed by how many enthusiasts ignore this invaluable technique. Ultimately, you can establish pretty much any inhale/exhale cadence that doesn't lead to hyperventilation or oxygen deprivation. But the general rule of thumb is to inhale deeply before the first rep, exhale slowly during the contraction, then inhale deeply again during the negative, exhale again during the next contraction, and so on. Try not to grunt or groan (please don't ever scream!), and make sure you're not holding your breath at any point during each rep.

The Not-So-Secret Weapon: Strength of Spirit

Even where BioLogic Workouts employ bodyweight exercises like push ups and weightless squats, you'll find yourself approaching the effort in not just a more focused way, but also a more spiritually minded way. If you're not a spiritual person, then consider it from the perspective of "team spirit," as surely you've seen how that sort of charismatic activity empowers champions in every sport, and many of the world's top charities and corporations as well. Even if you're an agnostic or atheist, this is where the *joy factor* finds the most fertile ground in our workouts. More than mere positive thinking, this supercharging of your mental enthusiasm sets the stage for you to exercise not just your mind and strength, but also the power of confidence and subconscious belief in the super-human potential designed into each cell of your body. You'll eventually find yourself encouraging your muscles, sometimes silently and sometimes audibly, always believing your muscles can flex with greater strength with each successive workout and doing all you can to make them believe the same. Much like the practice of motor imagery,[102] this sort of *muscle psychology* is key to how we stimulate the *super fast twitch cells* as they wait for a reason (and your command) to fire up their incomparable glycolytic, hypertrophic, fat-burning engines.

BioLogic Protocol 2: The Three F's Progression and Muscle Psychology

The physiological science behind this protocol is solidly rooted in long-held principles in neuromuscular research and cellular biology as noted throughout the book and further detailed in the Appendix. I'll continue writing of these subjects in the same simple terms that I've long used with great success when sparking the revelation in my students and clients. So have no fear of it getting too complex for you, though I am admittedly a nerd about such topics. My goal is to get your muscles working according to their genetic design ASAP, not to burden you with highly technical explanations that do little to inspire. Just as you don't need to understand the science behind how jets can get you across an ocean in hours, you don't need the ability to explain the science that triggers the *BioLogic Cascade*—though I'm confident many of you are already there.

All that said, I will be making liberal use of common psychological terms to teach this particular protocol, and you'll be best served to consider my terminology as metaphorical guides. This sort of terminology will help you fully grasp the progressions that satisfy the fiber type relay of *orderly recruitment*, and thereby more quickly leap out of the lobby and dash down the hallway to kick in the golden door that leads to proper stimulation of your *super fast twitch muscle cells*. After all, you only have ten minutes, and most of that is devoted to warm up and recovery. Here's how it works.

Fire, Fatigue, and Failure

The *Three F's* of *fire, fatigue, and failure* are the mental/physical markers that ensure you are quickly and effectively progressing through the *orderly recruitment* of all your target fiber types during your workout. As detailed below, these three markers will indicate the last repetition you should perform (when to stop) during each of the three sets. The basic *10 Minute Workout* recommended for most people consists of just three sets of six to twelve reps of an exercise that targets a single muscle group using the same amount of resistance for all three sets. Sounds simple I know, and that's a good thing, but what the workout lacks in difficulty it makes up in mental challenges. Once you have your isolation mechanics firmly set and your mind fully focused on the flexing of the target muscle group, you will progress to the golden door by employing the *Three F's* across the three sets as follows.

If you're wanting to scream out that three sets over ten minutes couldn't possibly do all I've promised, you'll find great irony in the following facts. A large body of research and decades of real world application indicate that we can effectively stimulate our *super fast twitch fibers* in a *single* set.[103] The single set approach requires tremendous discipline and a trainer or partner to assist in the final failure reps that kick in the golden door, and it tends to fall a bit short of the multi-set approach where results are concerned, but it can still get the job done.[104] I have highly respected colleagues that preach the single set approach. Having used the approach on many occasions while traveling or in an extreme hurry, I can attest that a single set can in fact apply effective stimuli to our *super fast twitch fibers*. As you know by now, results are not dependent upon the volume of the work, but the quality of stimuli, so among all the teachers who share the *low-volume* and *short-duration* school of thought, I'm actually among the most conservative.

As we continue, you'll see and feel why my clients and I prefer the three set approach, and the latest research demonstrates that specific aspects of the BioLogic Method—especially our specific long-term goals—establish superiority of our three-set approach.[105] While some will argue I'm splitting hairs in what amounts to the same cause and effect regardless of the number of sets, I also find the three-set approach to be far more enjoyable and accessible, especially when training without a partner. I'll further address this topic when discussing workout variations in Chapter 6, as the single-set approach is employed in the two most time-saving variations. Back to the *Three F's*.

Set 1: Fire

Where most strength training enthusiasts put far too much effort into the first set of a given exercise, its role in the BioLogic Method is simply to fire up the engines and warm up your tissues. Just as it's unhealthy to crank up a car and immediately race it to top speed, you never want to rush your body into any *fast twitch* activity, unless of course it's a matter of survival, in which case adrenaline covers most concerns. The fire set consists of six to twelve repetitions (no more, no less) and should be performed until you feel the target muscle begin to heat up and generate a mild burn at its central core during the final two to three reps, and never more than that. If you feel like two or three more reps would be impossible to perform with correct form at the end of this first set, then you've gone too far, as the feelings of fatigue and failure must be saved for the final two sets—thus the progression of fire, fatigue, and failure. The initial fire set serves four major purposes:

- It is the set where you properly fix your physical and mental techniques to ensure optimal isolation and continuous range of motion, with the fine tuning of the arc of this range being among the primary goals by the end of this set.

- It's the set where you dial your full focus onto flexing the target muscles rather than thinking about moving the weights or allowing anything else outside of that singular focus to ever distract you. Anything that pulls your attention away from the actual flexing of the target muscle must be purged during this set or you will stunt your progress.

- It is the set where you'll alert all three major fiber types to the fact that they will all be needed as you progress, especially the *fast* and *super fast twitch fibers*. In the early reps you're basically getting out of our metaphorical lobby by telling your *slow twitch fibers* that the work at hand is beyond their job description and capabilities. In the latter reps, you'll be telling your *fast twitch fibers* that the workout will challenge them to their fullest—a message that in turn alerts your *super fast twitch fibers* that they'll soon be needed.

- Finally, it's the set where your target muscles and their adjacent joints (bones, cartilage, tendons, ligaments) are lubricated and fired up. As I'll soon discuss, you will have performed very light dynamic stretching and other lubricating movements prior to the first set (see protocol 3). It's imperative to realize that only under the stress of the full weight of the selected resistance can you prepare your target muscles and joints for the task at hand. For this, while you should take liberty in reducing the range of motion and even the number of reps in this initial set, never reduce the resistance (weight) as a means to warming up (see protocol 4). So you should start with a reduced range of motion, flexing across just twenty-five percent or less of the full range of motion during the first rep (typically just a few inches of movement). Then gradually increase the range over the next several reps until your joints and muscles feel warmed up enough to cover the full range by the time you complete the final rep of this first set. Those of you who are blessed to have avoided major joint injuries during your life can generally use the full range of motion right from the start. But even if you are so blessed, don't hesitate to shorten the range during the first few reps of the initial fire set. There is virtually nothing to gain from rushing into the full range of motion until you're approaching the completion of this first set. No need to risk pushing yourself into the ranks of the rehab survivors, like me.

As I'll detail in the protocol 3 below, the rest between sets is the recovery period where the *slow twitch fibers* process the message to further step down their role during the next set, while the *fast* and *super fast twitch fibers* gear up to take over the full load as needed. This of course is a key process in *orderly recruitment*. Be reminded that all throughout the day your *slow twitch fibers* have been performing nearly all the mundane and menial tasks of moving you through life, while your *fast* and *super fast twitch fibers* have simply snoozed in the backseat for a free ride—doing virtually nothing but hanging out. If at this point you had ended this particular exercise to move on to work another muscle group—as so many do—your *fast twitch* and *super fast twitch fibers* would receive the message that they're simply not needed, and their resulting atrophy would reduce you to a *slow twitch* weakling as you age.[106]

During your rest between sets, you should relish the fact that the BioLogic Method ensures this sort of age-accelerating atrophy is being thwarted by the youth-sustaining hypertrophy you'll spark in your higher-order fibers as you proceed. Stay excited about that fact through every workout. While you prepare your mind for the final two sets, remind yourself that your *fast twitch muscle fibers* exist solely to do the work *slow twitch fibers* cannot handle, and that your *super fast twitch fibers* are likewise waiting for the *fast twitchers* to fail before they'll kick in to save the day. *Orderly recruitment* has begun, and *super fast twitch fiber* hypertrophy is just a few minutes away. This first set and its subsequent rest period should take about three minutes, total.

Set 2: Fatigue

During the second set of six to twelve reps, you should now move through the full range of motion during every rep, and you must continue your rep count until the fatigue becomes so acute that you honestly believe you can only accomplish one more very difficult rep without losing correct form (as detailed in protocol 1). This is what I consider to be the point of true fatigue during the set. The fatigue set could also be called the *success* set, as it gives your *fast twitch fibers* a sense of accomplishment for having successfully carried the bulk of a relatively intense load for all the reps leading up to this "just one more rep" threshold absent any sense of failure.

At this point your *slow twitch fibers* and the full spectrum of *fast twitch fibers* in the target muscle group will have reached this fatigue marker in proper order, well before the super fast twitch fibers fully take over, which is a measure of success in the lower-order fibers that should not be discounted. Just as your mental confidence is built upon success, the individual motor units that include these fibers will also have gained through both the optimal hypertrophy stimuli and the *motor learning* delivered through your mental focus on flexing the target muscle during the successful repetitions.[107]

This is the process I call *Muscle Psychology*. You can take it as a metaphor or as an actual neurological event occurring within your central nervous system (which directly controls all motor units). But don't ignore it, or you'll risk losing both the mind-body connection and the full benefits of the accelerated motor learning that occurs when you adhere to the four protocols. Once you implement this concept, not only will you find it much easier to fatigue your lower-order fibers, but your *super fast twitch fibers* as well; for they have been activated but not yet exhausted. The sudden halting of the set with "just one more rep" remaining in the tank, leaves these Superman cells wanting more, and fully prepared to succeed when the *fight or flight* stimuli is finally applied during the third and final set.[108] If this doesn't make sense now, I can promise you that after just a couple weeks of workouts it will. So let's press on.

In a truly successful fatigue set, you should ensure the final rep is legitimately difficult to complete, while building the confidence that you definitely could have completed just one more rep, but not a single rep more. Learning to recognize the point when you've reached this "penultimate rep" (second to last possible rep) is probably the most challenging skill in the BioLogic Method for novices to master, yet even this will become child's play in a matter of weeks. When you reach the penultimate rep, you'll feel a deep burn in the core of the target muscle group, but even if you struggle a bit to finish the rep, you'll still feel fuel in the tank to get "just one more rep." If not, you went too far—prematurely stimulating your super fast twitch fibers in a less effective manner—and would be best served to end the workout knowing you still achieved a modicum of success without risking the damage that would occur if you over-trained these precious fibers.

Like the psychology used by a drill sergeant training his soldiers, or a coach pushing his athletes, or a mother teaching her children, in the fatigue set you want to challenge the target muscle as far as you can without breaking its morale or "exasperating" it. In doing so, you send the message that greater strength is needed, while also ensuring you don't overwhelm the muscles' perceived threshold, which in turn conditions the target muscle group to also expect more from itself. Though I'm speaking metaphorically, it's very possible that this sort of motor unit "thought" process could in fact be happening at the cellular level, but we need a lot more research to support such a conclusion.

Meanwhile, thanks to *orderly recruitment,* the *slow twitch fibers* have pretty much bowed out of the battle, and now that you've conditioned the lower-order *fast twitch fibers* to recognize their limits, once they burn up all their stored glycogen as fuel during the final set, they'll be quick to call on Superman (their *super fast twitch* fibers) to take over. As long as you're not quitting on yourself mentally (the biggest challenge of all) and are holding firm to the mental techniques, the target muscle group will respond to your commanding encouragement, standing at the ready with *super fast twitch fibers* blazing. This is "operant conditioning" at the cellular level, and the ultimate goal of the *Three F's* progression in the *Muscle Psychology* protocol.

Set 3: Failure

This is when the ultimate stimulus is applied to exhaust the glucose stored in the highest order fibers of your target muscle group. For this, it's the set where the key is turned to unlock the hidden potential of your *fast twitch* and *super fast twitch muscle fibers* to spark the *BioLogic Cascade.* While you were resting before this final *Failure* set, you should already have felt a significant amount of burn and "pump" in the target muscle group. So after a minute or two of recovery (which I'll fully address in protocol 3), you and your *super fast twitch muscle fibers* should feel refreshed and inspired to attack the final set with greater isolation, greater focus, and greater effort than the previous sets. Not only have your target muscles and adjacent joints been fully fired up for this final challenge, but even more important, so has your confidence.

You'll start the final failure set just as you did the previous set. But once you reach the point of fatigue you felt in the second set (which will usually be on or about the same rep count), you will instead press on to complete not only the next rep but still another rep if possible. In fact, you'll want to continue with every possible rep until you reach the point that you can no longer complete another rep with proper mechanics. At that point, you should put extra emphasis on placing one-hundred percent of your mental focus on flexing the single muscle group as you compel your *super fast twitch fibers* to "believe" they can in fact finish and "flex" that seemingly impossible rep. Your *slow twitch fibers* are now acting as safety spotters (emergency brakes), while your *fast twitch fibers* have reached the limits of their ability and have finally handed off the bulk of the workload to your *super fast twitch fibers*. This is where your *10 Minute Workout* should be just one intensely focused *golden* failure rep away from completion.

Beginners may be surprised to discover they can actually perform several more reps during the final failure set than they thought possible when they ended the second (fatigue) set. Over time, you will learn where your true fatigue threshold exists, as it is surely beyond what most beginners expect. As long as you've been sure not to pause or allow your isolation techniques to break down during the final failure set, you should find great reward in your super fast twitch fibers' ability to exceed your strength expectations as you allow them to determine their actual point of failure, where they fully exhaust their glucose stores during the final *golden rep*.

The Golden Rep

If you have in fact maintained proper focus and mechanical techniques during the final failure set, you will feel your target muscles "give out" on you during this intense, seemingly impossible final rep (which is of course the goal of the final failure set). Once the target muscle group truly fails in its effort to flex through the full range of motion for the chosen exercise, you must then perform the negative lowering movement as slowly as possible (approx. five seconds), while you continue flexing the muscle group with one-hundred percent of your focus until you reach the point of zero resistance.

During these arduous final seconds of intense burn you should concentrate on the fact that you're not simply lowering the weight to attain and finish a quantifiable goal (total rep count in the final set), but are literally scorching every last molecule of glucose stored in your *super fast twitch fibers* as you seemingly flex in futility. And there is the key. Flexing the core of the target muscle group with maximum effort while the muscle fails—for as long as possible— stimulates hypertrophy in *super fast twitch fibers* in the most sustainably effective fashion. The better you can continue flexing at the core of the target muscle beyond the point the muscle begins to fail, the deeper the glycolytic burn. This is the "key node" in the cascade. Never diminish or forget the *golden rep*. The demonstration videos will show how simple the *golden rep* should be, so don't let any of this overwhelm you.

If you have a training partner or personal trainer, research has shown that adding resistance and otherwise gaining encouragement to continue focus on flexing to the very end of final negative can maximize the *golden rep's* effectiveness.[109] Don't forget that it's unlikely that you'll be able to break a sweat during the entire *10 Minute Workout*, so you know it can't be as difficult as it may sound. Yet it is without question an urgent skill to learn. It's worth repeating: the *golden rep's* final burn is the glycolytic catalyst that cranks up the full BioLogic effect and the resulting *BioLogic Cascade* of benefits.[110]

Over the course of ten minutes or less, you've A) established proper mechanics through isolation and mental focus, B) applied an ideal amount of "load" on your *slow twitch fibers* to prep them for an early exit from the final set, C) applied an effective amount of stimuli to trigger hypertrophy in your higher-order *fast twitch fibers*, and D) applied the proper amount of resistance to fire up and overload your *super fast twitch fibers* to the point that all stored glycogen is burned as fuel, thereby leaving all the higher-order fibers in the desired state of failure where the healing process immediately begins. In our *orderly recruitment* metaphor, you've gotten up from the couch, you've passed through the lobby, you've opened every door as you crossed to the end of the hallway, and you've entered through the golden door.

At this point—just ten minutes or less into the workout—you have programmed your *super fast twitch fiber cells* to enter hypertrophy as they heal, refuel, and begin the satellite stem cell recruitment process. All of this increases your insulin sensitivity as these fully glycolytic fibers attempt to store even larger quantities of glucose, in an effort to exceed your current performance threshold the next time you train their specific muscle group.

It's a wonderfully rewarding cycle. The *BioLogic Cascade* has begun in you just as it did in the alpha-humans who established most our gene pool, through millennia of adaptations triggered by naturally *occurring fight or flight* stimuli. Again, don't let the science distract you from the simplicity of this ten-minute process. The demonstration videos will prove all of this to be a piece of cake even if you've never even touched a dumbbell in your life. Trust the research, follow the protocols, eliminate all doubts, and your instincts will kick in and take over before you even know it.

CHAPTER 5

BioLogic Workout Protocols 3 & 4

BioLogic Protocol 3: R&R—Recovery and Recuperation

Recovery: Inter-Set Rest

If you're a beginner or someone who has burned out from exhausting traditional workout programs, *R&R* should be an exciting and welcome concept for you. As I continue to stress, proper rest and recovery are essential to optimally stimulate your *super fast twitch muscle fibers*—before, after, and *during* your workouts. This is due in part to the essential need for recovery between the three sets (fire, fatigue, and failure). These recovery periods generally last for two to five minutes, depending on your condition. Contrary to what most personal trainers and virtually all *CrossFit* and endurance training promoters teach these days, the overwhelming preponderance of research has established that frequent rest and recovery during the workout is mission critical. It's also perfectly logical.

Shortly before publication of this book, a team of thirteen scientists from the US and the Netherlands published their findings in the July 2016 *Journal of Strength and Conditioning Research*. Not only did the study provide definitive evidence that longer rest periods promote significantly greater increases in muscle strength and hypertrophy, but the research also revealed that the increases in muscle endurance were the same regardless of the length of intra-workout recovery periods.[111] This further reinforces previously cited research. Intervalized (short bursts, rest, repeat) strength and speed training enhances endurance commensurate with the goals of endurance training—minus the damage and significant time expense.

Furthermore, experienced male strength training enthusiasts should be the last to reject the importance of inter-set rest (intra-workout rest). Concurring research published in the July 2016 journal of *Experimental Physiology* and the October 2015 *Journal of Strength and Conditioning Research* prove this point. The two studies conclude respectively that *"short inter-set rest blunts resistance exercise-induced increases in myofibril protein synthesis and intracellular signaling"*[112] and that *"longer [inter-set] rest promoted a longer lasting elevation for both total testosterone and free testosterone."*[113] As detailed in *Section I*, the research has long demonstrated that BioLogic type workouts enhance proper levels of various hormones (and thereby slow the aging process while empowering the various metabolic processes they control). This is equally true for men and women of all demographics.

If you're still holding to the belief that sweat production is an indicator of an effective workout, follow the four BioLogic protocols and those misperceptions will be erased in a matter of weeks. Despite the relatively high-intensity short-burst effort required to properly isolate and flex your highest order fibers in each major muscle group, unless you're working out in an environment over seventy-five degrees, you shouldn't be able to break a real sweat during the entire *10 Minute Workout*. Of course, some folks sweat at the drop of a hat, so if that's you, I'm sure you won't be surprised if you start sweating before you finish the first set. But for the majority of us, heavy sweating in cool environments might be an indication of a failure to recover between sets. So make sure you're fully recovered before you start the next set no matter how long it takes.

Once you complete a set, the general rule is to ensure your breathing has returned to a semi-normal rate before you start the next set. You do yourself no favors to feel aerobic stress or shortness of breath at the beginning of a set. Remember, you're trying to stimulate very specific muscle fibers through simple scientific protocols, You're not trying to get an exhausting, sweaty, *no-pain no-gain* workout. If you make the mistake of beginning the next set too soon, you'll start taxing your *fast* and *super fast twitch muscle fibers* before they've been able to properly recover, and you'll thereby push them into prematurely shutting down.

In addition to the recovery of your breathing patterns, you should ensure your target muscle group has also sufficiently recovered before starting the next set. That doesn't mean you won't feel a pump and some fire in the target muscle group, as you definitely need to ensure you don't rest so long that your muscles have fallen asleep. If you are struggling to regain your breath, a *five-minute* inter-set rest period should do the trick, but that should be your maximum. Your target muscles should actually feel very ready (even hungry) to take on the next challenge, and in time you'll know firsthand what I mean, but as an additional indicator, that feeling of readiness can be most easily measured by your ability to talk normally without becoming breathless mid-sentence.

While you are recovering between sets, you should begin practicing what I call *resting movements,* which are similar to "dynamic stretching," but with even greater care when employing momentum. As you will see detailed in Chapter 6, these joint lubricating, flexibility enhancing movements are a required activity before, between, and after each set during the actual workouts. They help flush fresh blood into the muscles and flush out waste while bringing a host of physical and mental benefits that can be enjoyed anytime, day or night, even when you feel totally recuperated.[114] In addition to the subsection in Chapter 6, I'll fully explore *resting movements* in the demonstration videos. I believe that, like me and everyone else who performs BioLogic Workouts, you'll quickly grow to love them.

Recuperation: Rest for Your Soul

Where *recovery* deals with the re-energizing rest required between sets of a single workout, *recuperation* is the rejuvenating healing period of four to fourteen days *required* between successive workouts for each major muscle group. The recuperation rule helps explain why six *10 Minute Workouts* or less per week are all we need to trigger the *BioLogic Cascade.* If you train a particular muscle group before it has fully recuperated from its previous workout, you'll be beating on muscle fibers that are trying to heal, and need to heal. We must refrain from training our *super fast twitch muscle fibers* until after they have fully reloaded with glycogen and fully healed from the much-needed micro-tears (micro-injuries) we generated to stimulate hypertrophy during each workout.[115] Stunting this healing process is a strict no-no. You must give your muscles time to recuperate and heal into their stronger state before you throw them back into the fire.

If, however, you make the mistake of training that muscle group while it's still sore, you may in fact increase the size and strength of your lower-order *fast twitch fibers* and cause a lot of inflammation. Over the long-term, this form of overtraining will prove counterproductive and potentially destructive. Research has also revealed that women need to take these concerns even more seriously than men. A recent study conducted by a team of eleven scientists from the Human Performance Laboratory at the University of Connecticut addressed the effects of a short rest protocol for women. Published in the April 2014 *Journal of Strength and Conditioning Research*, in reference to the short rest protocol (between workouts) the team concluded:

> Overall, women demonstrated a faster inflammatory response with increased acute damage, whereas men demonstrated a greater prolonged damage response. Therefore, strength and conditioning professionals need to be aware of the level of stress imposed on individuals when creating such volitional high-intensity metabolic type workouts and allow for adequate progression and recovery from such workouts.[116]

Please take that to heart, especially the final sentence. Recovery and recuperation are without question mission critical, so ensure you train no muscle group before its time. When practicing BioLogic Workouts, micro-tears are the cause of the localized soreness you'll feel setting in within forty-eight hours after each effective workout. This soreness can be quite intense for a day or two, and you'll learn to love it—especially as you begin to see and feel the results kicking in. The intensity of the soreness you feel over the three to four days after each workout is a general indication of how successful you were in properly stimulating your *fast* and *super fast twitch fibers*. And just as is true for any type of injured tissue, while rehab movements can be greatly beneficial, actual loaded work on injured tissue (even for the much wanted micro-tears) should be considered taboo. Beginners often experience soreness in a specific muscle group that gradually fades over ten to fourteen days, so patience is a true virtue that should come easy to those short on time.

Some of you might find you need just twelve workouts per month to trigger the BioLogic effect. I personally feel fully recovered in about eight days, so I'll take a couple days off from the workouts to partake in other activities that keep me off the couch. Much more on that in *Section III.*

Once the *fast* and *super fast twitch fibers* in a specific muscle group are fully healed, they will become incrementally stronger and more numerous due to hypertrophy and satellite muscle stem cell activation. With each passing day that you continue with your *10 Minute Workouts*, the *BioLogic Cascade* of benefits will become increasingly evident, and your muscles (and your mind) will welcome the increases in resistance that comprise the fourth and final protocol detailed below. Trust this process, and please ensure that you never rush it or try to get ahead of it by training a target group before it is truly recuperated, which should take at least one week if you properly followed the four protocols. Research has shown there is no benefit in strength or hypertrophy from training a specific muscle group twice in a single week, especially if you're a beginner.[117] If all of this sounds entirely opposite to what you've been taught in the past, welcome to the revelation.

During recuperation, your *fast* and *super fast twitch muscle fibers* will be begging for rest. Don't forget that those same muscle bundles are loaded with *slow twitch fibers* that are more than ready to carry you through your normal lifestyle movements, minus all the acute pain you would have experienced had you stressed these lowest order fibers, your joints, and your spine through high-volume long-duration exercise. So don't let the localized soreness generated through BioLogic Workouts trick you into babying those muscle groups by sitting or lying around instead of finding something fun and active to do. Your higher-order fibers benefit greatly from the increased circulation and physical stimulation they gain when their co-mingled *slow twitch* counterparts do what they were designed to do.

With all my past sports related injuries, I stick to low impact activities like walking, hiking, swimming (along with various games that can be played while engaging in these *slow twitch* activities) whenever I'm itching for more activity immediately after or between my BioLogic Workouts. A *10 Minute Workout* affords me enough time to work fun back into my life, so I'm always brainstorming and researching fun activities I loved as a kid and an increasing number of games I've learned to love as an adult. I've especially enjoyed recruiting my friends and family to join in on the highly active fun. Doesn't this sound more fruitful than hours of sweating in the gym or lone wolfing it down an endless road? If not, give it time and I guarantee you'll change your mind.

The Taboo of Muscle Over-Training

It cannot be stressed enough that knowing the precise time to stop flexing during each set is crucial to ensure you never over-train a muscle group. That's exactly what you start to do when you try to push your muscles to continue working even after the *super fast twitch fibers* have burned all their fuel and thrown in the towel. In their landmark study, Andersen and Aagaard addressed this concern in the simplest of terms:

> The fact is that muscle fibers containing predominantly [super fast twitch cells] are also fibers that rely on a metabolism that enables them to produce very high amounts of energy in short time (i.e. exerting very high power), but only over a very limited period of time (seconds). Consequently, the [super fast twitch] fibers need to rest to avoid exhaustion.[118]

If you recall from the previous chapter, while the BioLogic Method trains all fiber types in the target muscle group, it isn't until the final *golden rep* that the failure (exhaustion) stimuli are applied to your *super fast twitch fibers*. This single rep takes just a few seconds, or as the dynamic duo put it, the "very limited period of time" that fulfills our highest goal and concludes the hard work involved in BioLogic Workouts. Recognition of this remarkable paradox within my own body was the epiphany that first sparked the BioLogic revelation back in the nineties.

Don't ever forget that the final seconds of your BioLogic Workouts are worth far more than all the minutes of work that lead up to that final *golden rep*. For further evidence, Andersen and Aagaard also noted that the typical bodybuilder's tendency to continue training a muscle group after the *super fast twitch fibers* have been exhausted will lead to their sharp decline. In fact, a 2008 study published in the *European Journal of Applied Physiology* revealed that traditional bodybuilding type protocols can totally eliminate these invaluable fibers in the over-trained muscles.[119]

If you make the mistake of continuing to train a specific muscle group immediately after reaching this point of exhaustion—which is actually quite easy to miss if you don't follow the protocols detailed in the previous chapter—you'll do far *more harm than good.* But don't be discouraged bodybuilders, as it appears there may be a way for you to redeem all your time in the gym. Not only does the literature indicate that your satellite muscle stem cells can revive and restore your *super fast twitch fiber* content once corrections are made, but the research shows that prolonged periods of detraining (rest periods lasting as long as three months) can actually revive *super fast twitch fibers* to a remarkable degree.[120] I know the thought of a three month sabbatical can be depressing to a bodybuilding enthusiast, but the rest of us can only envy your unique opportunity. More research is likely needed before this wondrous theory will become widely accepted, but so far all research points to its validity. *Less is more* in more ways than we know.

It's important to note that traditional *old school* three-set resistance training approaches promote failure as the goal in every set performed, even when performing twelve sets per workout. It is this error that leads to a feeling of dread in your conscious mind and a negative response in your target muscles. Like athletes who expend all their strength and energy in the first half of a game and leave nothing in the tank for the second half; or soldiers who are so beaten down and neglected by commanders that they become demoralized in the heat of battle; or children who are pushed so hard by their parents that they become "exasperated" and lose heart, these traditional approaches do far *more harm than good.* When you over-train your muscles, most of your body systems suffer right along with them. If you're wondering how the biggest bodybuilders at the gym seem to maintain their ability to move their weights even after failing over and over at the end of their earlier sweat soaked sets, the answer can be found in their use of momentum, pauses between reps, and assistance from peripheral muscles—each of which are taboo in the BioLogic Method.

I hope you're starting to see how *old school* practices can destroy your invaluable *super fast twitch fibers* during their crucial recuperation period that should last for days while hypertrophy and glucose refueling work their magic. Ignoring this scientific fact is like seeing Superman struggling to regain his strength after a Kryptonite bath, only to dump a ton of the green stuff on his now-fragile head. Those who make this mistake risk pounding their *super fast twitch cells* (and their equally valuable satellite stem cells) into a toxic fuel for the fire. Such a breakdown is an early stage of rhabdomyolysis, the potentially deadly syndrome made infamous by the creators of *CrossFit*.[121] But even if you stop short of liquefying your invaluable super fast twitch fibers into this cannibalized fuel, research has proven the post-exhaustion beating they endure still hurls them into atrophy, early death, or some other inactive or downgraded state that the scientific community has yet to clearly define.[122] If I was a bodybuilder reading this peer-reviewed, well-substantiated research, I'd be planning my three month sabbatical ASAP.

As discussed in the introduction, all the misinformation the fitness industry has flooded through the media over the past thirty years might make it difficult for many enthusiasts to accept that long layoffs could be a good thing, or that their one hour bodybuilding workouts could possibly be destroying their largest, most powerful muscle fibers. If that's you, let's allow one of the leading bodybuilding experts in the world to weigh in. Physiologist Jacob Wilson, a well-published research scientist who writes for *Bodybuilding.com* (the world's leader in the niche), pulls no punches despite being an avid bodybuilder. In the April 2016 edition of his *Ask the Muscle Prof* column, Wilson wrote:

> Fast-twitch muscle fibers are indeed the largest and most powerful muscular movers in your body. Unfortunately, they're also neglected in most bodybuilders' programs. It's time to change this! [123]

Amen, Doc. And that's the soft pitch. Be reminded that your *super fast twitch fibers* are ten times more powerful than your *slow twitch fibers,* and twice as powerful as your highest order *fast twitch fibers.* Absent the protocols used in the BioLogic Method, long-duration strength training will indeed swell you up and make you *look* more powerful. But due to the loss of your *super fast twitch fibers* and highest order *fast twitch fibers,* you'd actually be weaker, far slower, and a good bit less healthy and youthful than if you had properly triggered hypertrophy in your *"largest and most powerful"* muscle fibers. This is the pitfall most bodybuilders fall into all their lives; and once they enter their senior years, unless they take the prolonged sabbaticals the research recommends, they eventually pay a heavy price in pre-aging for their short-term fleshy gains.

This sort of negativity loop takes a significant toll on their glucose metabolism and other metabolic systems, and the *BioLogic Cascade* is virtually unplugged right along with their super-human glycolytic fibers. I can't quote some of the angry pushback I've received when trying to share this revelation with a few of the bodybuilders I've surveyed, so I hope Dr. Wilson can help the bodybuilding community open their eyes and ears to the preponderance of research. Nearly all strength training enthusiasts suffer from this misguided over-use abuse, so if that's you, rejoice in the revelation and change your ways by first opening your mind to the positive possibilities while taking a sober look at your current trajectory.

Have you ever seen a massive bodybuilder try to sprint or climb a tree or fight off a speedy attacker? It's not a pretty sight. Yet as we've established, our goal should be to condition our bodies for *fight or flight*. Any amount of over-development, regardless of the short-term or extrinsic benefits, is simply another case of doing *more harm than good*. Keep reminding yourself that optimizing your genetic design is the path to a longer stronger life, and you'll save yourself from a lot of self-inflicted heartache.

Occasional Layoffs Are a Good Thing for All

As addressed in Chapter 2, once you have developed a strong base of *fast* and *super fast twitch muscles*, you'll benefit from occasional layoffs that last weeks at a time. Research has even shown that effective hypertrophy can be sustained during many weeks of bed rest if ever necessitated by serious illness or injury.[124] This points to the youth-sustaining benefits of the *fight or flight* stimuli inherent to the BioLogic Method. When I miss several successive weeks due to a prolonged mission trip or other excursion, I always feel stronger when I return to my workouts, especially when I continue with my *resting movement* routines and active lifestyle while away. It's an awesome phenomenon, but once you fully understand the aforementioned science behind *R&R*, it will all make perfect sense.

Like a warrior resting up after a hard battle or a football player taking a prolonged break after an especially violent season, our bodies need periodic sabbaticals from the grind. Your *fast* and *super fast twitch fibers* simply do not want to be overworked, and they love to get extra rest after prolonged periods of work. So unless you're making the mistake of damaging these muscles by participating in high-stress endurance events or starving them of proper nutrition, they'll remain at the ready, just as they've been conditioned. Those are facts you should never forget.

BioLogic Protocol 4: The Scientific Method

This final protocol completes the logic in the BioLogic Method. By now I hope you recognize that most fitness programs are devoid of real science that supports their protocols. In contrast, my approach to the *scientific method* (as defined below) is the capstone among the four BioLogic protocols. Without it, sustainable success is virtually impossible. For the sake of this protocol as it applies to BioLogic Workouts, here's the definition of the *scientific method* that we'll use to optimize our results. The *scientific method,* according to *Merriam-Webster's Dictionary,* reads:

> Principles and procedures for the systematic pursuit of knowledge involving the recognition and formulation of a problem, the collection of data through observation and experiment, and the formulation and testing of hypotheses.[125]

Even among the programs developed by my colleagues that also target *fast* and *super fast twitch muscles*, the *scientific method* is mostly lacking from their protocols. No matter how you slice it, fitness is a science. The absence of experimentation, observation, and documentation will take the science out of the fitness, which results in diminishing returns or net zero gains over time. The collection of data from your close observations and occasional experimentation to determine the exercises, the amount of resistance, and the number of sets and repetitions employed to work each target muscle group are vital for you to identify, test, and prove the unique routine that is ideally suited to optimize *your* results. Use the BioLogic mobile app to collect, track, and analyze your progress and facilitate adjustments on the fly. Traditional journaling can also work, but nothing beats the ease and technology built into our app.

The Basic Muscle Groupings (Super Groups)

All six variations of the BioLogic Workout will be detailed in Chapter 6 where I will also note my top rated exercises to fit various levels of experience *or* strength in each target muscle group. The following are the six *"super groups"* my students and I (along with most of my colleagues) have found to be the most effective for the basic ten-minute, no-sweat variation of the BioLogic Workout. It's also called *The Healer.* As you'll see in Chapter 6, these are also the best groupings for the 20 minute variation appropriately named the *Once-a-Week'er* and the thirty-minute version named *The Weekender.* Both of these variations are designed for those of you who feel you can only keep up with your program once or twice every week or two (much more on variations later). The six *super groups* are:

1. **Buttocks and Front of Thighs** (Glutes and Quads)
2. **Chest** (Pectorals)
3. **Upper and Outer Back** (Lats)
4. **Back of Thighs** (Hamstrings)
5. **Mid and Lower Back** (Rhomboids and Erectors)
6. **Shoulders** (Deltoids)

While many who promote *fast twitch* training suggest a similar set of groupings, the BioLogic approach is rare in its separation of the hamstrings from the leg group (Butt and Quads). Sadly, most workout programs neglect or over-train legs, and I've found that this particular division is especially effective in reversing that trend. If by chance you are a sprinter interested in adding sprints to your program, you can drop the hamstring workout from your schedule, as proper sprinting (coupled with the proper glute/quad workout) will cover your legs beautifully. Advanced dancers can also consider their dance training to satisfy this adjustment, but please remember that despite dance being especially effective over the short run, it is unfortunately an unsustainable form of exercise. For those of you who are competitive athletes, I promise not to ignore your extreme needs. I'll begin introducing the advanced variations of the BioLogic Workout and their more defined target muscle groups later in this chapter.

The Steps within BioLogic's Scientific Method

In BioLogic Workouts, the *scientific method* is applied in a simple and logical set of steps. If you adhere to the following procedures, you will make the gains and attain the results I've promised. As is true with most missions that matter, you will reap in strength and longevity what you sow in discipline.

1. While keeping the *joy factor* firmly in mind (see Chapter 3), experiment with the exercises I recommend for each target muscle group to determine which is the most effective exercise for you.

2. If you have selected a weight bearing resistance exercise (free weights or machines, as will be the case for the majority of you), identify the proper starting weight that you can properly perform the BioLogic way for at least six to eight repetitions and no more than twelve repetitions during each set. To ensure you remain within this range for all three sets, move up or down in weight accordingly. Likewise, if you have selected a body weight resistance exercise (no free weights or machines), you must ensure that you can perform at least six to eight repetitions and no more than twelve repetitions during each set.

3. Track and document the number of repetitions you can complete during the final set (the *Failure* set). Once you can perform twelve reps during any of the three sets, you must move up in weight *by the smallest increment possible.* As a beginner, don't be surprised if you find yourself needing to move up in weight on a weekly basis. But again, we're all different, so it also may take several

workouts before you move up. While the increasing number of reps you can perform during the failure set is your primary means of measuring gains, the truest indication of hypertrophy will always be proven by increases in the amount of weight you can properly move for at least six reps.

4. As you progress and move up in weight or resistance (which is required over time), stick with each specific exercise indefinitely unless, A) you are unable to move up in weight over time, or B) you no longer feel soreness in the target muscle group forty-eight hours after the workout. In either case, you should first ensure you are properly adhering to all four BioLogic protocols. Then, if you are sure you have done so, change to a new exercise and repeat the previous three steps. Go to BioLogicWorkout.com for guidance in selecting new exercises from a robust list of options for each *super group*.

Important side note: please note that you should never let anyone convince you to mix up your exercises for the sake of the hapless practice known as "muscle confusion". You never want to "confuse" your muscles regardless of the short-term results this practice may bring, as this sort of confusion will hinder the *BioLogic Cascade* while stunting long-range results and greatly increasing the risk of injury. While your *super fast twitch muscle fibers* can handle confusion in an emergency or during play, they do not respond well to confusion during training. The above procedures of the *scientific method* properly achieve the goals that the proponents of muscle confusion misguidedly promote. Muscles respond to confusing changes in their hypertrophy training the way toddlers respond to confusing changes in their skills training—not very well. While there is no serious scientific literature or research on this subject (which in itself is evidence of its lack of credibility), the majority of fitness experts and journalists are in agreement.[126] Please trust my three decades of personal trial and independent research. I've observed many hundreds of men and women of all ages making no sustainable progress unless they adopted the *scientific method.* Muscle Confusion is indeed a myth, and it doesn't even line up with common sense, let alone science or logic.

Myth: The Muscle Confusion concept helps avoid plateaus while enhancing results.
Truth: Muscle Confusion simply does not work as advertised, creates a high-risk of injury, and thwarts the *BioLogic Cascade* of benefits while entirely dismissing the power of the *scientific method.*

5. The *scientific method* requires a modest measure of consistency and control of external factors in order to maximize our ability to effectively measure increases in strength and accurately make change decisions. For this, you should do your best to ensure you are:

    - Properly fueled up
    - Receiving proper sleep the night before each workout
    - Working out at or about the same time of the day if possible
    - Approaching each workout with a positive mindset and enthused spirit (how could you not get excited about a *10 Minute No-Sweat Workout*?)

6. If at any time you feel acute pain (as opposed to the desired deep burn effect) in the target muscle group, joints, or your spine/neck, move to another muscle group for that workout and give the original muscle group a few days before making another go at it with a different exercise (step 1 above). If the pain continues to persist—as is true for any persistent, acute pain regardless of its potential pre-existing nature—you should confer with a sports medicine professional or your personal physician.

Stay the Course!

As is true with all efforts that truly matter, whether it deals with your career or family life or spiritual life, the *scientific method* is invaluable when effectively applied, especially when stimulating hypertrophy of your *super fast twitch muscle fibers* in a sustainable fashion is the primary goal. Whether you're training with barbells like an Olympian or working out in your bedroom with nothing but your body weight and household items for resistance, your ability to understand, implement, and "take to heart" the fundamentals, cornerstones, and protocols of the BioLogic Method will guarantee your success. Let's press on for the prize!

CHAPTER 6

The Workouts

BioLogic Workout Scheduling Variations

While all beginners and the vast majority of current enthusiasts will utilize the *10 Minute No-Sweat Workout (The Healer)*, some of you will quickly see that one or more of the other five variations may better serve your tight schedule or competitive goals. All six variations build upon the fundamentals, cornerstones, and protocols discussed in previous chapters, so please don't let these scheduling twists confuse you. If you have these core concepts figured out, all you'll need is a cursory understanding of the target muscle *"super groups"* and familiarity with just one weight bearing exercise for each of these six groups, and you could head to the gym right now and start your transformation.

As you proceed, it's important to know the difference between the major muscles that comprise the primary *"super groups"* and the more specific *"advanced groups"* detailed below. As you'll see, beginners who use *The Healer or* the uber-efficient *Once-a-Week'er* or *Weekender* variations need only focus on the *super groups.* I expect as much as eighty percent of you will use one of these three variations. The remaining twenty percent will practice one of the three advanced variations or some combination of the three, and will generally focus on the more specific *advanced groups.* These folks will thereby follow a more robust workout schedule, but as you'll see, even the most advanced variation calls for a relatively short-duration, no-sweat workout when compared to non-BioLogic strength training programs. If you are a beginner, I suggest you save (or briefly review) the sections on advanced variations and advanced muscle groups for future reference, well after mastering the *10 Minute Healer* targeting just the six *super groups*.

For review, the six *super groups* include just glutes (buttocks) and quads (front thigh), pectorals (chest), lats (upper back), hamstrings (back thigh), rows (mid and lower back), and shoulders. Going forward I will use the terms in parentheses for each muscle group interchangeably with its common terminology, so don't be confused if I use buttocks and front thighs in one sentence then refer to the muscles as glutes and quads in another. It's important that you know how to name these groups in each of these synonymous "gym" names, so in my outline I've used them in a way that should help beginners quickly catch on to the various common names. These are the only anatomical terms I need you to commit to memory, so it's good to realize that most of you already have some level of familiarity with these relatively common terms, from high school biology class if not from past experience.

Whether you are planning to start off with the basic *super groups* of the *BioLogic 10 Minute Workout* or feel the need to jump up to one of the advanced variations, all will apply the *scientific method* as outlined in Chapter 5, so be sure to avoid confusing your muscles, and always document your progress!

Before Getting Started

The four BioLogic Protocols of 1) *Isolation and Focus*, 2) the *Three F's*, 3) *R&R*, and 4) the *scientific method* are especially important to fully understand before you can truly optimize your results. But don't fret if you're not able to master all the physical and mental skills that empower these four protocols right out the gate. With practice, you will begin to employ an increasing number of these skills with increasing precision.

For a quick reference guide to the combined protocols, you'll find them outlined in the BioLogic Mobile app. For a more detailed chronological review, look for the *Flight Checklist* in Chapter 7. As previously noted, even BioLogic Workouts can be stunted if you fail to obey the *Great Requirement*. So never forget to map out a more active lifestyle (especially more walking!), and maintain *proper* nutrition (add the good, eliminate the bad) to ensure the BioLogic approach proves fruitful no matter which variation you choose, no matter where you stand today. We'll take a solid dive into BioLogic strategies to fine-tune and enhance your adherence to the *Great Requirement* in *Section III*.

The BioLogic Workout Variations

The Healer

This is the classic BioL*ogic 10 Minute No-Sweat Workout* that eighty percent of us should stick with for the remainder of our earthly lives. No variation of this most basic BioLogic Workout more easily employs the four protocols or obeys the *Sustainability Axiom* better than *The Healer*. As mentioned in the previous chapter, the *10 Minute Workout* consists of three sets of a single exercise targeting a single muscle *super group*. For instance, on "glutes and quads" day you will perform three sets of leg press (or squats, or lunges, etc.), six to twelve repetitions per set, using the amount of resistance (weight) that satisfies the BioLogic protocols, even if the resistance is no more than your bodyweight.

As you progress, you will do your best to perform each of the six *"super group"* workouts once every seven to fourteen days, being sure to rest each target muscle group until it has fully recovered from all local soreness. Performing all six workouts once per week (with the seventh day set apart as a day of rest) should be your ultimate goal, but never force six successive days of training at the expense of the *full recuperation* rule. Some of you will find a specific muscle group needs ten days or more to fully recover even after practicing the BioLogic Workout for several years. If this is the case, bravo. You are clearly stimulating the *super fast twitch muscles* at their optimal level, so enjoy the many days of rest for that muscle group that your daily success affords you. On the other hand, if you're not feeling any soreness in the targeted muscle group two or three days after a workout, you are most likely failing to properly adhere to the four BioLogic protocols. If, after reviewing Chapter 4, this lack of deep local soreness persists, please refer to the demonstration videos *or* send me a note on the BioLogicWorkout.com blog. I'll personally help you troubleshoot what you're doing wrong.

A Note About Old School Stretching

The medical community and a majority of physical therapy experts have come to recognize that traditional long-hold stretching techniques, commonly referred to as static stretching (or passive stretching), can often cause *more harm than good* when performed as most were taught.[127] Same goes for the dangerous ballistic stretching routines that bounce damage into cold tissues and joints.[128] So unless you're a professional athlete who will be subjecting your joints to stresses that would tear essential tissues if they weren't loosened through extreme stretching routines, I implore you to bail on these *old school* approaches.

Instead, adopt *BioLogic resting movements* and other dynamic or active muscle stretching techniques that have been clinically proven to enhance performance while avoiding extreme stress on your ligaments and tendons.[129] I have no doubt that I caused many pulled/torn muscle injuries and exacerbated my joint injuries (especially the torn ligaments in my knees) by overstretching all the vulnerable soft tissues targeted by static stretching routines. It's no coincidence that my dramatic reduction of these injuries and chronic joint soreness lines up with my abandonment of *old school* stretching and my subsequent creation and deployment of BioLogic *resting movements* (dynamic stretching) as their replacement. This is still a controversial subject in some circles, but don't let that mislead you. Even the most common logic and observation have shown *old school* stretching to be an extreme athletic effort that only competitive athletes need for the battle at hand. Non-extremists should avoid these aggressive stretches. Though we'll dive deeper into this subject through live discussions at BioLogicWorkout.com, let's take a look at the far easier, far faster, far more effective, risk-free *resting movements.*

BioLogic Resting Movements

Second only to the *golden rep*, this is my favorite part of every BioLogic Workout regardless of the variation I choose. It's also the only form of stationary "warm ups" I perform before engaging in any casual sport. These movements are so therapeutic that I employ them all through the day, even on days I don't work out (more on that in Chapter 10). These invigorating movements should be employed before, between, and after each set of your workouts.

Resting movements are BioLogic's joint lubricating (rotation), muscle stretching, balance building, tissue flushing, circulation enhancing, re-oxygenating, mind clearing meditation in a fluid series of intuitive concentric and eccentric flexing movements. Never forget that every cell in your body wants to receive some sort of stimuli every day. Just as researchers have shown that we can trigger health in our muscle cells through mind-body bridging techniques like visualization and motor imagery,[130] mentally connecting with all your cells and vital body systems while involving them in fluid movements can have profoundly positive effects. If you work at a desk or stand around for most of your work day (like me), please recall the section of the introduction that deals with the epidemic that is sedentary living. Folks like us should feel a special brand of urgency to stimulate every precious cell in our bodies. And that's exactly what I attempt to do during my *resting movements*. Not only do I make an intentional effort to get my blood flowing through every joint and muscle in my body, but I also meditate during these movements, speaking health and life into every fiber of my being. Many of you will simply employ dynamic stretching movements, or simplified variations of yoga, Pilates, or Barre movements if you have experience with these disciplines. Some of my clients have humorously called *resting movements* their BioLogic Tai Chi, as that Chinese therapeutic art accomplishes similar goals and can even resemble our *resting movements*. They certainly share many of the same goals.[131]

Demonstration videos will indeed give you some visual ideas on how to approach *resting movements*, but I strongly encourage you to simply move as your body feels the need. Breathe deeply while connecting with the easing of tension and soreness (or the stiffness associated with impending atrophy) in your muscles and joints. Here are the general guidelines for you to follow as you create your own favorite *resting movements*.

- Identify the joints, and points in each joint, where your target muscles attach (points of insertion); or in simpler terms, identify the limbs *or* sections of your torso where you feel the most stress during each exercise.

- While breathing deeply and rhythmically, make slow, fluid, graceful movements and joint rotations in these areas of high stress as if "lubricating" the joints involved. Whatever feels good, do it, as long as it's slow and controlled. If it causes acute pain, work around it until the pain eases. If the acute pain persists, it's always wise to confer with a sports medicine professional or your doctor.

- While the joints involved in the exercise are most important, you will also "work out" the stress generated by soreness in other muscle groups from a previous workout. So be sure to involve them in your *resting movements* as well, and you'll surely grow to love the healing and pain relief these movements have on your sore muscles. This may include moving through a deep squat motion or grabbing an overhead bar to hang and slowly turn, or pretty much any other natural movement that feels therapeutic to your muscles.

- While it's easier to focus and meditate when sitting or standing firmly in place, feel free to walk around or pace back and forth during your *resting movements* (even while moving upper extremities).

- You should find that gently and rhythmically rotating your wrists, elbows, shoulder joints, and neck will release a noticeable amount of stress during your *resting movements,* even when you're training a lower body muscle group during that workout. By doing so, you might also release tension that is putting pressure on or possibly even pinching nerves. Try to remember that your central nervous system starves for this sort of safe stimulating movement, especially if you've been sitting all day.

Resting movements bring a host of benefits to the program, but don't ever forget that the highest purpose of this part of the workout is preparation for the next set *or* recovery from the previous set. The breaks between sets should seldom last more than three minutes, but beginners can extend to *five-minute* inter-set breaks if needed to achieve full recovery. As soon as your breathing returns to a normal rate, refocus your mind on the BioLogic protocols and *command* your target muscle group that it should be stronger in the next set than it was in the previous. This sort of mind-body connection will prove invaluable if you consistently remember to focus both during the actual reps and during your *resting movements*. The entire workout takes ten minutes or less, so please put away your phone during your workouts, unless you're using the BioLogic mobile app to document your session. It's worth repeating—what you sow in discipline you'll reap in results, so get your money's worth!

The Healer: Sample Super group Exercises

The following chart outlines my most highly recommended exercises for each of the six *super group* workouts.

Day | Targeted *Super Group*	In the Gym	At Home or Work
1 | Glutes and Quads	Leg Press	Squats or Lunges
2 | Chest	Chest Press	Push Ups
3 | Lats	Lat Pull Downs	Pull-ups (chair assisted)
4 | Hamstrings	Leg Curl Machine	Stiff-leg Deadlifts
5 | Mid and Lower Back	Parallel Cable Rows	Single-arm Dumbbell Rows
6 | Shoulders	Seated Shoulder Press	Seated Dumbbell Press

Doubles, Anyone?

While *The Healer's* goal is to perform each 10 Minute, three-set workout once every seven to fourteen days, you can always double up (perform two different *super group* workouts) on any given day as long as *R&R* and the *scientific method* are obeyed. If you're so enthused (or if your schedule is so tight) that you feel you must do a double on any given day, you'll want to take a healthy break (the longer the better) between each *10 Minute Workout*. Re-fueling/re-hydrating is strongly recommended.

The Once-a-Week'er

If you are one of those rare people who either A) can only squeeze in a single twenty to thirty-minute workout per week, or B) prefers just a single intense total body workout over six *10 Minute Workouts* spread across a week or two, this variation is for you. But there is one additional logistical challenge to this variation. If you don't have a training partner or personal trainer to assist you, as discussed in Chapter 4, it's unlikely that you'll be able to stimulate your *super fast twitch muscle fibers* to the degree you'd achieve following the basic *10 Minute Workout* approach. Partial stimulation is still better than nothing (as is the case for most workout programs), but please understand that this "all in one day" workout can be so intense for beginners that you will definitely want the moral and technical support from a partner or trainer who understands the BioLogic Method. The *Once-a-Week'er* packs the *Fire/Fatigue/Failure* progression of *Muscle Psychology* into a single set for each of the *super groups* (one set for each of the six groups for a total of six sets). The final three reps of each set serve the role of the *failure* set for each muscle group. For this, each of the six sets ends with a *golden rep*. If you read Chapter 4 you should be able to imagine why you'd want an educated voice to keep you from cheating yourself in the face of total body, *super fast twitch* exhaustion. If some of your exercises use free weights, a partner will also be needed to ensure safety during the six distinct golden reps.

While many will find the *Once-a-Week'er* variation exhilarating and highly rewarding even beyond the extreme efficiency, most of my friends and colleagues find it a bit overwhelming. The total body soreness that lingers for a week or more can be a bit restrictive to an average lifestyle. It's not that the workout is overly difficult, but the intensity of the total body approach is multiplied by the number of *true failure golden reps* your mind endures within a twenty-minute period. Not everyone has that kind of mental constitution. One potential sweetener is that the hamstrings group can be effectively stimulated during a properly spotted leg press or squat set; so you have the option of eliminating the hamstring exercise, thus reducing the workout to just five sets of five different exercises (and of course just five *golden reps*).

Colleagues Dr. Doug McGuff and John Little, authors of the groundbreaking book *Body by Science*, promote the five set approach as *"The Big 5 Workout,"* and it's the first variation they recommend to their readers. While I greatly respect the all-in-one approach and those who sincerely enjoy it, I personally dread it. Not because it's flawed, but because it misses the *joy factor* in my personal Motivational Paradigm. It's simply not a workout I can regularly stomach. That said, the clients I've surveyed who prefer *The Once-a-Week'er* have grown to love it, and they often express *The Healer* leaves them wanting more, so it's really a matter of personal preference. Otherwise, aside from the three set protocol, the *Once-a-Week'er* strictly adheres to all BioLogic fundamentals, cornerstones, and protocols including the *joy factor.* So if you find that you don't enjoy it, you are unlikely to stick with it, so be sure to count the cost before committing. Likewise, the full recuperation rule must be obeyed—even if it takes three weeks for your body to get fully healed up—before you can perform your next workout. And if you're feeling ready in less than six days, you're probably not following the four protocols to a satisfactory degree. If this variation truly is for you, within a few workouts you should be genuinely excited to do it again within seven to fourteen days.

The Weekender

This variation is the twice-a-week *split* version of The *Once-a-Week'er,* consisting of three exercises per workout. It's ideal for those who need the extreme time efficiency but are less inclined to enjoy five to six exercises in a single, highly intense twenty-minute workout. While many will want to free up the weekdays by performing both sessions over a single weekend, you can also spread the two sessions several days apart to best accommodate your schedule and increase your *joy factor.* Other than the two-day split, the *Weekender* and the *Once-a-Week'er* are identical in their one set per *super group* approach, and both require a BioLogic educated partner or trainer to spot you and push you through the failure zone during the final *golden rep* for each set.

If this is the variation for you, feel free to group and divvy up the six workouts to three plus three or four plus two with any grouping, but I recommend you split the *super groups* in the three plus three approach in the following manner. Day one: glutes and quads, hamstrings, and shoulders. Day two: chest, lats, and mid and lower back—just as indicated in the BioLogic mobile app. Since I train with my wife, who also teaches the BioLogic Method, I often enjoy *The Weekender*, especially while we're traveling together.

A Quick Note on BioLogic Interval Training Workouts

These speed-training approaches to the BioLogic Method are beyond the scope of this book, but since I've suggested their use as replacements for endurance training methods frequently enough to warrant a simple discussion, let's take a sufficient dive into the topic. If you are a runner, cyclist, cardiovascular machine enthusiast, endurance swimmer, or practitioner of any other type of endurance training, you can and should immediately replace your long-duration steady-state approaches with rest-infused intervalized sprinting methods. Though many of you may already insert rest periods and call these "intervals," this minor adjustment alone will not eliminate the damage and *more harm than good* nature of these exercises unless you sincerely know when to stop training.

To constitute *BioLogic Interval Training* you must first realize you are no longer applying the *fight of flight* stimuli by challenging your strength, but instead by challenging your speed. For that, you'll need to achieve between seventy-five percent and one-hundred percent of your maximum speed during the intervals if you hope to make effective inroads to triggering the *BioLogic Cascade* through *orderly recruitment* of your *fast twitch* and *super fast twitch fibers*. From there, you will need to follow all four of the BioLogic Protocols, but with even greater attention to *R&R* and the *Three F's* progression—especially the requirement to end the training session as soon as you hit the point of true failure in your final interval. There are of course many different variables depending on the type of "speed" exercise you perform, but a full understanding of the four protocols should help clear up any questions that may arise as you experiment with these sprint intervals. If you've become so addicted to the long-duration part of your endurance regimen, you can always add more intervals to the basic three of the BioLogic progression. But please ensure these constitute a repeat or lengthening of the *Fire* and

Fatigue goals of the first two sets in the *Three F's* progression, and never an extension of the *Failure* goal of the final interval (set). Once your *super fast twitch muscle fibers* truly fail, if you try to force them into action again, you will without question begin damaging them. If you've read the full book up to this point, I know I might sound like a broken record about this issue, but this scientific fact is so critical to the BioLogic Method that it's worth repeating, and repeating.

So study up on the four BioLogic protocols, and until we produce the handbook *or* video series exploring these approaches in great detail, please send me a note if you have any questions. And as previously noted in the Chapter 2 discussion of HIIT training, nothing can replace the unrivaled benefits gained from hypertrophy strength training, so please be sure to interlace your high-intensity interval training (HIIT) with *BioLogic 10 Minute Workouts* (*The Healer*). By doing so, you will in effect be performing a "high-intensity interval resistance training" program (HIIRT) that will without question make greater inroads toward triggering the full *BioLogic Cascade*.

Advanced Workout Variations

If you are a professional or amateur competitive athlete, or if you have a short-term need for greater immediate aesthetic or performance related results for other reasons, the three *advanced variations* will meet all your strength training goals while still sparking the *BioLogic Cascade*. But please note that each of these can constitute examples of "over-training" if performed too frequently or for too many successive years, so the temporary advanced results come at the expense of the *Sustainability Axiom*. That said, I often employ the variation I call *The Builder* whenever I crave more time in the gym or want to see some of my minor muscle groups gain a bit more size (old habits are hard to break). Aside from the additional time investment (fifteen to twenty minutes per workout), as long as I return to the ten-minute *Healer* within a few months, I'm able to avoid any setbacks and have never suffered any significant wear and tear. So definitely do not fear *The Builder!*

The Twelve Advanced Muscle Groups

The following *advanced groups* employed in the advanced workout variations will be familiar to most enthusiasts. For those of you who for competitive or professional reasons need greater strength or size (more than is necessary to effectively stimulate your *super fast twitch fibers* to trigger the *BioLogic Cascade*), you will likely appreciate how these variations ensure you meet your extraordinary goals while minimizing the negatives. The advanced groups are:

1. **Glutes** (Can be divided into various exercises that target glute subgroups)
2. **Quads** (Can be divided to target inner and outer quadriceps)
3. **Hamstrings** (Can also be divided to target subgroups)
4. **Calves** (Can be divided to target inner and outer calves)
5. **Pectorals** (Can be divided to target upper, mid, lower, inner, and outer subgroups)
6. **Shoulders** (Can be divided to target front, outer, and rear delts as well as trapezius)
7. **Lats** (Can be divided to target upper, mid, and lower latissimus dorsi)
8. **Rhomboids** (Inner upper back)
9. **Triceps** (Can be divided to target all three major "heads" of the triceps group)
10. **Biceps** (Can be divided to target the two major heads of the biceps group)
11. **Abs** (Typically over-trained through exercises that can injure and weaken your back, abs should only be targeted for competitive or professional reasons)
12. **Lower Back** (Erectors)

The Builder

The Builder is identical to *The Healer* in its adherence to all BioLogic fundamentals and protocols but is ideal for enthusiasts who want to maintain larger muscle size *or* increased cut lines within the *advanced muscle groupings. The Builder* is pretty well described as the "pumped up" version of the basic ten-minute *Healer* workout. It typically takes about twenty minutes but can run as long as thirty minutes if extended resting/recovery and more advanced *resting movements* are employed. *The Builder* variation trains the twelve *advanced muscle groups* by pairing them up to create six workouts where you strictly follow the four protocols, just as you would if you were performing a "double" (two separate three set workouts back to back). As long as you're using the *scientific method* to track results and make change decisions, you can freely adjust these pairings to generate greater targeted results *or* to boost the *joy factor.*

For those of you who feel that your target muscles are still hungry for more after the failure rep in your second muscle group exercise, *The Builder* also allows for optional sub-group (secondary or polishing) exercises that you can also add to a workout after the final failure set of the primary exercise. These add-on exercises will still target the advanced muscle group trained in the primary exercise, but they must target a subset of secondary fiber bundles that will have performed a supporting role during the primary exercise. A prime example would be training your chest with bench press as the primary exercise, then polishing up with the pectoral butterfly machine. Because the primary three set exercise has already fired up or even fatigued the supporting muscle bundles without actually driving them to the point of failure, you will only need to perform one or two sets of the secondary exercise, as only the *failure* set need be performed to ensure the supporting muscle bundles gain the *golden rep* experience. You will of course still have the option of performing a double workout if you're feeling inspired or if your schedule requires you to do so. In this case, you would complete both chest exercises, for a total of four to five sets on chest, then take a full recovery break before doubling with another advanced muscle group workout.

From there you could, of course, add another secondary exercise, which would net a total of eight to ten sets for the entire double workout. So in this four or five set, two-exercise approach per advanced muscle group, you will have one true failure *golden rep* for each of the two exercises. The increase in gains depend entirely on these final *golden reps,* and as is always true with the BioLogic Method, optimizing the *super fast twitch* stimuli during that final *golden rep* requires absolute mental engagement. This is much simpler than it may read, so review the four protocols as often as needed, and refer to the demonstration videos for detailed demonstration and instruction.

Let's take a quick look at the potential scheduling of *The Builder* if performed in its most advanced format, featuring a double workout approach along with secondary exercises for each advanced muscle group.

The Builder: Sample Advanced Group Exercises

Day | Double Pairings	1st Primary/Secondary	2nd Primary/Secondary
1 | Glutes & Quads	Squats/Lunges	Outer/Inner Leg Extensions
2 | Chest & Triceps	Bench Press/Pectoral Fly	Nose Breakers/Kickbacks
3 | Lats & Shoulders	Pull-ups/Lat Pull	Shoulder Press/Shoulder Fly
4 | Hamstrings & Calves	Stiff-leg Deadlifts/ Leg Curl	Outer/Inner Seated Calf
5 | Rhomboids & Low Back	High/Low Parallel Rows	Full Cable Rows/Hyperextensions
6 | Biceps & Abs	Preacher Curl/Dumbbells	Plate Loaded Crunch/ Vertical Lifts

Again, as long as you are adhering to the *scientific method*, you can jumble up these pairings however you'd like. You can even reduce the pairings to just four or five *Builder* workouts by combining three groups for a modified, less exhaustive *triple workout*. For example, some of you will want to combine Lats, Rhomboids, and Low Back, in which case you could modify the 2nd and 3rd primary groups to a single, three set exercise per group, and then perform just one set of the optional secondary exercise.

Where you see Outer/Inner for the leg *super groups* in the sample chart above, this denotes two different exercises using the same machine to target different sub-groups simply by turning your feet outward or inward respectively during the entirety of the exercise. Never forget to follow the four BioLogic protocols as closely as possible at all times. I'll explain this option in greater detail in future discussions and texts, and it's really quite simple. But deep-dive discussions of the advanced variations are beyond the scope of this book, so I'll continue with brief overviews of each.

The Extremist

As you might expect, *The Extremist* variation is a more intense version of *The Builder* and is only recommended for those of you who—after a year or two of great results—feel you've hit a plateau and want to add even greater muscle size and muscle cut. *The Extremist* is also ideal for those who want more than just thirty minutes in the gym for *joy factor* reasons alone. *The Extremist* will generally incorporate more secondary/polishing exercises and more frequent midsection (and core) exercises. Like all BioLogic variations, *The Extremist* adheres to all BioLogic mental and physical techniques, but with even greater exploration and precision in the execution of each.

With the increased training time and increased use of *slow twitch* and lower-order *fast twitch muscle fibers*, you will develop larger muscle mass, but there are a few significant costs. Most notable among these *Extremist* trade-offs are the likely decrease in *super fast twitch muscle fiber* percentage, but not to a devastating degree. This is a trade-off the extremist is willing to make to get "larger than life." Never forget that—in contrast to *The Builder* and the three basic variations—*The Extremist* (and *The Competitor*) can increase the risk of damage to your joints and body systems to an escalating degree, so it's important to take extra care to strictly follow the technique protocols. That said, where stimulating *super fast twitch fiber* hypertrophy and triggering the *BioLogic Cascade* of benefits are concerned, *The Extremist* variation is far superior to the programs most gym rats are following.

The Competitor

This variation is an adaptation of *The Extremist* that is customized for various professional or seriously competitive amateur athletes (including those in the warrior class). These are the types of athletes who are more than willing to accept less than optimal adherence to the *Sustainability Axiom,* the health motivator (mostly talking joint damage), and the aesthetics motivator, all for the sake of their professional or amateur sports goals or greater emphasis on the *joy factor.* While *Isolation and Focus*, the *Three F's,* and the *scientific method* protocols are still strictly followed in every variation, the recovery and recuperation rules of the

R&R protocol are minimized in this variation. *The Competitor* is willing to make numerous concessions in BioLogic long-range benefits in exchange for greater short-term performance in their sport or greater short-term muscle mass, albeit with a lower *super fast/slow twitch* ratio.

The good news is that practitioners of this variation can revert to *The Healer* or *The Builder* when they stop competing and can, for the most part, correct the twitch ratio in a relatively short time frame. The higher potential for joint, bone, organ, and skin damage is a high price for living (muscularly) large. So I hope you won't remain in this group for more than five years of your life. These advanced training approaches are beyond the scope of this book, but feel free to post your questions and demonstration requests to our Facebook page or the BioLogicWorkout.com community blog for the fastest response. In all, please remember to count the cost before committing to this workout, and be sure to listen to your body along the way.

CHAPTER 7

BioLogic Exercises

The Healer's 10 Minute Super Group Exercises

In this chapter, for each of the six super group workouts, you'll see demonstration photo pairings of three different exercises. For each muscle group, the first pairing of photos shows the "selectorized" and "plate-loaded" machines most recommended for safety in a health club environment. You will find these machines (sometimes several versions of each) in virtually all health clubs. You'll also find most of these even in the smallest gyms (like those found in hotels and corporate centers). The second pairing of photos show a common weight-lifting exercise using free-weight equipment found in nearly all health clubs and small gyms. This sort of free-weight equipment is also well suited for home gyms due to its low cost and modest space requirements. The third and final pairing of demonstration photos show the simplest exercises that can be performed at home, at work, or while traveling. Most of these exercises don't require weights or special equipment.

"Selectorized" and "plate-loaded" strength machines come in all shapes and sizes, but the ones shown in the first set of demonstration photos for each muscle super group are the most common styles you'll find in most health clubs. These are the exercises I recommend for most novices and first-time strength trainers. However, due to the higher level of focus and isolation that free weights require (i.e., barbells and dumbbells), the free weight exercises shown in the second pairings of photos offer a measurable increase in effectiveness over the machines. But they also add a few obvious safety concerns, and often necessitate a trainer or partner to serve as a spotter. For this, I recommend that all beginners with access to gym equipment start with the machine exercises and advance to free weight exercises only when needed to satisfy the goals of protocol 4 of the BioLogic Method (see the *Scientific Method* in Chapter 5). Similarly, all who plan to begin with at-home exercises will eventually need to graduate to machines in a gym or similar home-grade variations (or free weights) as they progress. Visit BioLogicWorkout.com for my recommendations of the most effective and afforable home equipment available on the market today, from the simplest free weights to the most sophisticated machines. I will update these recommendations monthly, so be sure to check back often as new equipment designs and BioLogic "members only" pricing becomes available.

While the simple instructions and photos found in this chapter should serve as a satisfactory guide for those of you with even the most modest strength training experience, many of you will need to see the four protocols and the various physical and mental techniques in action before you can effectively apply the proper stimuli generated through the full BioLogic Method—especially the golden rep. If that's you, be sure to visit BioLogicWorkout.com for the demonstration videos for each muscle super group.

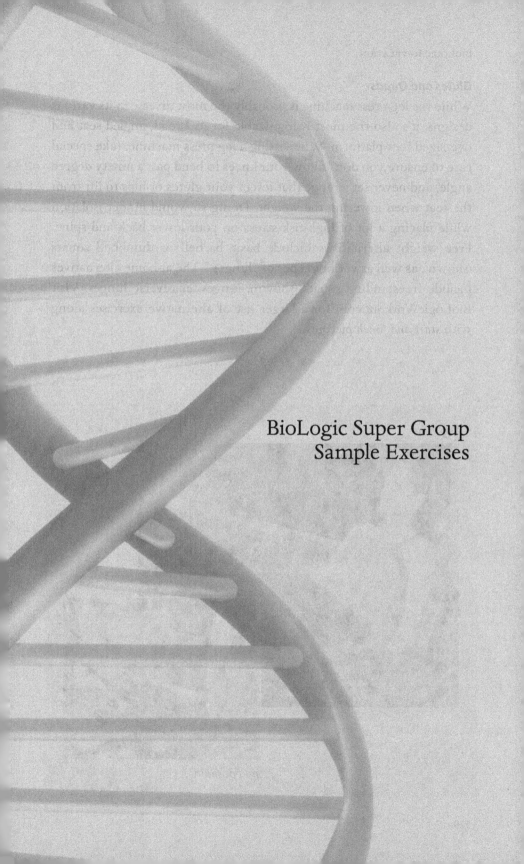

BioLogic Super Group
Sample Exercises

Glutes and Quads

While the leg press machine is probably the most diverse in its various designs, it's also the most recognizable for its broad, angled seat and oversized foot platform. When using a leg press machine, take special care to ensure you don't allow your knees to bend past a ninety degree angle, and never set a range that forces your glutes or hips to lift from the seat when lowering the weight. Doing so would hinder isolation while placing a lot of high-risk stress on your lower back and spine. Free weight alternatives include basic barbell or dumbbell squats (shown), as well as various types of "lunges." The at-home alternatives include freestanding squats (shown), lunges, *or* reverse lunges. Visit BioLogicWorkout.com for a larger list of alternative exercises along with *start and finish* pictures.

Leg Press

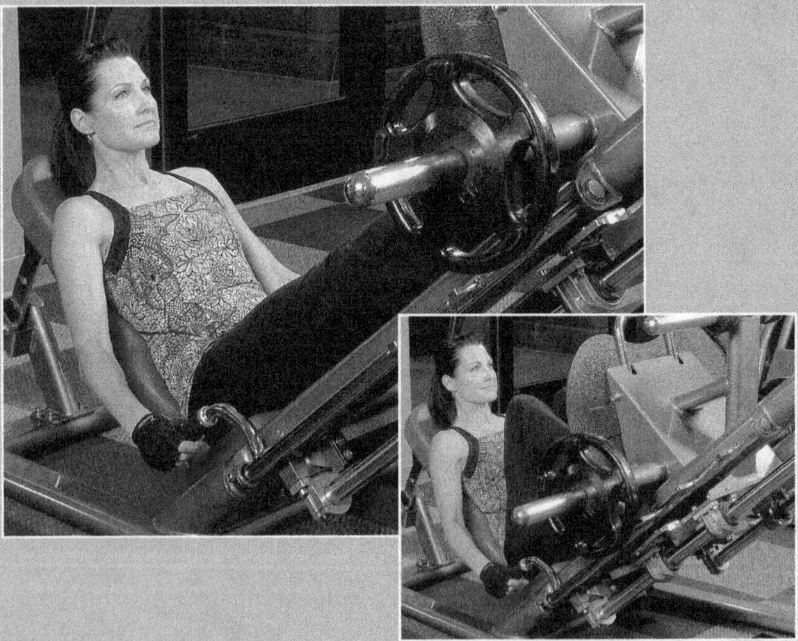

mid position

Dumbbell Squats

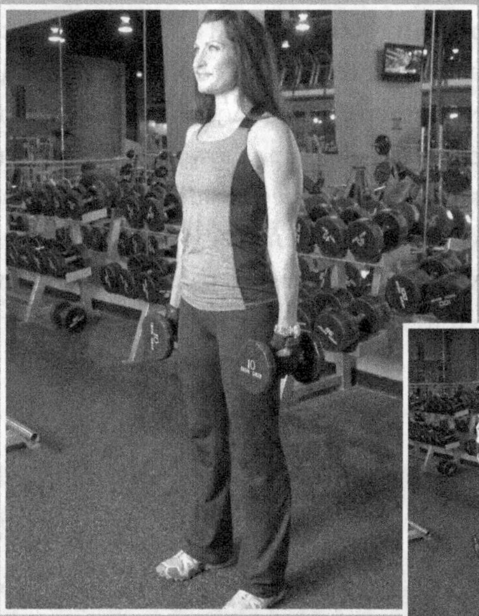

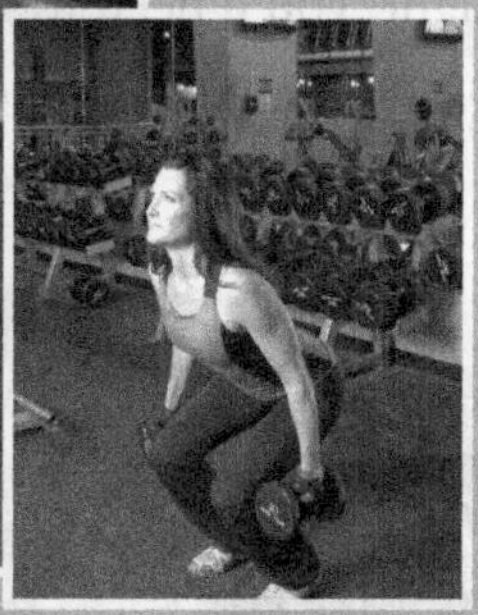

mid position

Freestanding Squats

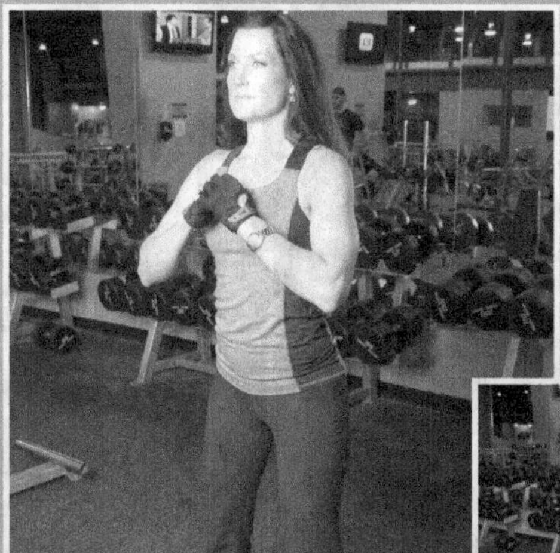

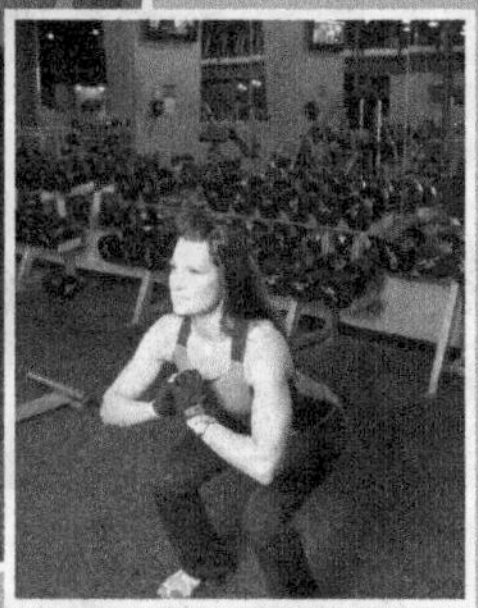

mid position

Chest

The chest press is another machine that has a wide diversity of designs; but as is true of all such machines, they should be clearly marked as chest press or bench press machines. Free weight alternatives include barbell or dumbbell bench press (shown). The at-home alternative is the good old-fashioned push up or safety push up (shown). In order to maintain the twelve rep limit, many men will need to add some sort of weight to their backs for push ups. This can be done using a backpack loaded with heavy objects (or free weights). If twelve reps are too easy even with added weight, you'll need to go into "super slow" mode to compensate, or else it's time to join a gym or get some free weights for your home.

Chest Press

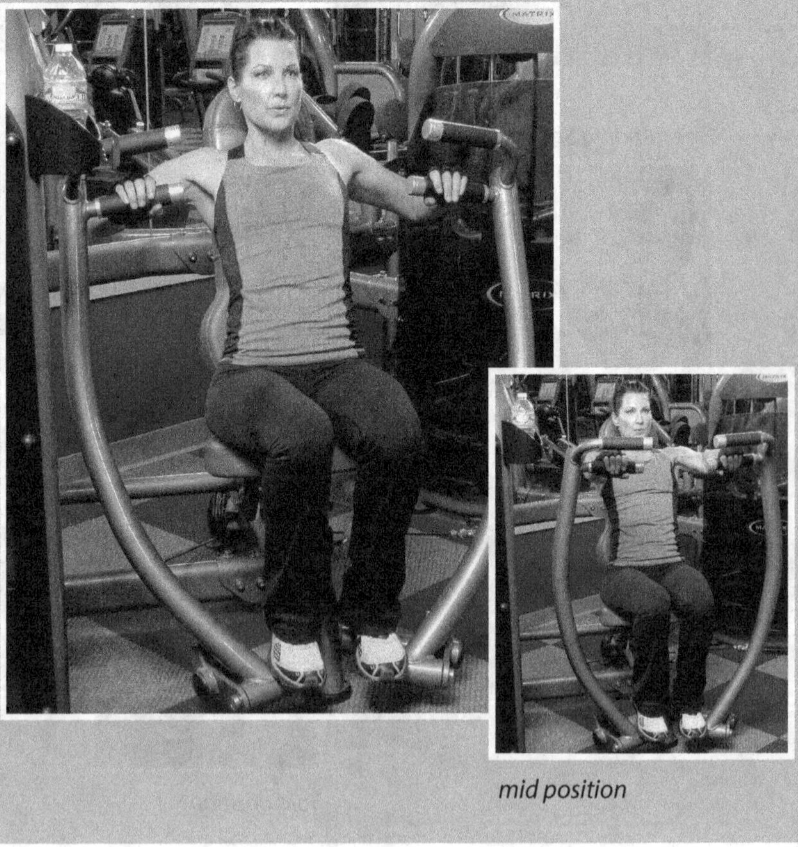

mid position

Dumbbell Bench Press

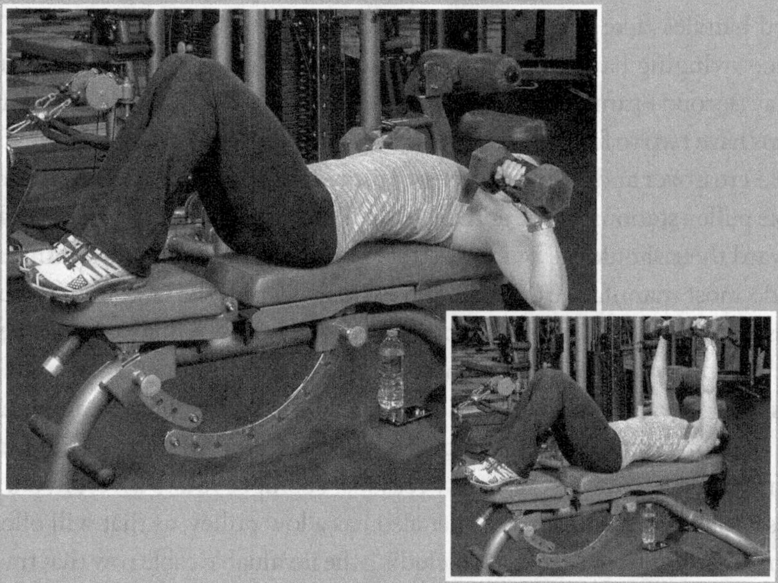

mid position

Safety Push up

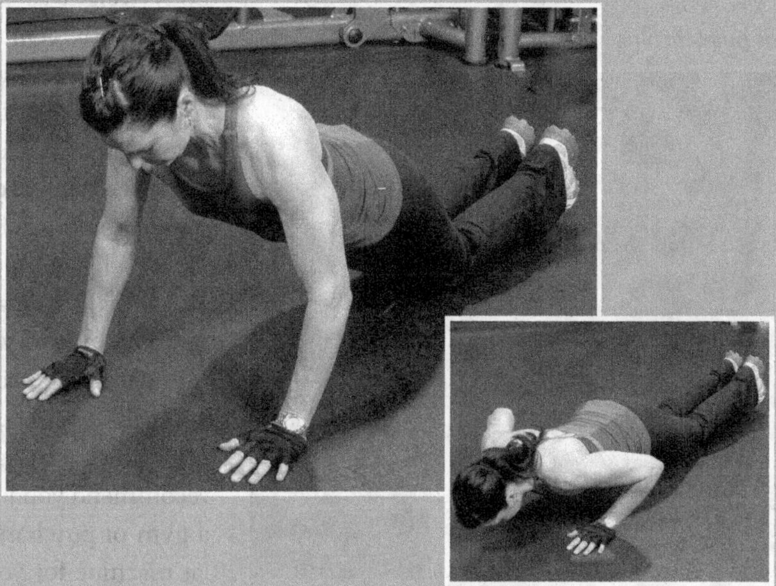

mid position

Lats

While most health clubs now have very safe lat pulldown machines with fixed handles (like the first example below), the cable lat pulldown with a free swinging bar is one of the most common machines found in gyms today (second example shown). Sometimes they stand alone, but most large gyms have two to four lat machines of the cable variety bolted together with cable-crossover and pull-up structures to create a large array of high and low cable pulley stations. Some enthusiasts pull the bar down behind their heads toward their shoulders, but for better spine and joint safety, I recommend (as do most manufacturers) that you exclusively pull the bar down to your chest. Good old-fashioned pull-ups (palms aimed away, pulling to your chest) are the only common free weight (or body weight) alternative exercise. For this, the at-home alternative will require some sort of home equipment. Lat pulldown machines made for the home are getting cheaper and more numerous every day, so for safety reasons, I compel you to invest in one of these. Make sure you get one that also has a low pulley, as that will offer a number of additional exercises including the invaluable cable row that trains your mid and lower back (see below). Another at-home alternative is a pull-up station or a door frame pull up bar. For most, performing pull-ups will require a chair, stool, bench, or rubber training straps to help reduce your body weight as you attempt to achieve the six repetition minimum. In the third demonstration exercise, you'll see a stepping stool is being used. Sadly, your lats are difficult to train at home even if you master self-spotting yourself during pull-ups, so I strongly recommend you join a gym or purchase a lat machine for your home.

Lat-pull Machine

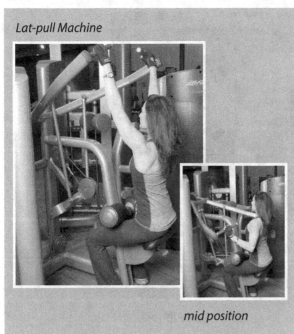

mid position

Cable Lat-pull

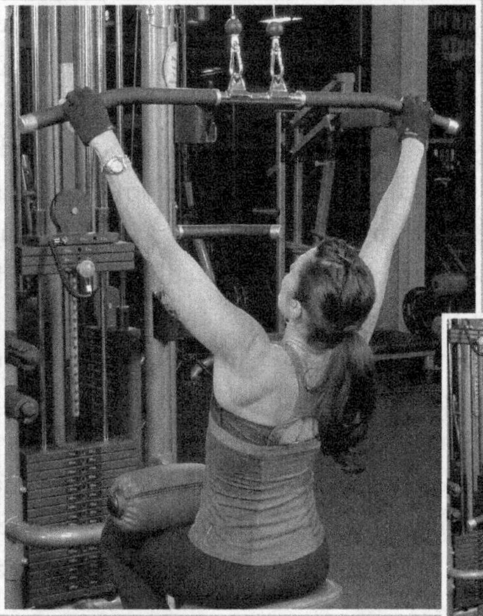

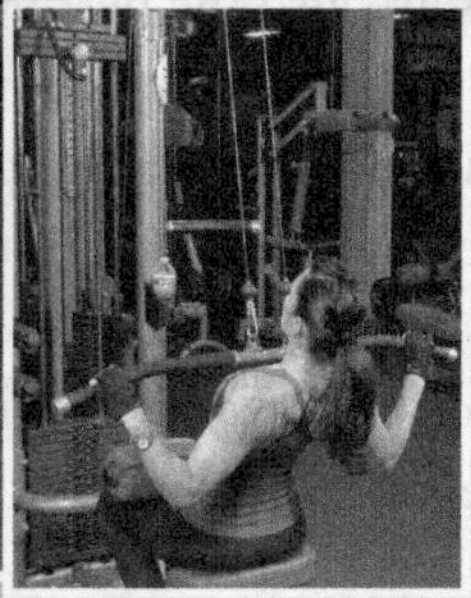

mid position

Pull-up (stool assist)

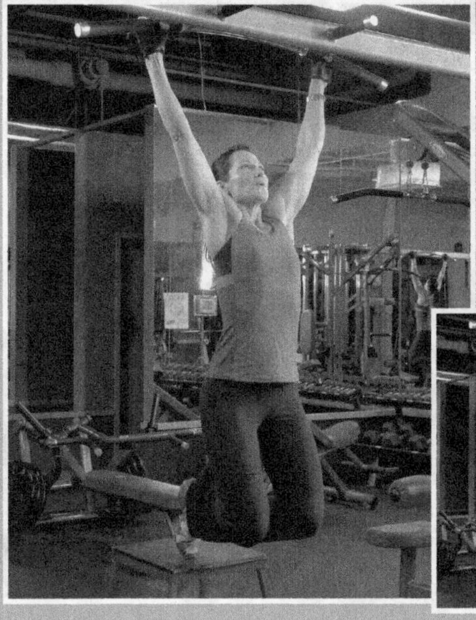

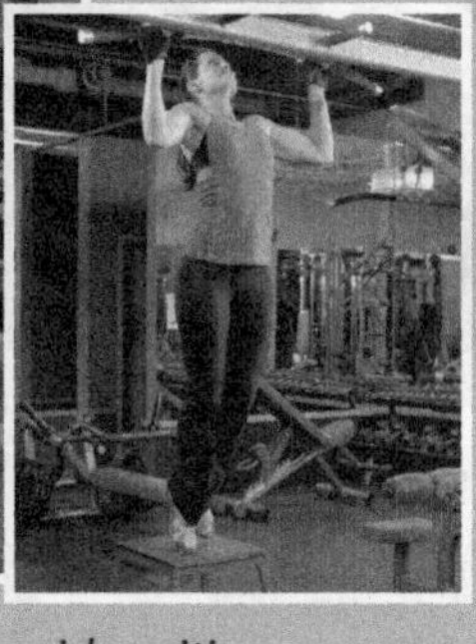

mid position

Hamstrings

The leg curl machine is another very common piece of equipment in both health clubs and small gyms. The most popular versions are the seated design (shown), the standing single-leg design, and the prone (lying down) design that was far more common before the turn of the century. Each works well when properly used, and though most feel the prone design is a tad bit more effective, it's also among the more uncomfortable machines (no one likes to stick their butt up in the air at a gym). Alternate gym exercises include barbell or dumbbell stiff leg deadlifts (shown). Stiff leg deadlifts are also the best home exercise and can be performed with or without weights (also shown). If you've been inactive for a very long time or if you're overweight, for the first month or so you'll have all you need to trigger effective stimuli standing right where you are (see *Free Stiff-leg Deadlifts* on page 177). There are also several low-cost leg curl machines and bench attachments designed for home use, but the cheap ones aren't very effective, so please visit our website for our latest recommendations.

Seated Leg Curl

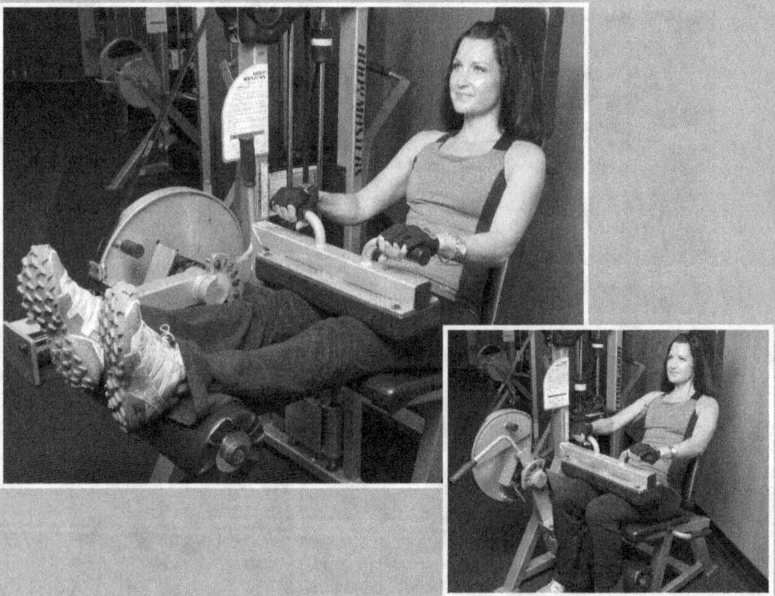

mid position

Stiff-leg Deadlifts

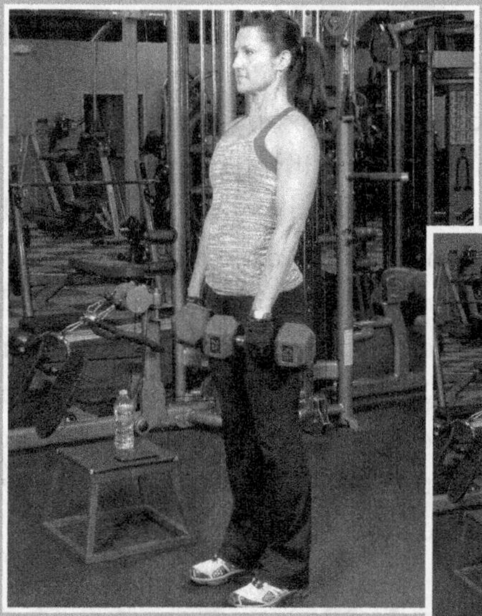

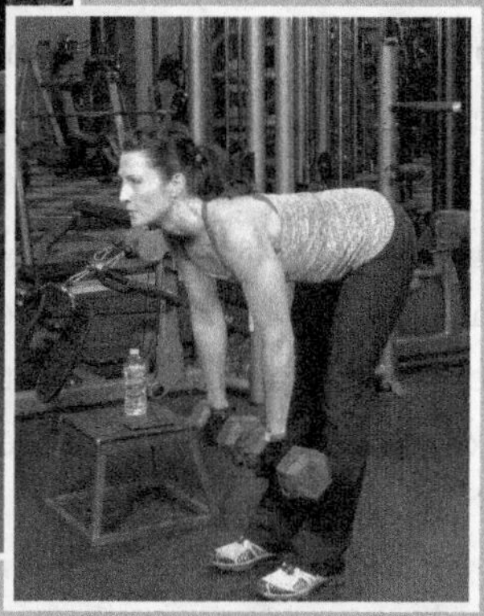

mid position

Free Stiff-leg Deadlifts

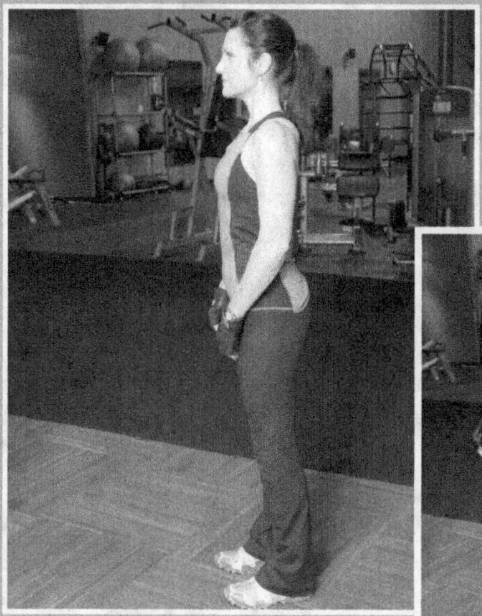

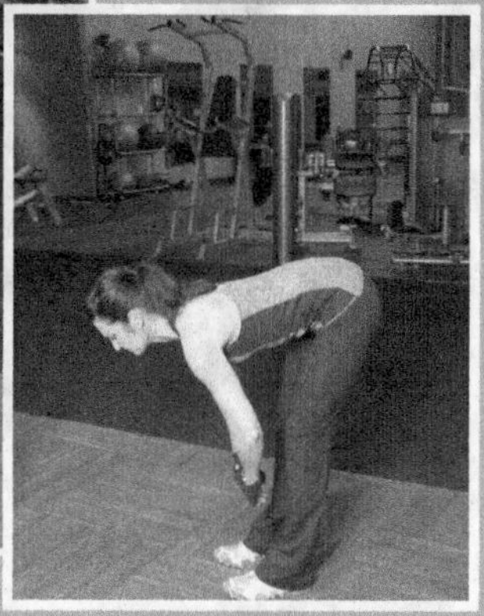

mid position

Mid and Lower Back

Most health clubs have a rowing machine similar to the one shown below, and it is by far my top recommendation. Cable row machines with parallel grips like the one shown to the right are a common piece of equipment in gyms of all sizes. As noted under "Lats" above, I highly recommend securing a home-grade machine like this if you plan to conduct all your workouts at home. If you use a low cable machine of any sort, be sure to maintain fixed hip and leg angles and a fixed back curve during the exercise. Free weight alternatives include single arm dumbbell rows (using a flat bench as shown) where you'll perform three alternating sets per arm for a rare 6 set workout. In addition to the lat pulldown machine (also known as a high-low cable machine), a simple home bench and dumbbells are an affordable solution for single arm dumbbell rows and a variety of exercises as you progress.

Rowing Machine

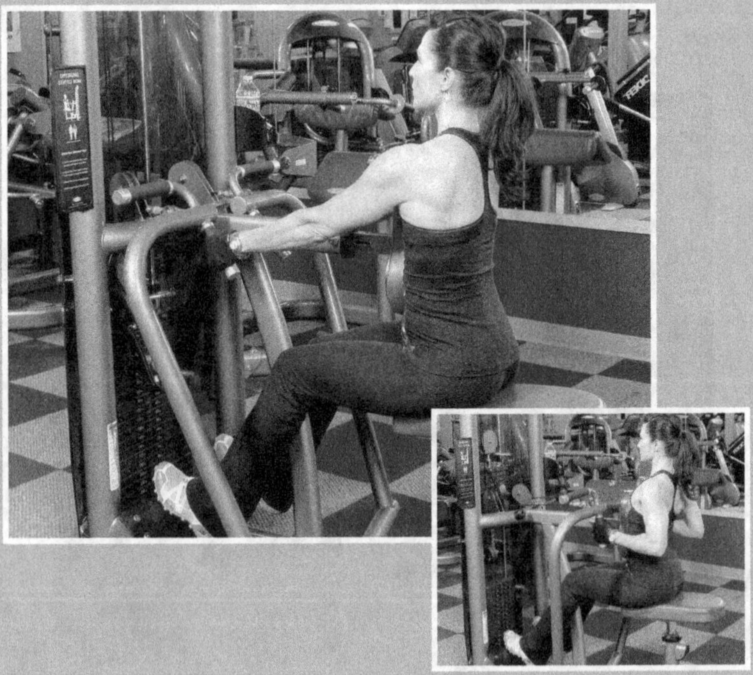

mid position

Cable Row

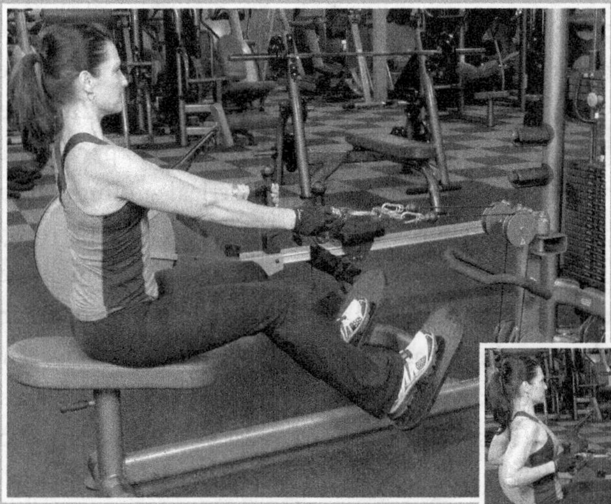

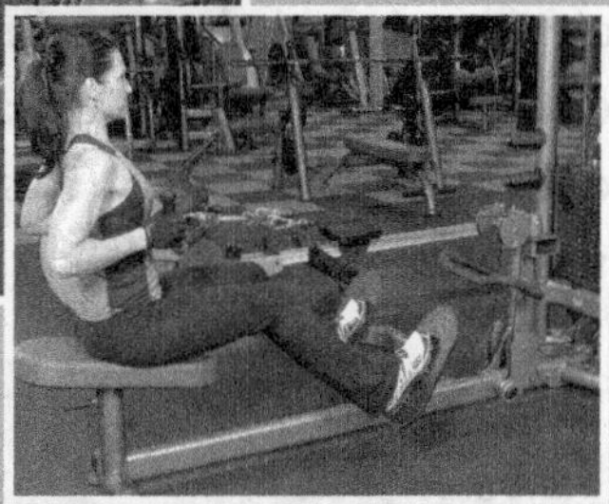

mid position

Dumbbell Rows

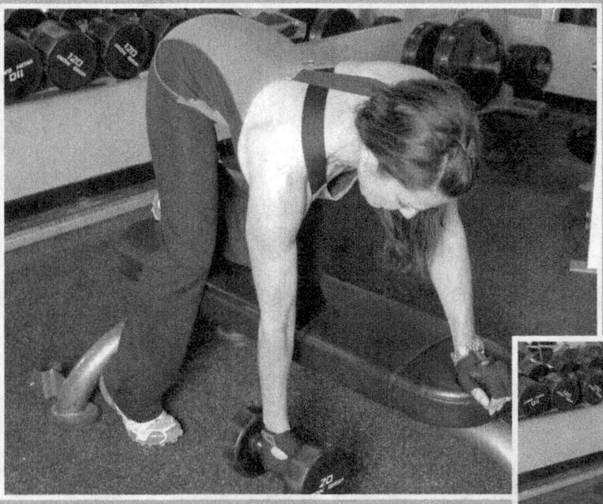

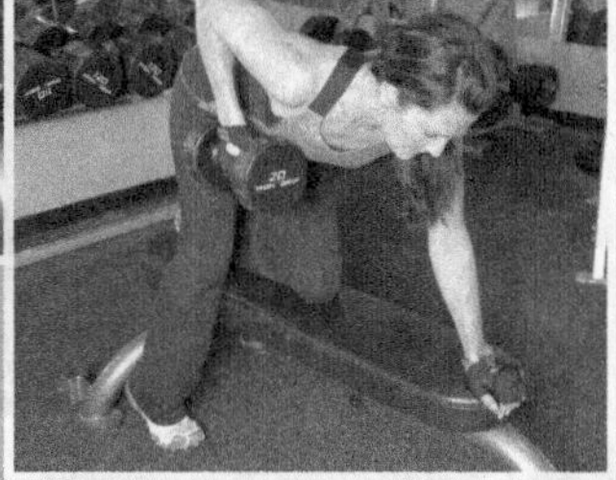

mid position

Shoulders: Seated Shoulder Press

Similar to the Chest Press, there are many different designs for the Shoulder Press like the one shown below, and you'll typically find this machine even in the smallest gyms. Similarly, there are numerous free weight alternatives, including seated and standing barbell or dumbbell presses (shown to the right). This is also a great exercise to perform on a Smith Press machine, which is an ultra-safe vertical gliding barbell system. You can stand or sit when using a Smith Press, but I strongly recommend sitting for safety reasons above all else. The home-based alternatives require some light dumbbells and a weight bench or strong chair. You should always take great care whenever lifting free weights over your head, so try to use a very stable home bench with a back rest, and try to have a partner or spotter ready to assist you or monitor you as needed.

Shoulder Press

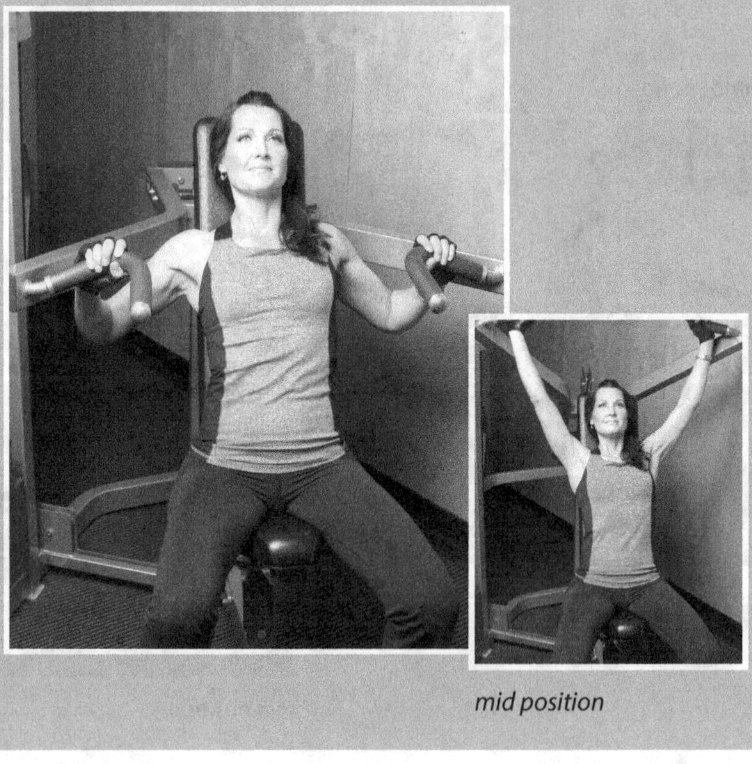

mid position

Dumbbell Shoulder Press

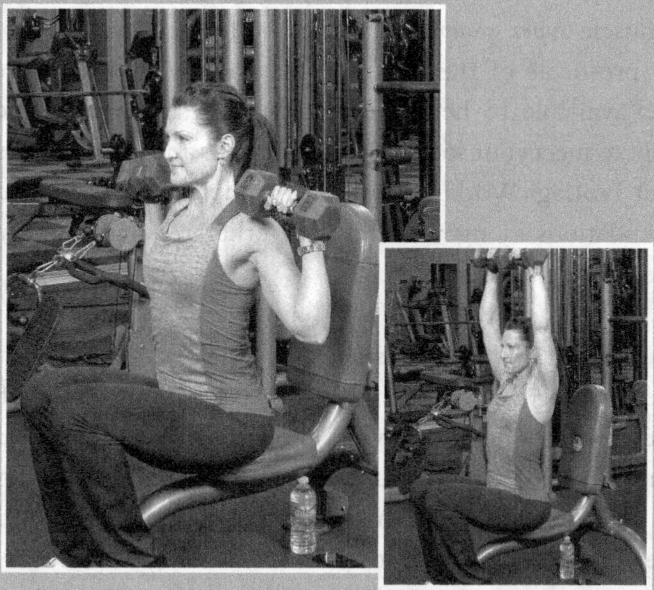

mid position

Dumbbell Shoulder Flies

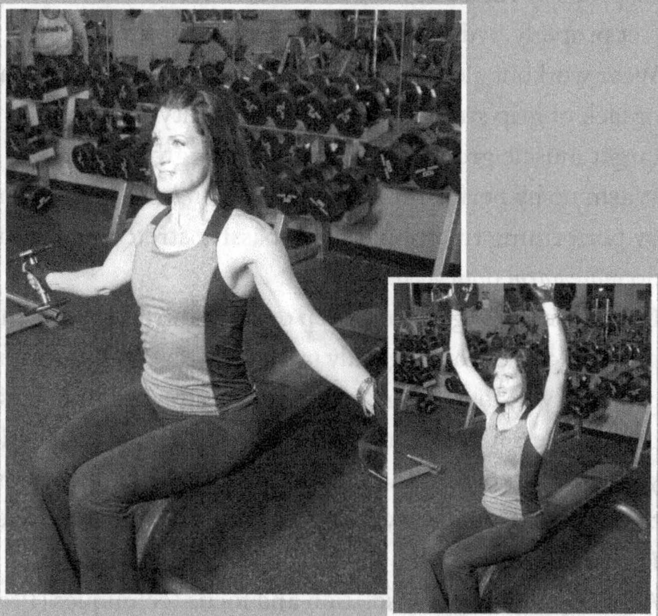

mid position

A Wealth of Options

As previously noted, there are many dozens of exercises that target the six muscle *super groups* and can be performed in accordance with the four protocols of the BioLogic Method. While there are many resources available to help you select the best exercises and home equipment to meet your specific logistical needs and physical constraints, visit us at BioLogicWorkout.com for a complete outline of our latest recommendations along with links to other reputable websites and resources relating to these topics.

BioLogic Workout Flight Checklist

When performing the BioLogic Workout as a beginner, you'll find this simple review very helpful in your effort to follow the principles and techniques of the four protocols. Like a pilot preparing for a flight with precious cargo on board, the more seriously you follow this checklist the better prepared you'll be to quickly and safely reach your desired destination.

1. Be properly fueled at least 30 minutes before your workout.
2. Get properly hydrated and stay that way 24/7.
3. Wear workout gloves if needed. Do your best to ensure hand pain or lack of grip strength thwart your ability to focus and flex the target muscle group with your full strength.
4. Warm up by performing *resting movements* (Chapter 5) and never by performing traditional static/passive stretching routines that do *more harm than good*.
5. Check the BioLogic mobile app or your journal for which muscle group is due chronologically (and to review your notes from the previous workout using that muscle group), and train this muscle group unless it's still sore. If so, make the mental connection with your body to determine the muscle group that feels most ready to be trained and prep your mind to flex only that muscle group.
6. **During Set 1**
   A. Mentally fix your isolation and focus techniques (Protocol 1, Chapter 4). Recognize that the real source of your strength

starts with your brain and nervous system. As you've come to recognize, the BioLogic approach is far more mental than physical. Bring every thought into focus as you mentally fire messages from your brain directly into each muscle bundle. Clear your mind, relax, and focus.

B. Ensure your core is firm but relaxed, and that your face and neck remain relaxed throughout. Never strain, clench, or wrinkle your face during the exercise. Ensure your movements are controlled, balanced, and entirely absent momentum in both the positive and negative (flex and unflex) directions.

C. Set 1 is the *Fire* set where you fire up your engines (Protocol 2, Chapter 4). Don't be surprised by early discomfort in your joints as they will be lubricating and warming up during Set 1. If you take care to start with a very small range of motion in the first rep and gradually increase it to full range of motion in the final rep, your joints should feel progressively warmer and stronger through the progression.

D. Immediately after the set, return to your *resting movements* and follow the resting movement techniques with your full focus. Document or commit to memory how many reps it took to achieve the burn. If it took more than twelve reps despite using proper form, add resistance in set two.

E. When your breathing returns to a relatively normal rate (after at least one minute but no more than five minutes), begin the next set.

7. **During Set 2:** Repeat the steps outlined for set 1, but since this is the *Fatigue* set, you must stop when you feel you can perform just one more successful rep.
8. **During Set 3:** Again, repeat the steps outlined above; but since this is the *Failure set,* you must continue until you have fully failed and finished with the *golden rep,* consisting of focused flexing while moving much more slowly through the negative (release movement) for approximately five seconds. Since it's the final set, you should find it relatively easy to increase your isolation and focus.

9. Wrap up your workout with *resting movements* and some light abdominal crunch work if desired.
10. If you're feeling especially hungry for more, perform a double (see Chapter 6).
11. Remain "locked and loaded" throughout your day, walking with a centered spine and a fluid gait of strength and grace. Move like an athlete before during and between your workouts and you will constantly send messages to your muscle fibers to develop accordingly. Otherwise, you are telling them to slouch and slack, and so they will obey. What you sow in discipline you reap in results!
12. Get at least seven to eight hours of sleep. Never forget that you will be healing your target muscle groups for a greater *super fast twitch* ratio while burning blood sugar and fat to fuel the workouts and the healing process respectively—all of which in turn triggers the *BioLogic Cascade* of benefits across all your body systems.
13. If you ever start to lose your sense of purpose, re-read chapters 1 and 2. If the list of *BioLogic Cascade* benefits still leaves you uninspired, you need an accountability partner. Recruit a friend in similar need!

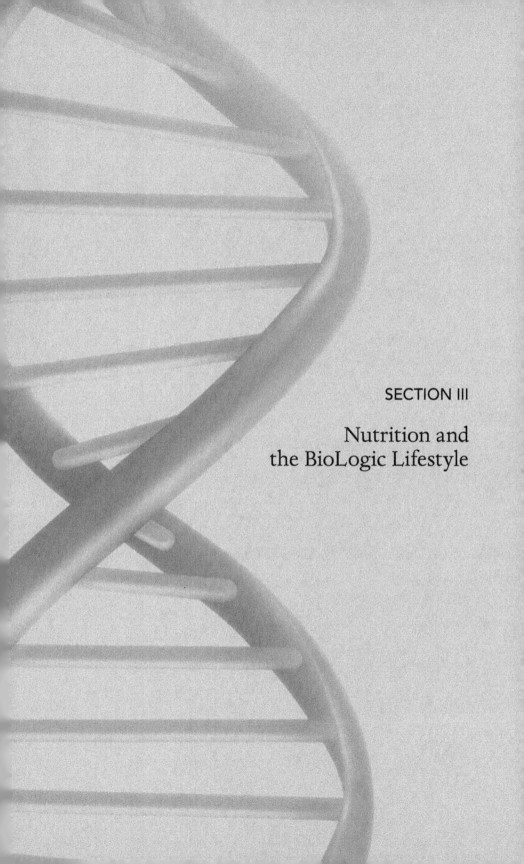

SECTION III

Nutrition and the BioLogic Lifestyle

CHAPTER 8

BioLogic Approach to Nutrition

Take It Easy

As is the case for virtually everything going on in the world today, proper nutrition and dietary strategies are simpler and far more instinctive than the industrial food complex, the government, and the snake oil salesmen want you to believe. Though I could fill several chapters debunking all the ever-changing nutrition myths and lifestyle fads flooding the Internet, I'll take a more practical approach to help you make changes as quickly and as easily as possible. In *Section III*, I'll present the known absolutes with brevity in the most encouraging fashion and let the real-time research resources and discussion threads you'll find at BioLogicWorkout.com do the rest. Those of you who are well-versed on these subjects will find this to be an easy-to-read review, but a good bit of the vital information I'll share throughout this section has been buried away by the establishment, so I hope you don't speed-read your way through it. The content in this three-chapter section is commonly accepted among a consensus of nutrition and lifestyle experts in the public domain, so I'll only cite sources where fresh research brings relatively new theories to light.

In this chapter, I'll address the delicious, nutritious foods you probably need more often. In Chapter 9 I'll follow up with an outline of the most common foods you should avoid and load you up with an arsenal of highly practical strategies to help correct your diet with ease. Then we'll wrap it all up with the highly sustainable BioLogic lifestyle strategies in Chapter 10.

The Motivational Paradigm Returns

It would be impossible to count the number of people I've witnessed experimenting with each new fad diet or miracle supplement, only to go back to square one over and over again simply because they failed to count the cost where sustainability and enjoyability were concerned. With these next few chapters I hope to spark conversations that help you and everyone you know break that trend once and for all.

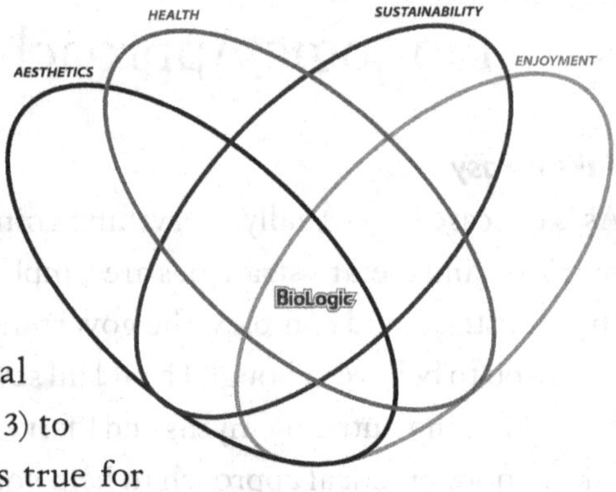

For starters, before you can make changes in your diet you first have to make changes in your decision-making processes, so I hope you already realize you should apply the Motivational Paradigm (detailed in Chapter 3) to start getting it right. Just as is true for fitness activity decisions, most people make dietary choices based on just one or two of these cornerstones while completely ignoring the role of the others. But finding the sweet spot (where all four motivators overlap) is more imperative with food choices than any other concern, including your workouts.

For instance, many diet gurus tend to promote foods and supplements that feed on your fears, which for most are related either to insecurities about your aesthetics or to your concerns about the most dreaded diseases. They tell you to start eating certain foods and supplements and advise you to avoid others, while excitedly rattling on and on about the mostly unproven set of benefits you'll gain by consuming these products. Most lead you to believe that some element of your body composition will surely improve (abs are especially popular these days), and many have the audacity to "guarantee" results. Most skip right over the *joy factor* in their sales pitch and seldom if ever address whether or not you stand a reasonable chance to integrate these products into a sustainable (forever) diet. Others offer little to no advice on how to let go of the foods you've grown to love (or become addicted to) over the course of your life.

I'm grateful for my colleagues in the nutrition field who understand that all is lost if we fail to obey the *Sustainability Axiom,* and that the *joy factor* is especially important in this regard. We're part of a growing community that fully agrees that proper nutrition is far more obvious than the industrial food complex and the snake oil salesmen have been leading you to believe, and for that, you are much closer to turning major corners than you may think.

Attacking the Obesity Epidemic

Before proceeding, it would benefit you greatly to go back and read the subsection titled *Fat Burning, Body Shaping, and Your Metabolism* in Chapter 2—especially if you jumped ahead and have yet to read it. Your ability to understand the truth about calories and how the human body really burns fat (as opposed to all the myths and outright lies) is invaluable to your quest to conquer the food issue. So please get the truth fresh in your mind and these last three chapters will surely become more practical and far more enjoyable to read.

Most of us struggle with our diets. That's a fact. The Centers for Disease Control (CDC) reports that 34.9 percent of U.S. adults (nearly seventy-nine million) are clinically obese. That's more than one in every three adults. It should come as no surprise to those of us who live in the South, where fried foods and starchy carbohydrates and triple sugar desserts are standard fare, that we are even more vulnerable.[132] Far more alarming, since my high school graduation in 1981, childhood obesity has increased by nearly three-hundred percent for children under twelve and has increased more than four-hundred percent among American teenagers (yes, that's *tripled* and *quadrupled*, respectively). So while my generation grew up in an era where fewer than one of every ten children suffered from obesity, in 2012 the CDC reported that more than thirty-three percent of children are obese or overweight.[133]

That's a shocking statistic, but if you've had your eyes open the past thirty years, in retrospect, it's no big surprise. We should make sacrifices and deny our selfish desires for the betterment of our children, not to lead them down a path where they suffer obesity by giving them no option but to eat what we eat. Consider the following: upwards of sixty percent of American adults are *considerably* overweight. Yes, that's six out of every ten of American adults, most of whom grew up in the days where less than one in ten of us were overweight as children. So if current generations are three-hundred to four-hundred percent more likely to suffer childhood obesity, where will they be when they reach adulthood? Even more, consider where this trend will lead if we don't stop it now. While this is clearly an epidemic among adults, it's a national tragedy among our youth.

But Fear Not

Yes, physical activity plays a crucial role no matter your age, but we unquestionably are what we eat, so proper nutrition should be our highest concern. Until you can discipline your appetites, your intake will hold the greatest sway over your health and aesthetics. That reality should set off an alarm. But fear not, there are indeed simple ways for you to bring your nutrition plan (for you and your kids) into alignment with the latest scientific research. Likewise, brand new research has shown that BioLogic Workouts and others with similar protocols will without question suppress your appetite, so you'll have that additional benefit to enjoy.[134]

We're all creatures of habit, and most of us have appetites that we can't just wish away—some of which we, in fact, should never wish away. So the trick isn't to learn what works for others or even which of the latest research darlings might prove beneficial for you and in turn trigger dramatic shifts in your diet. Instead, make small, sustainable adjustments toward the known absolutes, starting with the ones you're probably already anxious to try. Once you feel inspired to further refine your appetites, start experimenting with the *good* foods you find appealing or intriguing, and commit only to those you believe you can enjoy for the long-term. As long as it fits the sweet spot in your personal cornerstone paradigm, that particular correction to your diet or lifestyle should eventually take hold as one of your personalized absolutes thanks to the *joy factor* alone. Few of us can discipline ourselves to make corrections that suck the joy out of our lives. Let's start with the ones you know you can sustain *and* enjoy, and drop the ones you know you can live without.

Does Organic Matter?

Does it *really* matter whether your food is produced organically? The answer is an emphatic YES. For each of the foods detailed below, I strongly recommend certified organic products with zero synthetic food ingredients, and only non-genetically modified (non-GMO) foods wherever possible. Similarly, whenever possible your beef products should be organically raised, grass-fed, and grass-finished, while your poultry (and the eggs they produce) should also be organically raised in a free-range (or at least a cage-free) environment. But don't let my strong recommendations derail you if scarcity or cost make these foods prohibitive. If these "ultra clean" food factors thwart your ability to consume them on a regular basis, you'll never sustain them in your diet, so be smart and realistic about it. Likewise, make sure you truly enjoy (or will grow to enjoy) the foods you add, even if you have to buy non-organic more often than not.

I suggest you take the organic question to an absolute degree where plant foods with edible skin are concerned, as this is where we find the highest concentrations of toxic chemicals including pesticides and herbicides (more on this below). If you don't eat the skin, shell, or outer leaves of a fruit or vegetable, you can feel a good bit safer eating non-organic options. Otherwise, do all you can to avoid eating the skin of any non-organically grown produce, and avoid non-organic berries altogether. If you set a sustainable course with attainable short-term goals, you're bound to get there—if you remember to take it one day at a time. It's important to note that the terms "All Natural" or "Natural" or "one-hundred percent Natural" are not to be trusted, as government agencies allow these marketing terms for nearly every food that doesn't include entirely synthetic ingredients. But with little enforcement in place, not even that can be guaranteed so let the buyer beware.

Foods We Need More Often

Speaking of absolutes, if all you do is start eating the most nutritious, delicious foods that you've been denying your body all your life, you'll gain significant health and aesthetic benefits. This alone may not help you escape obesity, but those strategies are coming up next. Let's focus first on recommended additions (or better yet, *replacements*). For many of you, the list of these ultra-healthy foods are common knowledge, but that doesn't mean you've tried to add any of them lately. Maybe you've tried some new foods in the past and vowed to start eating them, but then your life continues in patterns of habits (especially on shopping days), and before you know it you no longer eat these healthy foods. If you sincerely enjoyed a particular healthy food product, you simply need some new approaches to serve as reminders, so I suggest you make note of which are best for you. A good old-fashioned grocery list or sticky note on your fridge should help immensely. Now that you have a new workout program that truly works, I hope you'll be inspired to finally start to eat these foods on a measured and consistent basis. Let's turn this thing around!

1. **LOVE clean water and drink it often.** I almost put this at the end of the list, not because it's the least important but because everyone knows good clean water is our most vital beverage—and, of course, it isn't a food. In all honesty, even a nutrition geek like me can get spotty in my water consumption, and with this being the single most important consumable, that just shouldn't be. In fact, the very first physical act of each day, immediately after waking up, should be drinking a tall glass of clean room temperature spring water. The health benefits from this single act are profound and numerous, which should be obvious after a night of dehydration. So just do it and we'll delve deeper into the metabolic and life-sustaining benefits of this "top of the morning" rehydration in future discussions. Not only do most of us get far too little water each day, but we get far too much of every other sort of beverage. Contrary to the long-standing advice that "three glasses a day" is sufficient (which is less than two liters), recent research indicates that men need roughly three liters per day, and women need about 2.2 liters daily.[135] Likewise, we need to increase this intake when a variety of environmental and physical factors are present, including very hot weather, times of illness, and times of intense work or play. For a bit of good news (and contrary to the long-believed myth that somehow keeps hanging

on), everything that contains water does, in fact, deliver water to your body regardless of its caffeine content, coffee and tea included. I simply ensure my coffee is made with clean spring water and I minimize or avoid added sugar. These hot beverages have earned a special place among water bearers; first for being wrongly demonized for so many decades as "contra-waters" due to the diuretic properties of caffeine, and second for the double-edged nature of phytochemicals (plant-based chemicals) both contain. Due to lack of sufficient research, the jury is still out on how much of these beverages one should consume for improved health. I love both immensely, both make me feel better, and both fit the sweet spot in my cornerstone paradigm, that's for sure. Look for deeper discussions about these topics at BioLogicWorkout.com. But don't be mistaken; nothing beats good old-fashioned unadulterated spring water. As for tap water, there are pros and cons, but for the sake of brevity, I suggest you avoid it as much as possible. We'll discuss these ever-evolving topics in great detail at BioLogicWorkout.com.

2. **Eat more healthy fats.** If you can't find something on this list you love, you're not from around here. I remember in the eighties when the food industry was pushing a no-fat diet to create demand for new highly processed foods. Millions of enthusiasts swallowed it hook, line, and sinker. Your body desperately need healthy fats, and it's not fat in general that is our primary enemy, but sugar, starchy carbs, and *bad fats* that are the actual body fattening culprits. You, without question, need good fat for a long list of health reasons including heart health, brain health, and body fat reduction. The amount of healthy fat you should consume each day is unique to each one of us, but I suggest you make sure about one-quarter of your caloric intake consist of healthy fats (and no more than one-third). So to translate that to numbers you can read on a label, I suggest you get at least forty grams but no more than eighty grams of fat each day. Reading labels is a practice everyone needs to adopt, as it will help you figure out a good daily target for your major nutrient consumption. Feast

your eyes on these delicious foods you should keep or add to your diet, many of which are also high in fiber (something we all need more of). And as always, eat these in moderation, and avoid eating too many of these fatty foods in a single meal, as eighty grams can add up quickly!

Whole organic eggs: The incredible edible undeservedly demonized egg deserves a book to itself. This is one of our true miracle foods. Eat them with joy!

Avocados: Some would argue this is the single most nutritious food on earth, and I thank God for that because I can't get enough of this buttery *superfood* fruit.

Dark chocolate: This food is virtually a must for too many reasons to list. The higher the cocoa percentage, the better. I don't buy bars that are less than seventy-five percent pure (organic) cocoa.

Raw or dry-roasted nuts and nut butters: Try to limit the peanut butter (you likely know they're not really nuts). Almond butter is far tastier anyway.

Seeds: Sunflower, pumpkin, flax, sesame and chia seeds are easy to find.

Extra virgin olive oil: It's hard to get more "old world" than this precious oil, which is most nutritious when not overheated.

Coconuts and coconut oil: One of my personal favorites for too many reasons to list. More on the added benefits of coconut oil later.

Full-fat "no sugar added" yogurt: I used to hate it. That was before I had my second spoonful.

Good fatty fish: Three to four ounces, no more than once per week (see Chapter 10). Salmon is king.

Cheese: As always, moderation rules. Unless you are lactose intolerant, you're very glad to see cheese on the list.

Grass fed dairy butter: As always, look for certified organic and ensure the cows were grass-fed whenever possible, especially for butter. It's not much more expensive than the less healthful grain-fed varieties.

There are, of course, many more foods I could add to this list, but I stuck to the ones I know you could easily find in most grocery stores. Visit BioLogicWorkout.com for the ever growing list of healthy delicious fatty foods.

3. **Eat the healthiest proteins.** Sadly, we don't get to eat the relatively clean animal proteins our ancient ancestors ate, especially not the fish. The toxins and disease we risk when consuming industrially raised species of fish in high quantities are simply not worth it. While the food industry is slowly creeping toward the certified organic bandwagon, they have a long way to go before I'd trust their mass produced products. I strongly recommend you increase your intake of alternative protein sources while cutting back on the beef, pork, poultry, and seafood. But if you're a meat junkie like me, always try to get certified, organic, grass-fed grass-finished beef (one serving per week) and free-range certified organic poultry to satisfy your meat fix. These are the two easiest "clean" meats to find and both are fairly affordable. The most highly recommended among these alternative proteins sources include organic free-range eggs and organic grass-fed dairy proteins, especially goat and sheep kefir (a cultured dairy beverage with a yogurt-like taste), as each contains complete proteins (a sufficient proportion of all nine essential amino acids) and are loaded with nutrients.

   If you're a vegan you'll obviously be avoiding these, but vegetarians should at very least add kefir to your diets, as it is proving to be a true *superfood* with greater nutrients than nearly all other animal-source non-meat products. Kefir has been all the rage among nutrition gurus in recent years, and though most Americans have yet to try the thick beverage, it's starting to show up in even the most common grocery stores. Otherwise, regardless of your stance on animal source proteins, we all need to add or increase the following plant source alternatives, especially since most deliver invaluable fiber as well. Men need about fifty-six grams of complete proteins per day, and women need about forty-six grams,[136] so I hope you can ensure at least half of those grams come from plant sources. Even if you don't track your calorie intake, I strongly encourage you to keep track of your daily protein intake along with your fat intake. Most people get too much or too little of each, so make sure you take steps to start getting your numbers in order. As you should know by now, muscle development depends on proper protein intake, so try never to skip proteins, especially while training the BioLogic way. Here are my most highly recommended plant source proteins:

Quinoa: As recently as 2013 hardly anyone was eating this delicious ancient pseudo-cereal (a seed that is not a grass plant like most grains). Quinoa is a relative of spinach, beets, and chard, and the word is getting out about this nutrient packed complete protein. Even NASA published a report touting the ancient grain for production on interplanetary space flights. As always, seek out certified organic, non-GMO options if possible.

Beans and Rice: While individually both fail the "complete protein" test, once combined in a single meal you've got all your essential amino acids covered. Whenever my wife and I talk about how we'd survive a cataclysmic disaster, I can always count on her to smile and say, *"beans and rice and Jesus Christ."* Amen. Black, kidney, mung, and pinto beans are our favorites.

Lentils or Chickpeas and Rice: Same story here as stated above for the beans. I'm a third-generation Bostonian, so lentils have long been a staple in my family. Love them!

Hemp Seeds and Chia Seeds: Both of these formerly exotic seeds deliver complete proteins, and both are packed with *superfood* nutrients. While they may be awkward for you to eat as a stand-alone staple, both make for excellent ingredients in salads and other combo dishes. I find hemp seeds to be so nutty and tasty that I eat them by the mouthful straight out the bag. Give it a try.

Buckwheat: First, buckwheat is not a wheat at all, but rather a pseudo-cereal related to rhubarb. Made famous as the main ingredient in their namesake pancakes, buckwheat is a gluten free high protein food that is known to lower blood cholesterol and blood glucose levels while also improving circulation. So if you've been craving pancakes but (like me) are trying to cut back on wheat, you're welcome.

There are many additional non-animal complete protein foods I could add to this list, but I've kept my recommendations to the ones I know you could easily get into your diet today. Like the healthy fats noted above, You'll find the larger list of complete protein plants at BioLogicWorkout.com.

4. **Eat more colorful vegetables, greens, and dark berries.** All fruit and vegetables have nutrients, but the most colorful veggies and the darkest berries pack the most punch. Many of these are considered to be *superfoods* (see below), and all are famous for their high fiber content, so be sure to target your favorites. These particular veggies also avoid the *more harm than good* pitfall, while many of the most popular food plants fail our litmus test for containing limited nutrients and unwanted quantities of starchy, simple carbohydrates and sugars. Where the organic issue is concerned, I again suggest you avoid all plants whose exterior surfaces (exposed to chemicals and the elements) are an edible component unless it is certified organic. It's worth repeating that most of the pesticides and other chemicals that non-organic farmers spray on their crops coat the skin *or* leaves of these plants. So unless you want to ingest all these dangerous chemicals—toxins that certainly aren't naturally occurring in our foods—either peel the skins, seriously wash the leaves, or avoid them altogether. This is a major concern for berries that can't be peeled, so do your best to buy only organics in this category. It also benefits you in numerous ways to buy local whenever possible, so support your local farmers, especially if

they're certified organic! All in all, eat non-organics with great care. Concerning all the nutritious fruits besides dark berries, as much as I crave all varieties of fruits, due to the extremely high sugar content, we have to discipline ourselves in how often we eat them. The nutrients in most fruits are simply not worth all the sugar you'd have to consume to get the health benefits of these phytochemicals (most of which are only found in trace amounts anyway). So if like me you have developed a mild addiction to these sugar-packed fruits, eat them sparingly, mix up the varieties frequently, try only to buy organic (especially if you eat the skin), and try to deploy the next strategy.

5. **Eat sweet vegetables to tame your sweet tooth.** The highly nutritious carrots, peas in the pod, sweet potatoes, squash, and beets are the most popular sweet vegetables. Not only are these vegetables packed with nutrients and high in fiber, but they can also help cut or eliminate sugar cravings. Excess sugars are the greatest taboo of all foods (especially if you're trying to burn fat), and in their most commonly available forms are literally toxic. For this, everyone should have a strategy in place to overcome sugar addictions, and this one should be utilized as soon as possible. If you're thinking that fruit juices can serve this purpose, please scratch that option. Our bodies definitely need sugar to survive, but only when consumed in their naturally occurring states and in their historically common quantities (the relatively small amount our ancestors could access) can the harms of excessive fruit sugar (fructose) be minimized. Being a nutrient rich *superfood*, I give a rare pass to whole organic apples, but apple juice is hardly better than Kool-Aid, so I suggest ditching fruit juices altogether. Make sweet veggies a part of your balanced diet and over time you'll lose or reduce your craving for the toxic sugars and the even more toxic artificial sweeteners. As always, eat these sweet veggies in reasonable quantities, and try not to bundle them together too often.

6. **Add or increase your favorite *superfoods*.** While the term *superfood* is a non-scientific slang term used mostly for marketing purposes, the fact that this unofficial category includes the most nutrient-rich disease-fighting natural foods should pique your interest. As you'll see, most all *superfoods* fit into other categories on this list, and that should make those particular foods all the more attractive to you. Most *superfoods* are vegetables and fruits that are already known for their healthful potency and high fiber content. Others are animal sourced protein foods that have ironically been unjustly maligned over the years. The incredible edible whole egg is number one among them. While you can find resources at BioLogicWorkout.com that identify and describe all the foods that are rightly gaining the *superfood* adjective of honor, here's a short list of *superfoods* that I have long enjoyed. I recommend each in their certified organic form if at all possible. They are: dark chocolate with at least seventy-five percent cocoa content (pure cocoa powder is best), avocados, tomatoes and tomato sauce, garlic, dark leafy greens, turmeric, almonds, walnuts, bell peppers, black pepper, beans, onions, salmon (see The Fish Crisis in Chapter 10), most seed foods, cabbage, red wine, most dark berries, and of course, apples. Few surprises, I'd guess, but make sure you add the ones you lack and always eat them in moderation—particularly salmon, red wine, the high-sugar fruits, and the dark chocolates.

Supplementation

This is another subject that would require a dedicated book to fully explore. To ensure we don't neglect the subject, we'll post a steady stream of related video and written content on supplements to the BioLogicWorkout.com blog, and I'll stick to the simplest essentials in this chapter. Taking all the food related advice in this chapter would, in theory, give your body all the nutrition it needs. However, some nutrients are so important or so difficult to maintain in our modern diets that supplementation becomes an important consideration. Quality whole food supplements (as opposed to products that include synthetic *or* processed ingredients) can also be very expensive, so if you're on a tight budget let your food intake fill all your nutrition needs. Start investing time into learning how to target the essential vitamins, minerals, antioxidants, adaptogens, and other nutrients in your daily diet (see BioLogic.com for a full listing of recommended food-source dosages).

Over the three years leading up to the time this book was published, the supplements listed below have earned a consistent place in my pantry, so I obviously encourage you to try them. Please note that research on the pros and cons of supplementation is all over the map and has thereby produced very few scientifically proven absolutes. I'll simply offer the following examples as a brief survey of what I currently recommend to friends and readers looking for a starting point that generally produces positive results for most, including my family and me.

1. **Organic grass-based green *superfood* powder:** Aside from serving as a truly green alternative to vitamin and mineral supplementation, the best of these grass-based powder supplements are chock full of whole food nutrition, potent phytochemicals, and in many cases dietary fiber to a greater degree than most any other food product on the market today. Some of these powders boast that a single serving mixed with water accounts for three to five servings of whole food vegetables per day. So (if true), they can also help ensure your children who hate vegetables can more easily drink some down every day. Honestly, if I could take just one supplement, this is it. As is true for all supplements, go to BioLogicWorkout.com for a list of our most highly recommended *superfood* powder options.

2. **Vitamin D:** According to the highly respected natural health expert, Dr. Joseph Mercola (and a throng of research scientists around the globe), vitamin D deficiency has reached pandemic status. Some estimate more than half of the US population are lacking this important nutrient. D isn't really a vitamin, but a hormone, which helps explain why the crisis is gaining so much traction in the medical community, and I hope the same becomes true for you as well.[137] Over the past decade, improved testing

protocols and increased research has revealed that as much as fifty percent of men, women, and children are D deficient according to FDA standards, and the number approaches seventy percent and higher for children and seniors alike. So please talk to your physician and get tested to see where your levels are, and do the same with your children's pediatrician, as some studies show them to be the most vulnerable. The cultural and environmental reasons for this pandemic are pervasive. Although I'm tempted to write a full chapter on this issue, I'll instead encourage you to do your own research, starting with the sources I cite in the notated bibliography (of the Appendix). I hope you'll continue accessing these sources as new nutrition research breaks every week. You might be amazed to learn the nagging ache or unexplained malady that's been plaguing you (many of which may be life-threatening) might be the result of a D deficiency. In the meantime, get a daily vitamin D supplement for every member of your family, and think of it as sunshine in a gel-cap!

3. **Omega-3 Oil supplement:** Very few of us get enough essential oils and fatty acids in our diet, so this is arguably the most important supplement of all. The large variety of health benefits are difficult to dispute and range from boosting blood health to fighting Alzheimer's and dementia. While I suggest avoiding fish oils despite their rich omega-3 content (just like the fish that are their source, see the "Fish Crisis" in Chapter 9), these oils are potentially too toxic for me to recommend. Thank goodness there are plenty of plant based omega-3 supplements. But even more, there's also krill oil, which is my personal favorite for its higher nutritional value and immediate potency. Krill are the tiny shrimp that are unique in their role near the very bottom of the food chain. And unlike most crustaceans, they are not bottom feeders, but instead feed on ultra-clean single-celled phytoplankton that live at that surface of oceans where they feast on a diet of sunlight and carbon dioxide. How's that for clean eating? A far cry from the toxic waste sitting on the bottom of

our modern oceans. If you're allergic to krill, go for flax, but do not ignore your need for more omega-3!

4. **Organic whole food multi-vitamins:** Yes, this is basically a "cover your bases" supplement, and though most of the old-school multivitamins have been proven ineffective or mostly non-digestible, the new whole food organics are starting to overcome a lot of these objections. Many of the best are also augmented with antioxidants, probiotics, and other potent phytochemicals, and there's no doubt that I feel more energized when I'm consistent with my multi-vitamin consumption. Some still argue this is mostly a placebo effect, but I don't agree. Nonetheless, I'll take a good old-fashioned placebo effect over zero benefits from doing nothing. That's a bio-logical truth that's impossible to dismiss when dealing with proper dosages of non-toxic whole food nutrients.

5. **Magnesium & Calcium supplement:** While both genders tend to suffer from a magnesium deficiency, men are especially susceptible. And though both also suffer from a calcium deficiency, you likely already know that most women are in greatest danger from their lack of this necessary mineral. I've found that a quality "Cal-Mag" combo supplement is the most effective and affordable way to ensure we get enough of these truly crucial nutrients.

6. **Turmeric (aka Curcumin):** This nutrient is historically known as a primary spice in curry. While I seek out and constantly test a variety of natural herbs and spices for health and healing (yes, nearly all are considered *superfoods*), I've included this particular spice among my most highly recommended supplements for two reasons. First, I want to encourage you to also test a variety of these ultra-natural plant-sourced supplements for yourself, and second, turmeric has proven its benefits to me and the scientific community. While it's relatively new to the supplement scene, this wonder plant is widely known for its ability to battle many common ailments. If you need an effective natural remedy for

inflammation, chronic pain, arthritis, or digestive issues, until further notice, this is my most highly recommended herbal supplement. Research has also shown it to combat a large number of ailments ranging from fibromyalgia to cancer.[138] Stay posted at BioLogicWorkout.com for updates on this potent spice and others that have shown promise in recent studies.

With nearly everything you consume or are exposed to, it is hugely beneficial (if not imperative) that you know the proper dose for your age, weight, and gender, so I implore you to always err to the side of conservatism, especially where concentrated supplements are concerned. Read the labels and instructions thoughtfully. I tend to keep my dosages between one-third to one-half the recommended dose until I've had a few weeks to measure results, and I strongly suggest you do the same. As always, if you have any health concerns at all—including allergies, pre-existing conditions, and especially pregnancy—confer with a trusted doctor before adding supplements of any type to your diet.

CHAPTER 9

BioLogic Nutrition Strategies: Reeling it In

The Fish Crisis

Early in my adult life I ate fish as often as I could get it, but not so today. The mercury levels (in the form of methylmercury) found in most fish are beyond alarming, and though it has always been present in seafood, the earth has never been as toxic as it is in the twenty-first century. The Environmental Protection Agency (EPA) recently reported that women living in US coastal communities had higher average blood levels of dangerous methylmercury, and many had methylmercury levels that the EPA considers unsafe for adults.[139] As noted above, today's fish varieties are not the same fish on which our ancestors feasted. Thankfully there are still a few low-mercury seafood options, but they are very few, so let's pray fish farms eventually produce ultra-clean versions of the most popular species. Until then, I strongly suggest you keep your fish intake to one serving per week or less. Since mercury and many other toxins build up to the highest levels in predatory fish who are near the top of the food chain, try to avoid the larger fish species (in adult size). Go to BioLogicWorkout.com for resources to determine where your favorites rank.

As for shellfish, the issues are generally the same but with the added concern that comes with eating bottom feeding scavengers, especially in today's toxic waters. If you can't give up these delicacies, at very least cut back, and please ensure you buy only ocean caught (non-farmed) American produced shellfish, especially when buying shrimp. You won't find this information on most labels so be sure to ask the management at your grocery store or fish market exactly where they get the shellfish you will buy. Shrimp raised in Asian countries (especially Vietnam) are especially suspect of conducting disgusting feed and packaging practices, so beware. For a wealth of easy reading research and recommendations on this fast evolving topic, a *Special Report* published in Consumereports.org on April 24, 2015 is the most comprehensive and timely multi-media report on shrimp safety available.[140] For shrimp junkies like me it's sort of a "read it and weep" report, so please do everything you can to cut back on these crustaceans. Let's face it, a bottom feeder likely has fecal matter, bacteria-laden rotting food sources, and toxic waste laced throughout their bodies, so please remember that we're not the only creatures that "are what we eat."

The Soy Paradox

Back in the nineties, I conducted an interview with Dr. Earl Mindell, author of the bestselling *Vitamin Bible* and his subsequent text *The Soy Miracle*. I joined a growing chorus of fitness writers who excitedly reported that if continued research proved soy to be as beneficial to Westerners as it is to folks from the Far East, it would and should one day find a role in many American diets. Despite Dr. Mindell's high hopes for the once lowly bean, he admitted the high concentration of phytochemicals in soy coupled with the lack of substantive time-proven research gave reason for caution and moderation and therefore recommended a maximum of three ounces per day. Sadly, few tofu feasters took heed. Two decades later, the jury is in, and no food has drawn more dramatic criticism concerning its *more harm than good* identity than the now pervasive hormone-wrecking soybean. Soy foods must be handled with great care or, better yet, not at all. So if you're hooked on tofu or soymilk as I once was, cut back dramatically or cut it out completely.

We simply have too many good meatless options (see above) to get hooked on enigmatic soy foods, especially for women and children. Yes, most soy products have been adulterated by the Western industrial food complex, so that's part of the net-loss equation. And yes, Asian soy has long proven to be a far *more good than harm* miracle food for Asians with Asian diets, which explains the research confusion. But with all the variables involved, until the scientific community gets it all sorted out and farmers start producing ancient strains of soybeans suitable for Western consumption, they're pretty much off my menu. So if you can't cut it out, please cut back. For the sake of full disclosure, I still love to steam up a fresh batch of edamame (soy beans in the pod), but that's all about the *joy factor* for me. On the bright side, fermented soy foods like tempeh, natto and miso soup have evaded most of the negatives, so if you're a true soy junkie stick to the fermented varieties and cut out the rest.

Cut It Out or Cut Back!

If I listed every product the average American consumes daily or weekly but shouldn't, I'd need several more pages. The industrial food complex and the pharmaceutical industry have a lot in common. You can count on ongoing updates at BioLogicWorkout.com to expose the harm of these foods and drugs as new research is made available. For the scope and intent of this book, however, I'll try to keep it short by addressing the foods and ingredient types that are the most dangerous, whether to your biochemical health, your fight against high blood sugar and obesity, or both. In all cases please remember, if you can't cut it out, at very least cut back.

The White Stuff: As you might recall from Chapter 2, dietary sugar is without question public enemy number one in the fight against obesity and collapse of our glucose metabolism; so I simply refer to it as poison. But what you may not know is that the consumption of naturally occurring sugars in more than moderate quantities (even in their whole food source) can be equally toxic to our bodies. The list of immediate and potential health risks is long, and if you've read the preceding chapters you now know them well. That list alone should give you cause to take heed. Moreover, don't be fooled by fruit juice (regardless of its source or organic nature). Once the juice is removed from its whole food fiber-rich source, it's not much better than a can of Coke. I suggest you stop serving fruit juices, sweetened sodas, and all other sweetened beverages (including sweetened tea). Also, stop adding extra sugar to your foods, and please spread the word.

While it is true that our bodies require sugar (as it naturally occurs in whole food*s*—see my list of sweet vegetables in the previous chapter), even minor over-consumption is dangerous. I shudder when I see a child licking a lollipop or eating other sugar-laden snacks and candies with glee. Their regular consumption of the sweet stuff is not merely wrecking their young bodies during their developmental years, but it's also brainwashing them to develop a dangerously addictive appetite for this exceedingly destructive substance. If you follow no other advice in this chapter, follow this one. When we consume more than our bodies get from natural food sources, sugar has a devastatingly negative impact on our health no matter the source. There are some great books on this subject, and several powerful short documentaries available on YouTube and other video sites. Visit our website for a recommended reading list and web links if you're struggling with this topic. If you really must partake of high-calorie natural sugars, I suggest raw honey and agave nectar. Both are generally sweeter than the more common sugars like cane sugar and corn syrup and therefore require fewer calories for equal sweetness. Both are also widely considered to be *superfoods* with a variety of health benefits you'll never get from the white stuff. But even so, please consume these sugars not merely in moderation, but with great conservatism.

The Other White Stuff: Wheat, white potatoes, white rice, and corn products are the most insidious Trojan Horse foods we consume. They seem so healthy, and surely the government worked hard (with the industrial food complex lobby) to ensure they're the foundation of their traditional Nutrition Pyramid. But these simple carbohydrates are merely sugars waiting to shed their disguise after you've swallowed them. And contrary to all the lies we were fed in the last half of the 20th century, these simple carbs have very little nutritional value compared to the negatives, especially the non-organic and GMO versions. So though you are likely addicted to one or more of these (I'm a recovering bread, pasta, and corn junkie), please wean off of them as soon as possible if you really want to slow the aging process and bring your body weight to healthy levels. If you must, save them only for special occasions, or at least cut the size of each serving in half if you're not ready to let go.

I still bounce into that zone from time to time, and thanks to my strong blood sugar and fat-burning metabolism, my body can handle it with ease. But the daily consumption of simple starchy carbs and sugars is, in my opinion, the most destructive enemy to our health and aesthetics. Simple empty carbs can obviously come in very handy during times of famine, especially in their original organic form. But in this era of plenty, these should be avoided—since they're otherwise worthless calories—if you really want to get in shape and reverse the aging process. I recently spoke with a major wheat farmer who confirmed that the highly toxic, chemical weed killers like Roundup are used profusely to make wheat and other grains easier to harvest. So, until the government steps up, please avoid non-organic wheat at all cost.[141]

Artificial Sweeteners: Avoid these like the dangerous chemicals most are. Until further notice, drop them like a cancer causing rock. If you have a sweet tooth and the sweet vegetables listed in the previous chapter don't satisfy every need, there are finally some tasty organic sweeteners that are simply low-to-no calorie sugar alcohols from healthy plant sources. Among these, I enjoy Stevia in foods, Erythritol frozen treats, and Xylitol is my favorite chewing gum sweetener. Yet even these have some unknowns due to lack of history and scientific research in their current form, natural as they may be. We need a few more years of research before I'll feel comfortable consuming any of these sugar alcohols on a daily basis.

Vegetable Cooking Oils: Aside from the healthy fats noted above, there are very few cooking oils readily available in grocery stores that are good for you. It's easier to name the good rather than rattle off all the bad oils and fats out there. For that growing list and other fat and oil related resources, you can look them up to BioLogicWorkout.com. The known harms of these bad oils have been long publicized. I hope it suffices to know that humankind should never have started deep frying with vegetable oil, as extreme heat can change an oil's chemistry even in its most natural form. For this, it stands to reason that processed vegetable oil is even more dangerous once heated. This might be the toughest change for some of you to make in your diet, especially in the South, but please start weaning off the common cooking oils as soon as you can. Use more coconut oil, grass fed butter, olive oil (the lower the temperature the better), and even animal lard to help with the transition. But avoid the most highly processed oils like corn oil, soybean oil, canola oil, and peanut oil, etc. Even more, unless you're eager to play lab rat for the food industry, avoid manufactured oils like margarine and Olestra (Olean).

Synthetic and Artificial Ingredients: If you're not yet reading the ingredients labels on the foods you buy, please start today. No matter what the front of the package says (especially if you see the words "natural" or "lite"), you have no clue what is in the product until you read the label. Many of the most popular ingredients are known to cause innumerable harms, including cancer. I have an ever growing list of FDA approved ingredients to avoid posted at BioLogicWorkout.com, so if you see any words on a label you don't recognize make sure it's not on our food label blacklist.

While most products labeled as "certified organic" are generally trustworthy, I still implore you to read the label, especially if it's not made by a long trusted manufacturer. Label reading is a practice that should become as common to your shopping experience as inspecting your fruits and vegetables for bad bruises before putting them in your cart. If you don't have access to our blacklist while shopping, do your best to stick to organic products. And please avoid products with food colorings and dyes (especially Yellow 5 and Yellow 6 used in processed mac and cheese), and artificial sweeteners (aspartame and sucralose are most common). Also avoid any of the following blacklisted terms: artificial, hydrogenated, trans fats, high-fructose, MSG (monosodium glutamate, maltodextrin, sodium caseinate), enriched, benzoate, BHA, BHT, preservative, chloride, sodium nitrate/nitrite, propyl, and—believe it or not—soy in any form, even if it's an organic product (see The Soy Paradox above). Again, if you don't readily recognize the ingredient as being natural and healthy, don't buy the product.

Processed Foods: If you read the five categories above, you already realize that most, if not all processed foods you commonly consume violate one or more of those BioLogic nutrition guidelines. This is a major concern, particularly if you're eating them at a non-organic restaurant, of which there are few (visit our website for a list of organic restaurant chains). While you'll also find an ever-growing "processed food blacklist" at BioLogicWorkout.com, here's a short list of the most common processed foods I hope you'll immediately replace with healthy alternatives. And again, if you can't cut it out, at least cut back!

Cow Milk: I grew up loving this stuff. I wish it weren't so. A growing mountain of research is proving that modern cow milk, even in its most natural/organic form, does far *more harm than good* when used as a staple in the human diet.[142] Though it's still a controversial subject in some circles—especially with the dairy lobby fighting hard to protect their profits—the chorus of experts pleading that we give up on this "liquid white stuff" grows larger every year. My daughter's elementary school was just a mile from my first big health club, so I used to spend lunch with her and her first-grade class nearly every day. The first time I told a table of seven- year-olds what was in the cow milk they were gleefully guzzling down, and how "bad" it was for their little bodies, you would have thought I canceled Christmas. Forever. That was twenty years ago. Americans have simply been brainwashed into "loving" milk, yet historically, most of our ancient ancestors (who established our gene pool) weren't even cow milk drinkers—and they had access to the clean stuff. Many are startled to learn that the Bible doesn't even mention cow's milk a single time as a beverage, and scholars are in agreement that the patriarchs drank lots and lots of goat milk, sheep milk, and even camel milk, but seldom (if ever) cow milk. And to add injury to insult, the milk we get today is so laden with toxins and so stripped of its mythical nutritional value that it's even worse than I told that table of first-graders two decades ago. So if you simply cannot give up animal milk, switch to the far healthier goat or sheep alternatives. Otherwise, let almond milk, coconut milk, hemp milk, and rice milk products replace your dairy needs. You might have noticed I left soymilk out of my recommendations, and if you read *The Soy Paradox* above, you know why.

Processed (non-organic) Fast Food, Snacks, & Candies: Surely you saw this one coming. Few processed foods more heinously violate our blacklist than these processed foods. If cleaning up your diet is a new consideration for you, this might prove to be your toughest sacrifice, especially if you use candy as a treat or reward for yourself or the kids in your life. The sugar issue alone should have us bailing on these processed foods. Knowing that they're packed with proven toxins and other cancer causing agents should at least be a wake-up call. In the nineties I unwittingly allowed my young daughter to eat all of the above in moderation, but I'm embarrassed to admit that one of our birthday traditions was to "treat" her to a shopping spree at one of her favorite candy stores, and of course, I joined in on the "childlike" fun. Today, though we both still have an affection for these confections, we know that no amount of processed sugar is worth the cost. If the goal is to avoid its toxic metabolism-destroying effects, then processed sugar is the first food we need to cut from our diets. This is especially true now that there are so many healthy/organic alternatives on the market today; too many to continue making excuses. Let's repent together, and get the word out to our friends and loved ones. I believe the day is coming when the thought of giving a child snacks and candy made of pure processed sugar will be likened to giving them addictive toxic medications or forcing them to breathe second-hand cigarette smoke. The sooner we wake up to that reality the easier it will be to turn the tide.

Bad Meats: If you anticipated I would recommend only organic "naturally raised" meats and declare all other meats to cause *more harm than good*, you're right. For this, as noted above, we should be replacing as much of our meat intake with organic meatless alternatives as possible. I'll admit I make exceptions far too often, mostly when I rationalize that I'm left with no options (i.e. when I'm "starving" while traveling or at a ball game), and I frequently let the *joy factor* trump my legitimate desire to avoid bad meat. Nonetheless, there are some meats we should keep on our blacklist at all cost. These include pork bacon, shellfish, pork sausage, hot dogs, fast food burgers, other fatty beef, deli meats, dirty fish, and any meats that are charred or cooked at very high temperatures, regardless of their organic nature. Again, if you're going to cheat on any of the above, do it sparingly. Over time, try to allow regret to override the *joy factor*, and let your desire for discipline overtake your weakness in the face of temptation. I was once a voracious meat addict, so if I can do it, you can too.

Alcoholic Beverages

I occasionally enjoy a quality beer, and though wine and hard liquor tend to give me headaches, I'll still have a taste from time to time, as it is widely believed that most alcoholic beverages have health benefits when consumed in small doses per day. But in the modern era, these are some of the most destructive consumables known to man. Sadly, *many* people over-consume alcohol today; the same way folks smoked cigarettes in the sixties. The chemical and addictive risks and high-calorie properties of alcohol are common knowledge, so I won't belabor the topic here. To balance all the concerns, let's be realistic. If you are a regular wine drinker or social drinker, please exercise wisdom and restraint, especially around children. I've lost too many friends and loved ones to the disease of alcoholism, and it is surely a major modern-day plague.

Beginning to Fulfill the Great Requirement: Remove Temptations

Now that you have a solid knowledge base identifying the good, the bad, and the ugly of the modern fitness lifestyle and diet, let's take a look at the eating habits and logistical strategies that will empower you to A) reduce your overall caloric intake and B) enhance your metabolic rate—without stealing your joy. Be reminded that discipline and joy are not mutually exclusive. Several times in the book I've identified the prerequisite of "proper nutrition and a more active lifestyle" as the *Great Requirement* that must be met for any health related program to fully succeed. The BioLogic Workout is no exception to that rule. In the following sections, I'll present strategies that have proven to help many people make the changes necessary to fulfill this overarching requirement. With proper nutrition accounting for 80% or more of the battle, I'll start with food related strategies and wrap up with the much easier "active lifestyle" strategies in Chapter 10.

Nothing can help you succeed in your goals more powerfully than removing the stumbling blocks that undermine you, and it's up to us to remove them. You know where you are weak, and by now you should know which dietary temptations are most destructive to your health, aesthetics, sustainability, and joy. Don't ever doubt that you *can* make the lifestyle changes that break the stronghold of these temptations. Over time, you will begin to wonder how you ever could have been so easily tempted by foods or lifestyle practices that you knew were leading you to damage your one and only body. To that end, take as many of these strategies to heart as you can today, then add more as needed tomorrow.

Diet Strategies: How, When, and Where

The following tips can help you gain control of your eating habits even before you correct the foods you eat. As you move forward, take on as many of these strategies as you can, but don't become so obsessive that you try to adopt every one of them at the same time—unless of course you're already almost there. The rest of us don't in any way benefit from that sort of pressure, so let's not set ourselves up for failure. When you adopt the strategies below that can immediately fit your personal cornerstone paradigm, especially sustainability and its best-friend the *joy factor*, you will find it increasingly easy to adopt more and more of them over time. But please don't find yourself disregarding these disciplines, or self-loathing will surely rise up to undermine everything you do. Heed all the recommendations you can, and before you know it you too will be teaching these strategies to your friends and loved ones.

Concerning Calories

As early in the previous chapter, for a factual understanding of calorie-consumption and how it affects fat-storage, please refer to the critically important subsection titled *Fat Burning, Body Shaping, and Your Metabolism* in Chapter 2. While the ideal caloric intake is different for each of us, unless you are on a rare fast, adults should seldom if ever get less than one thousand calories per day. As detailed in the above mentioned subsection, if you try to lose fat stores by dipping below your daily calorie requirements, your metabolism will simply gear down and go into a fat-storing famine defense. And you never want to happen. So if you think you can effectively lose weight by starving yourself, you are sadly mistaken, and likely could have shed more pounds of fat while eating more healthy foods instead of living in denial. Though an occasional fast has real benefits, please don't consider weight loss among them, as that practice is another example of doing *more harm than good*. And of course, unless you're a professional athlete with a legitimate need to grow larger than your ideal weight, you should take great care to avoid consuming more calories than needed to sustain your target body weight.

While it's far from an exact science, a general rule of thumb is to consume between ten and fifteen calories per pound of target body weight. So if your target weight is 180 pounds, you should aim for 1,800 to 2700 calories per day. That's merely dinner for some of you, but if you follow the guidelines in Chapter 8 you can easily satisfy your hunger despite those reduced numbers. A highly active lifestyle will allow you to consume a few more calories, but for all the reasons learned in *Sections I* and *II*, nothing will boost your calorie-burning efficiency and your fat-burning metabolism better than a consistent approach to your BioLogic Workouts. Thanks to the long-term consistency of my workout regimen and clean eating habits, my various metabolic processes are so efficient that I can regularly consume twice as many calories as my sedentary friends. So if you're hoping to fudge up on your daily calorie intake, stay disciplined with your *BioLogic 10 Minute Workouts* and employ as many of the strategies detailed in *Section III* as possible!

Food Consumption Strategies

Consider your caloric intake, not your caloric burn: After completing Chapter 8, you may have planned some food changes and calculated the calories you'd consume in an enjoyable, sustainable diet, but landed on a calorie count that's a good bit higher than the "ten to fifteen calories per pound" rule of thumb. Don't sweat it. Just consider it your starting point. Trust that your consistent practice of your BioLogic Workouts and the active lifestyle strategies you'll learn in Chapter 10 will spark a significantly higher calorie burn, and thereby move you toward your target weight nonetheless. If not, make adjustments accordingly, starting with the garbage—sugar and simple carbs. If all you do is cut back on all the white stuff (the consumables that pack the largest quantity of empty calories) and replace them with my lower calorie recommendations, you'll see a dramatic drop in your caloric intake—and you won't have to walk away unsatisfied. Try never to practice denial without an enjoyable replacement, or you risk setting yourself up for failure. You are far more likely to succeed in reaching your target weight if you focus on the joy of eating nutrient-rich foods and the satisfaction that comes when you eliminate the garbage, so scratch the white stuff from your meals as often as you can and start reaping immediate benefits.

Plate food with meat as the minority item: We Americans are notorious for making meat the centerpiece of our dinner, and we typically consume unhealthy amounts of meat and animal fat. While expert opinions differ widely, I suggest you eat no more meat than you could fit in the palm of your hand (3 to 6 ounces). That portion should take up no more than a quarter of your dish, so fill the rest with veggies and the other good foods detailed in the previous chapter.

Never skip protein! As you begin to reduce your intake of meat, don't let your protein intake drop below healthy levels. Be sure to add as many of the meatless protein options (listed in Chapter 8) as needed to satisfy your protein requirements. You simply can't build muscle without protein.

If you can't cut it out, cut back: If you've read the entire book so far, you realize that I will repeat a mantra as often as possible to ensure it sticks with you. Likewise, by now you know I empathize with the reality of food addictions and sincerely want to help you avoid attaching negative feelings to a healthy decision. So if you can't go cold turkey on a bad food, just cut back on frequency and serving size as much as you can. In time, especially after seeing visible results from your BioLogic Workouts, you should be able to give up your former addictions altogether.

Portion Control Strategies: These portion strategies should prove far easier to implement than most of the strategies outlined through chapters 8 and 9, so try to adopt the ones you know you can stick with, and save the rest for future consideration. Take it all one day at a time, and never lose your joy!

- **Eat a healthy breakfast**, and follow the guidelines in the previous chapter!
- **Pack your own lunch**. There is no easier way to ensure proper portions.

- **Plate your food in the kitchen**, not at the table. It's a great way to cut back on seconds.
- **Eat salads and greens first**. There are many great reasons for this one… just do it!
- **Boost flavor using organic spices**, but avoid adding salt. Spices help curb hunger.
- **Chew slowly, enjoy the flavor in every bite**. Reduces hunger and helps digestion.
- **Cut your food into smaller pieces**. This goes hand in hand with the above strategy.
- **Put down your fork every few bites.** It's another slow down tactic to reduce hunger.
- **Brush your teeth immediately after every meal.** Good hygiene curbs snacking.
- **Pack up leftovers before you eat.** This removes the temptation of eating seconds.
- **Use smaller plates and bowls at home.** Sounds elementary, but it definitely works.
- **Don't eat while watching TV or surfing the web.** Avoid distractions, taste your food!
- **Use organic protein shakes as your secret weapon.** Curb hunger with easy protein!
- **Don't buy bargain sizes**, unless you deliberately repackage into smaller containers.
- **When dining out, start splitting your entree with others.** It's healthy AND economical.
- **If you don't share your entree, pre-plan a take home portion.** Leftovers rock.
- **Don't clean your plate.** It's not just good manners, but good consumption control.
- **If you must have dessert (sugar), sample just a taste or eat just half.** Cut back!
- **Drink water from bigger bottles and taller glasses**. More water equals less hunger.
- **Eliminate sugary beverages.** Sugar isn't just toxic, it also increases your hunger.

Timing Strategies

Even in nutrition, timing can be everything, especially when it comes to the evening hours. These may not be as easy as the portion strategies above, but they can have a profound positive effect if you employ them consistently. You can do it!

- **No starchy carbs or sugar after lunch.** This may be the easiest way to cut back.
- **Never go to bed with a full stomach.** Burn fat rather than storing fat while sleeping.
- **Eat dinner as early as possible.** The sooner you digest dinner the better.
- **Eliminate late night snacking.** Easier said than done, but magic if you can do it!
- **Snack Healthy between meals to curb your appetite.** But don't sneak any sugar.
- **Grocery shop only after a full meal.** This *old school* strategy is golden.
- **Prepare healthy meals and snacks for weekdays on the weekends.** This ensures fast easy access all week long and helps push unhealthy foods out of your diet.

Psychological Strategies

The late Yogi Berra said, *"baseball is 90% mental and the other half is physical."* While this hyperbolic Yogi-ism is famously funny, it's ultimate meaning is nonetheless true, especially when we replace "baseball" with "nutrition." Implement as many of these psychological strategies as possible, and the "other half" of the battle will become increasingly easy over time. You've probably noticed that some of these strategies hit on other categories as well, so I hope you agree these are especially effective if taken seriously. Enjoy!

- **Focus on eating new foods** you enjoy, not on denial of your favorite bad foods.
- **Learn to recognize cravings** that aren't hunger, and admit when you're not hungry.
- **Celebrate your sacrifices**, and feel gratitude for your clean meals.

- **Plan a cheat day** every week or two and keep it modest… one serving, one slice!
- **Avoid denial** of your favorite foods when someone else serves them to you. Instead, sample a very small piece or a couple bites and enjoy the flavors.
- **Constantly remind others** that the white stuff is fattening and toxic. Teaching works.
- **Chew healthy gum** sweetened with Xylitol or Stevia to curb hunger. This truly works.
- **Shop with a rock solid budget** and use a calculator while shopping. This both saves you money and keeps you from buying the bad stuff.
- **Read the labels**, shop slowly and thoughtfully, and enjoy the education.
- **Find an accountability partne**r who will hold you accountable to all of the above.
- **Journal your experiences** and "gold star" your victories over old food addictions.

There are obviously many other strategies out there, so be sure to check in frequently at BioLogicWorkout.com for a growing list of proven ideas. You're sure to find many that will work for you.

CHAPTER 10

BioLogic Active Lifestyle Strategies

Keep an Open Mind and Seek Wise Counsel

Even when your workout activities and nutrition plan hit the sweet spot of your personal cornerstone paradigm, you will still need to seek advice from your doctor to ensure your new course isn't hindered by any pre-existing conditions, past injuries, allergies or issues with your current state of health. Of course, the low-stress nature of the BioLogic approach removes many of these concerns, but be sure to have these discussions nonetheless. You may even find yourself being the bearer of good news in your sharing of the BioLogic approach with the health professionals you know.

Many of these pros are so disenchanted with *old school* forms of exercise and are so busy keeping up with research in their own fields that it's unlikely they've caught on to our revelation. Some of them will be among the most receptive folks you know, so seeking their advice could produce fruit for both of you. The same goes for spouses, co-workers, close friends, pastors, or any mentors you may have. Seeking their feedback should prove beneficial for both of you, especially as one or more may become invaluable accountability partners or training partners for the workouts, nutrition strategies, and the active lifestyle strategies outlined below. You'll never "need" a partner to make any of these lifestyle tweaks, but teamwork definitely helps.

Walk the Walk

As you've journeyed through *BioLogic Revelation* with me, I hope you've been inspired never to forget that your enjoyment of the *10 Minute Workout* and its realistic approach to nutrition are required if this simple lifestyle is ever to remain sustainable. And though you'll never stimulate your *super fast twitch fibers* while walking, we are clearly designed to walk. Until the mid-twentieth century, walking was by far the primary means of travel for all of humankind, especially for the nomadic peoples who populated the earth. If you've ever walked any amount of significant distance with others you've surely recognized that the social, physical, mental, and spiritual benefits are refreshing and immediate. Walking with others is a beautiful thing. If by chance you or a loved one have a disability that limits or entirely eliminates the ability to walk, fear not. If you're wheelchair bound, I trust you (and your doctors) have developed strategies to help you increase your activity level and compensate with other activities. Just do your best to adapt as many of my walking strategies as possible, and I hope most if not all of the other active lifestyle strategies will prove entirely accessible to you. God bless you as you run the good race and persevere over obstacles most of us will never face.

Don't Enjoy Walking?

If you're simply not yet a walker, now is the time to give it a try. Unless a pre-existing health issue or disability takes walking off the table, I promise you will learn to love it, especially once you begin to see and feel the remarkable benefits of your BioLogic Workouts. That said, as is true for all the BioLogic nutrition and lifestyle strategies, just do what you can, and never let my plea for you to start walking feel like a requirement to gain positive results. So if you cannot or will not walk more often, at very least adopt as many of the alternative walking strategies listed below, and you will still enhance the cascade in equal measure.

As for power-walking, I suggest avoiding it. While there are conflicting studies on the negatives and benefits, I personally feel zero benefits from high-speed power walking, and even less from power walking while carrying weights. In fact I find that practice to be dangerous for our joints. Just establish a strong, steady, and consistent stride that you can maintain while still being able to carry on a conversation without totally running out of breath.

Walking your neighborhood, a nearby park, or even a shopping mall for fifteen to twenty minutes at a time as often as possible is the leading active lifestyle component of the BioLogic approach. Though it's futile to count the calories you burn during a workout (see Chapter 2, *Fat Burning, Body Shaping, and Our Metabolism*), I strongly encourage you to realize and celebrate the how you will be supercharging your metabolism by following the BioLogic lifestyle activities outlined in this chapter, as each of these can greatly enhance the 24/7 fat-burning power of the actual BioLogic Workouts. That said, the cascade of benefits from BioLogic Workouts will still be activated even if you struggle with these lifestyle and nutrition chapters (notice I said "struggle with," not "ignore"), but these additional strategies will greatly multiply the power of the cascade and the scope and depth of its benefits.

Though I'm not a fan of cardiovascular equipment as a primary workout device (never jog on a treadmill!), they can definitely serve you well where walking is concerned. So if you have a treadmill, stationary bike, or quality stepper, use them to simulate walking and hiking as often as you can, especially during inclement weather or after dark. You'll lose the benefits of fresh air and the inspiring nature of the great outdoors. But if you've learned to love these machines, as long as you're using them solely to increase your daily activity level and not as your workout unto itself, I encourage you to enjoy them.

Speaking of machines, I encourage you to adopt strategies that will get you walking and hiking to and from the machines that move us around as much as possible. All of the BioLogic lifestyle strategies in this chapter have one primary goal in common—to ensure you become more active for a variety of healthful reasons—and all are in line with our genetic "*fight or flight*" design. We weren't designed to spend the prime hours of our day sitting on our butts or riding around in transport vehicles. In a culture where most have little choice but to succumb to these sedentary activities, we have to take advantage of every opportunity to walk. To that end, try to adopt as many of these as possible for the rest of your life.

- **Park your car at a greater distance from the entrance** while still feeling safe. Imagine the miles you will have walked after doing this for a full year! Yes, it might cost you a few minutes every day, but surely you need the activity more than you need more time to sit. Ladies, while I compel you to take greater care to practice personal safety in all parking situations, please skip this particular parking tip once the sun sets. Park only in well-lit areas, try to ensure there are other folks within earshot when exiting your vehicle and walk circumspectly with your finger on the panic button of your car key fob no matter your distance from the entrance. Safety first!

- **Skip the elevators and take the stairs** every chance you get. Stair climbing is golden!
- **If you like shopping, hike through malls and shopping centers,** and be sure to hit *all* the levels using only stairs to move from floor to floor. No more riding lazy escalators for you.
- **If you use mass transit, get off a few stops earlier.** Adding a block or two of walking will prove invaluable over time and the mental and spiritual benefits will be immediate.
- **Sign up for charity walks** and participate as a walker in charity runs, especially if they're events sponsored by your employer, as you will further inspire your co-workers. These highly social, especially rewarding events should override any aversion you may have for a daily walking regimen.
- **Get out of the workplace and enjoy walking meetings** from time to time. Not everyone has the authority to do this, so if you do, please take advantage of your power and bless your staff along the way.
- **At home, sweep the driveway or rake the leaves** instead of using a leaf-blower. I know time is valuable, but this sort of activity on a regular basis can prove invaluable.
- **Start and finish "do it yourself" (DIY) projects** around the house, garden, and yard. This one pays dividends. For many of you, these efforts are already the core of your "fitness" program. Good job. Now add your *10 Minute BioLogic Workouts* and you'll be right as rain!
- **Trade your self-propelled mower for a push version**. It's still a mystery how we've been lulled into paying extra for the right to become less active, but let's all agree we need to reverse these

trends. Visit BioLogicWorkout.com for an ever-growing list of alternative walking strategies. The more you adopt the merrier!

- **Walk your dog** even if it's just around your yard. "Pokey" will love you for it.
- **Crank the music** and "get your dance on" the next time you mop or vacuum or perform any other repetitive chore. Music is good for your soul, especially when it gets you moving.

Move with Balance, Strength, and Grace

As you walk throughout your day, do so with balance, strength, and grace with your head held high. You might have noticed that people walk in a way that reflects their health. Most walk with poor posture, or with a limp, or simply exhibit weakness in their stride. Don't be like them. The more intentional you become in maintaining a straight uplifted posture, confident balance, and a strong graceful gate, the more these attitudes will translate over to every aspect of your life—your BioLogic Workouts included. This goes for your seated posture and attitude as well. So no more slouching, imbalanced tilting, or neck-straining forward hunch as you lean toward your computer monitor. Straighten up and raise your head! In doing this, not only will you benefit but you'll also shine before all who see you, surely inspiring many.

Don't Skip Recess . . . Play Like a Kid!

Even if you're an active walker into your upper adult years, don't dismiss your need for good old-fashioned play time out in the fresh air of the great outdoors, especially if you have kids. Find a low-impact low-stress sport or game that you can fall in love with, and weave these activities into each month as much as you like. If you're in love with high-impact or high-stress games like basketball, tennis, or golf, be sure you take care to gear down on the impact and stress these place on your joints. Listen to your body in order to curtail the activity if you start to feel joint strains or aches. These play time activities will bring a host of mind, body, and spirit benefits despite the potential cost in wear and tear. Much like the advanced BioLogic Workout variations, sometimes we need to accept these trade-offs to meet other goals or to answer to the *joy factor*. As you age you'll undoubtedly have to give up on the sports or games that have proven most threatening to your joints, so the more care you take while you're young, the more years you'll have to play them.

Though the traditional ball sports I passionately enjoyed in my youth were the first I had to give up in my mid-thirties, somehow I can still play tennis without feeling any significant wear and tear, so you may be surprised which sports remain safe for your joints as you age. We're all unique in this regard, so as long as you approach them with caution, don't fear testing some of your old favorites. But never push yourself beyond seventy-five percent of your perceived physical ability. It's not worth the risk, and absent the adrenaline you'd produce in a *fight or flight* situation, your tissues are especially vulnerable as you approach your limits.

While golf would seem a safe sport for most, it's far too stressful on my back, neck, and knees (I'm definitely not alone in this regard), so I've traded in my clubs for the flying discs we use in disc golf, my preferred outdoor game. In stark contrast to traditional golf, most disc golf courses are built on public parks and are free to use, and the discs are relatively cheap as well. Disc golf is without question the favorite outdoor excursion for nearly every member of my family and closest friend group, from the little kids to the seniors. I've never found a more socially interactive outdoor game or sport. I've seen large families that initially showed trepidation and disinterest in giving it a try, share lots of real laughs, high-fives, and sincere bonding moments during their very first time playing the game; especially when they split into two large teams in a "captain's choice" format. It's also an emerging professional sport. So though both of my boys dream of playing college and pro football, they also take disc golf very seriously as another potential professional effort. But for most of us, the game is best characterized as hiking the great outdoors with a higher sense of purpose—and lots of thrills and laughs along the way.

Another low-cost game that my family has grown to love Bocce ball. It's quite addictive, especially when played on a beach. We also love playing catch with all sorts of balls, street and mountain biking are always exciting, and various man-powered boating and water sports are awesome fresh air outings. Good old-fashioned hill and mountain hiking is still a favorite (though I often find myself wishing there was a disc golf course laid out along the way). And while swimming is famous for its low impact benefits, it's not the most accessible activity and it often forces you indoors, so if that's one of your favorites I still compel you to find at least one more sport you can play outside in the sunshine and fresh air.

While raw sunlight is much maligned for its UV dangers, we still benefit greatly from about ten to fifteen minutes of semi-direct sunlight several days per week for mental health and nutrient stimulation (especially vitamin D, see Chapter 8), so this particular lifestyle strategy is important even beyond the benefits of additional activity. But if you're heading outdoors for more than a few minutes, don't you dare forget to use one of the many organic, low-chemical sunscreens on the market, especially where your precious children are concerned. Though I have a large percentage of Pacific Islander genes (thanks to my Filipino father), you might be surprised to learn that I contracted and overcame melanoma skin cancer just after turning thirty. Though I'm sure the absence of sunscreens during my beach-boy childhood was mostly to blame, my dermatologist and I were both convinced that my use of artificial tanning beds during my twenties was a major accelerator of this especially deadly form of cancer. So please learn from my mistakes. Slather up your babies (and yourself) with organic high-SPF sunscreens when playing outdoors, *or* wear UV-blocking clothing and large brim hats. And I implore you . . . please stay clear of artificial tanning of any type. If an Islander like me can contract melanoma, anyone can. I thank God daily for the watchful eyes of my personal physician, and I hope my cancer scare serves as a wake-up call for all who read this.

Love to Run? Don't Jog . . . SPRINT!

I spent a lot of time cautioning against the heel-striking, joint abusing, *super fast twitch* diminishing effects of endurance running in *Section I*, so I won't belabor that here. Knowing that many millions are addicted to this counter-productive form of exercise, let me again offer up what I've found to be the ideal approach to weaning off this addiction. Stop running and start sprinting. Those of you who have yet to read *Section II*, see BioLogic Interval Training in Chapter 6 for greater detail on this subject. Whether you employ traditional short sprint workouts (utilizing all four BioLogic Protocols) or merely transform your continuous distance runs into intervals of sprints interlaced with periods of walking or resting, you can greatly reduce the damage to your joints and your *fast* and *super twitch muscle fibers*. I love to sprint, especially up hills, and even in my fifties I gain great joy from sprinting. But, despite being the most inherent form of *fast twitch muscle* training, the risks have greatly tempered my enthusiasm. I seldom run sprints more than twice per week, and never push myself beyond seventy-five percent of my perceived maximum. Like Jen, the sprinter from the true parable in Chapter 3, what I couldn't cut out for sake of the *joy factor*, I have significantly cut back. If however, you are a competitive runner who just can't give it up, at the very least please start training with sprint intervals over the distance, and reserve the heel-striking abuse only for race days.

Get More Sleep!

If there's anything we neglect as much as our nutrition and our physical fitness, it's our sleep. This is an ironic trio to neglect, as they're the three primary measures of good health. While eight hours of solid nocturnal sleep is the general rule of thumb for most adults, according to the National Sleep Foundation, most children over six years old need between nine and eleven hours, while adults need a solid seven hours and occasionally as much as nine hours.[143] In other words, kids typically don't get enough sleep, seniors tend to get too much sleep, and most adults are all over the map from week to week. While we all have different sleep needs and sleep habits, if you're an adult you should set a goal to get seven solid (non-drug-assisted) hours of sleep, and you should add more if you begin to run out of steam before the sun sets on your day. Most Americans get far too little sleep, so if you're struggling in this area, a ten to twenty-minute power nap at lunch or in the late afternoon can help you get through the day, but nothing replaces uninterrupted sleep during night time hours. This is another subject that warrants a dedicated text to fully explore it, so be sure to visit BioLogicWorkout.com for ongoing discussions concerning this urgent topic.

Don't Forget Your 10 Minute Workouts!

As you begin to feel the immediate benefits of your more active, more nutritious lifestyle (especially the weight loss many of you will experience through these changes alone), don't be lulled into missing out on the BioLogic effect! Believe it or not, those of us who practice the *10 Minute Workout* often find it difficult to remember to schedule the workouts. This oversight is partly due to their extraordinary convenience. But it's also a byproduct of the many days of recuperation required while our bodies adapt to *super fast twitch muscle fiber* hypertrophy and healing process, as these gaps create the need for a bit of long-range and day-to-day scheduling discipline. It's far from the burdensome "every day possible" fitness scheduling you've known in the past. Unless you have a personal trainer or serious training partner who can help you with our atypical scheduling needs, I strongly suggest you determine the best AM and PM time slots for each day of the week (twenty to thirty-minute slots should cover both the workout and travel/transition time). Ensure you train the muscle group that is due during the most convenient of those two slots (or both if your body feels hungry for a double). The BioLogic mobile phone app will take all the confusion out of your scheduling and documentation efforts, but even the simplest calendar app or journal should suffice. No matter how active you are, and no matter how clean your diet, if you neglect your scheduling discipline you'll risk failing to properly stimulate and develop your *fast* and *super fast twitch muscle fibers*. So don't let your short-term success derail your long-term goals of a longer, stronger life!

Find an Active Service Project or Ministry

If you want to find the perfect way to develop a less sedentary, far less TV-watching lifestyle, serve someone in need through your church, through other ministries like the Fellowship of Christian Athletes (my personal favorite), or any other services providing help to the sick, the poor, and the needy. Otherwise, any constructive effort to love on the kids in your family and community with a real sense of purpose can be life changing. When you volunteer for something that gets you out of your house you'll start engaging your head, heart, soul, and body in a noble and joy-filled way.

Not-So-Secret Weapon pt. 2: Meditate and Pray Throughout the Day

No matter your position on spirituality, many of you already know the power of meditation, prayer, quiet time, and gratitude even if you seldom practice it. If you're not into prayer, you should at least recognize the benefits of a hopeful mindset and the stress reduction hope-filled meditation and prayer can bring. No matter where you work or where you spend your day, you have the time to pause and clear your mind, even if for only a minute at a time. Do it. Even if you have to set your phone alarm to remind you, make sure you set time aside to get away from the noise (even if you have to step out to your car or escape to a restroom) and mediate with gratitude for your life and everything else for which you're thankful. The health benefits can be profound. I've learned I can stay at my desk and still tune out the noise just by closing my eyes, and the wave of gratitude and awe that often washes over me is a healing balm with legitimate biological impact. Perhaps you've felt this in times of prayer or meditation, or maybe while listening to beautiful music. All I'm asking is that you become intentional in finding daily quiet time, even on the job, and enjoy the immediate rewards of a clearer mind and more grateful spirit. Likewise, there's no more powerful way to start and end each day than to wake up with gratitude on your lips and fall asleep with peace and gratitude on your mind. While you'll find an invaluable list of resources on this subject at BioLogicWorkout.com, this is another topic I hope to discuss often in our blog threads and Facebook page.

Perform Resting Movements Often

If you recall from Chapter 6, where I discussed BioLogic *resting movements* in detail, these meditative, joint lubricating, circulation enhancing, tissue flushing, safe muscle stretching, total body cell stimulating movements bring all these benefits even if you're not working out. I spend two to five minutes performing these movements first thing in the morning, last thing before hitting the sack, and at various times throughout the day—especially when I've been sitting at my desk for a prolonged time. Go back to Chapter 6 to brush up on these techniques and be sure to watch the companion instruction videos to see some demonstrations. When I'm my most dialed-in with my breathing and focus, I often find my *resting movements* help me meditate, pray, and speak life and strength into every cell in my body. This, in turn, strikes up a feeling of potential power in every vital system. If we were ancient warriors preparing for battle or hunters preparing to take on a dangerous predator, we would likely practice these by instinct. This is another example of high-powered low hanging fruit, so seize yours hourly if possible.

Limit TV, Computer, and Mobile Device Time

Okay, for full disclosure, I confess that this is a strategy I need to better manage. As a writer and communicator, my computers often get more time with me than my wife and kids, especially while in research mode. Everything about sitting in front of these high energy electronics for extended periods is potentially unhealthy, and new studies are starting to reveal that the health dangers are probably far worse than anyone would want to risk. So if there's ever a case where playing it safe pays broad ranging dividends, it's this one. If all we consider is the harm of sitting (with typically terrible posture) for hours with our brains Wi-Fi connected to a powerfully influential mood-altering medium, that should be enough to get us to cut back. There is very little you can do with your time that is more sedentary than sitting with an electronic device, but again, I'm as guilty as anyone so I'm constantly developing new strategies to stay active even in my restful states. For starters, I've begun playing board games and card games with more frequency. Backgammon is my favorite, and nearly everyone in my close circle of friends has taken it on as an excellent alternative to sedentary digital activities. This may be another example of something that you can't immediately cut out but can surely cut back. So brainstorm a few alternatives, starting with the things you loved to do as a kid and start working them back into your life. We're avid film watchers in my family, as we always have long fruitful discussions after any movie or show, and we often pause the TV for midstream discussions. But that's still a step down from the four of us gathering around a board game or home project to truly engage each other.

Read More During Late Evening Hours

I'm amazed by how many people seldom if ever read in the evening anymore, despite the fact that reading was once the most widely practiced way to healthfully gear down one's mind, body, and soul at the end of a long day, particularly by reading inspirational texts. This tip also ties directly to the one above, as televisions and other light emitting digital devices have been proven to cause insomnia. Though some of you may use the television to help you fall asleep, I encourage you to wean off the tube and start winding down by reading more often.

CONCLUSION

Be Encouraged!

Make this commitment to the depth of your soul and you will begin to transform your entire being. You will spark the anti-aging power of the BioLogic fundamentals and protocols to trigger the full *BioLogic Cascade* of health benefits, and in doing so you will be strengthening your heart, mind, body, and soul. Your full-faceted, holistic response to the simple BioLogic stimuli will indeed seem *too good to be true,* but how else could an average person accomplish so much with a *10 Minute No-Sweat Workout,* if not for the scientific truth that proves the veracity of the revelation? If you've taken hold of the BioLogic fundamentals, cornerstones, and protocols, the science within the *BioLogic Revelation* should surely turn on the "AHA!" light bulb—if not now, within thirty days of practicing the BioLogic Workouts in proper form. Once there, you'll be seeing and feeling real and lasting results, maybe for the first time in your life. You'll start having days where the energy of your youth returns, you'll be joyfully craving your next BioLogic Workout, and I'll continue to be your guide if you engage me in our BioLogic blog and social media. My staff and I plan to do all we can to ensure you attain that "ideal you."

Now in my mid-fifties and heading toward my third decade using the BioLogic approach, I'm exceedingly grateful that I am without question in the best shape of my post-injury life. As I move towards my sixties, I'm more confident than ever that I'll continue winning the battle against unnecessary aging. I'm still getting stronger with every passing year, and I hope the same becomes true for you. Commit yourself to trying. Right now. Just commit! You *can* stick with this. Anyone can. And don't forget to spread the word among your friends and family. One day they'll thank you for it, and there's almost always more joy in the process when you're not going it alone.

In *BioLogic Revelation* we've considered a scientifically and historically based method to heal us, build our strength, combat our most dreaded diseases, burn unwanted fat, and delay the aging process in the simplest, safest, and most sustainable way possible. Like all action-based revelation, if you don't try it, you'll never know what you're missing, and will likely lose much more than your physical health. Come on friends . . . ten minutes? A piece of cake, right? En-JOY!

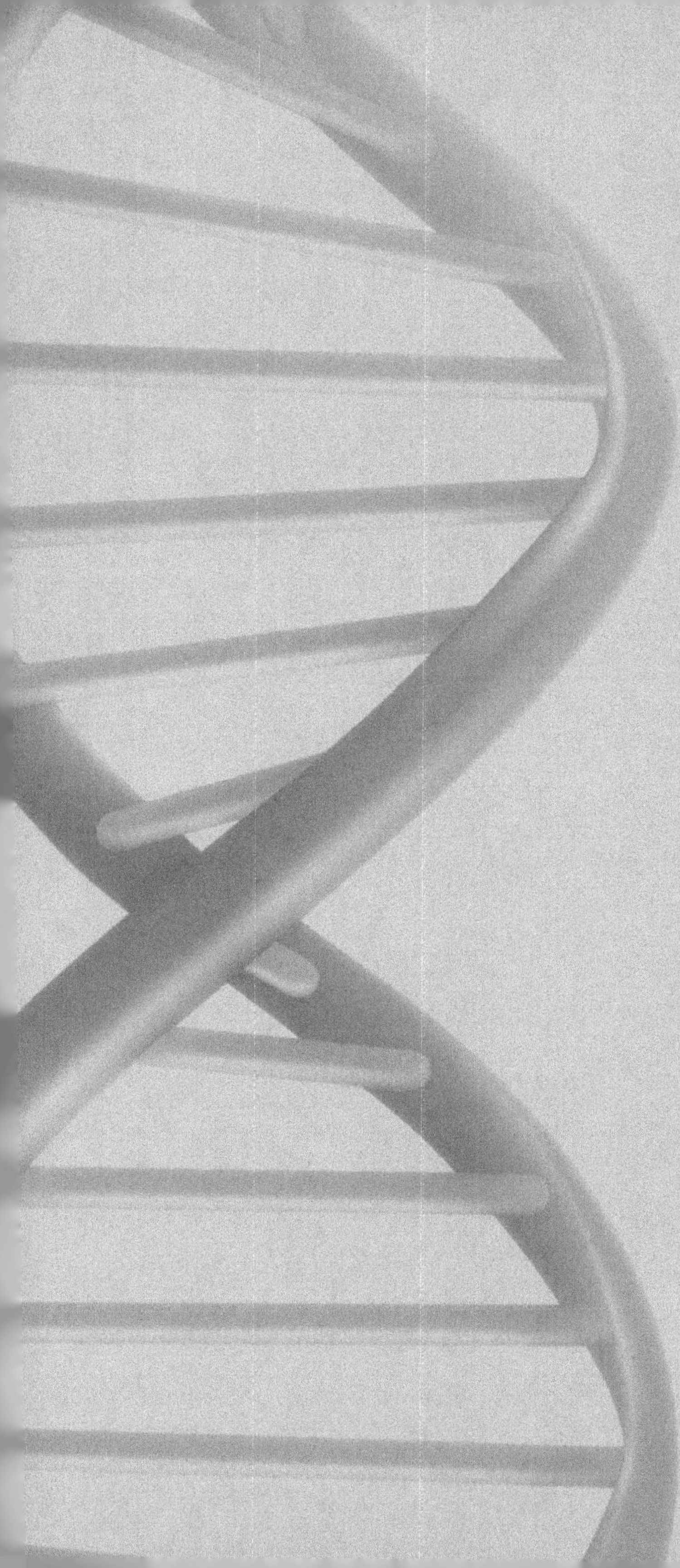

APPENDIX

APPENDIX I

Notated Bibliography with Excerpts

Many notes cited throughout the book are supported by multiple sources. To further aid in your study, a large number of these sources will also include excerpts in italics that were taken directly from the published study *or* the published abstract. Where sources support multiple notes, the latter notes refer to initial note.

1. **LeBrasseur NK, Walsh K, Arany Z.** (**Mayo Clinic**)
"Metabolic benefits of resistance training and fast glycolytic skeletal muscle." *American Journal of Physiology, Endocrinology and Metabolism.* 2011 January. Review.

Skeletal muscle exhibits remarkable plasticity with respect to its metabolic properties. Recent work has shown that interventions such as resistance training, genetic alterations and pharmacological strategies that increase muscle mass and glycolytic capacity, and not necessarily oxidative [aerobic] competence, can improve body composition and systemic metabolism . . . Collectively, these data suggest that even modest increases in skeletal muscle mass, the growth of [fast and super fast twitch] glycolytic fibers, and modest changes in glycolytic capacity can have remarkable effects on metabolic homeostasis. They also suggest that interventions targeting skeletal muscle may directly or indirectly alter the metabolic profile of other organs affected by insulin resistance and [type 2 diabetes mellitus]. It is now evident that skeletal muscle is a key node in the powerful and complex cross-talk between metabolically active tissues . . . In view of the coordinated responses of muscle, liver, adipose tissue [fat], and the vasculature highlighted in these models, it is likely that 1) increasing skeletal muscle mass will have favorable effects on affected tissues of [type 2 diabetes mellitus] and cardiovascular disease; and 2) a network of hormonal communication exists between muscle and other metabolically important organs . . . It is now recommended that resistance training be incorporated into the exercise regimen of patients with [type 2 diabetes mellitus]. Similarly, complementary resistance training is also recommended for patients with cardiovascular disease. Although a growing body of experimental evidence suggests that resistance training improves metabolic homeostasis in a manner distinct from endurance training, our understanding of how this precisely occurs is rudimentary.

Akasaki Y, Ouchi N, Izumiya Y, Bernardo BL, LeBrasseur NK, Walsh K.
"Glycolytic fast-twitch muscle fiber restoration counters adverse age-related changes in body composition and metabolism."
Anatomical Society: Aging Cell. 2014 February.

Aging is associated with the development of insulin resistance, increased adiposity [body fat stores], and accumulation of ectopic lipid deposits in tissues and organs. Starting in mid-life there is a progressive decline in lean muscle mass associated with the preferential loss of glycolytic, fast-twitch [and super fast-twitch] myofibers . . . the loss of lean muscle mass is a significant contributor to the development of age-related metabolic dysfunction and interventions that preserve or restore fast/glycolytic muscle may delay the onset of metabolic disease.

Wang Y, Pessin JE.
"Mechanisms for fiber-type specificity of skeletal muscle atrophy."
Current Opinions in Clinical Nutrition and Metabolic Care. 2013 May. Review.

Fast-twitch glycolytic fibers are more vulnerable than slow-twitch oxidative fibers under a variety of atrophic conditions . . . nutrient-related atrophy such as cancer/aging cachexia, sepsis, and diabetes are more directed to [fast and super fast twitch] glycolytic fiber wasting.

2. Sanchis-Gomar F, Pérez LM, Joyner MJ, Löllgen H, Lucia A.
"Endurance Exercise and the Heart: Friend or Foe?"
Sports Medicine. 2016 April. Epub 2015 November.

Although low- to moderate-intensity exercise has well-known cardiovascular benefits, it has been increasingly suggested that prolonged strenuous endurance exercise (SEE) could have potential deleterious cardiac effects. In effect, the term "cardiac overuse injury" (or "over-exercise") has been recently reported to group all the possible deleterious cardiac consequences of repeated exposure to SEE or "over-exercise".

Park A.
"When Exercise Does More Harm than Good,"
Time Magazine, 2015. Retrieved from http://time.com/3692668/when-exercise-does-more-harm-than-good/ Accessed June 22, 2016.

In a 2015 report published in the Journal of the American College of Cardiology, researchers say that "those who ran at a fast pace more than four hours a week for more than three days a week had about the same risk of dying during the study's 12-year follow up as those who were sedentary and hardly exercised at all.

Knapik JJ.
"Extreme Conditioning Programs: Potential Benefits and Potential Risks."
Journal of Special Operations Medicine. 2015, Fall.

Several cases of rhabdomyolysis and cervical carotid artery dissections have been reported during CrossFit training.

3. **Koehne K.**
A New "Threat to the Nursing Workforce: Take a Stand!"
Creative Nursing. 2015; Volume 21, Number 4, pp. 234-241(8).

The consequences of a sedentary lifestyle have been extensively studied, and the findings have been broadly reported in scientific journals as well as all forms of media. The development of cancer, cardiovascular disease, metabolic syndrome, venous thromboembolism, and extensive musculoskeletal strain can all result from prolonged immobility and repetitive computer use.

Younger AM, Pettitt RW, Sexton PJ, Maass WJ, Pettitt CD.
"Acute moderate exercise does not attenuate cardiometabolic function associated with a bout of prolonged sitting."
Journal of Sports Sciences. 2016; April. Epub 2015 Jul 17.

Epidemiological studies suggest that prolonged sitting increases all-cause mortality; yet, physiological causes underpinning prolonged sitting remain elusive." "We conclude prolonged sitting may be related to decreased posterior tibial artery blood velocity. Moreover, an acute bout of moderate exercise does not seem to attenuate cardiometabolic function during prolonged sitting in healthy, young adults.

Gao Y, Cronin NJ, Pesola AJ, Finni T.
"Muscle activity patterns and spinal shrinkage in office workers using a sit-stand workstation versus a sit workstation."
Ergonomics. 2016 February. [Epub ahead of print]

This cross-sectional study compared the effects of using a sit-stand workstation to a sit workstation on muscle activity patterns and spinal shrinkage in office workers. It provides evidence that working with a sit-stand workstation can promote more light muscle activity time and less inactivity without negative effects on spinal shrinkage.

Bailey DP, Locke CD.
"Breaking up prolonged sitting with light-intensity walking improves postprandial glycemia, but breaking up sitting with standing does not."
Journal of Science in Medicine in Sport. 2015 May. Epub 2014 Mar 20.

This study suggests that interrupting sitting time with frequent brief bouts of light-intensity activity, but not standing, imparts beneficial postprandial responses that may enhance cardiometabolic health.

Restaino RM, Holwerda SW, Credeur DP, Fadel PJ, Padilla J.
"Impact of prolonged sitting on lower and upper limb micro- and macrovascular dilator function."
Experimental Physiology. 2015 July. Epub 2015 Jun 10.

Collectively, these data suggest that prolonged sitting markedly reduces lower leg micro- and macrovascular dilator function, but these impairments can be fully normalized with a short bout of walking. In contrast, upper arm microvascular reactivity is selectively impaired with prolonged sitting, and walking does not influence this effect.

Keum N, Cao Y, Oh H, Smith-Warner SA, et al.
"Sedentary behaviors and light-intensity activities in relation to colorectal cancer risk." *International Journal of Cancer.* 2015 Dec 9. [Epub ahead of print]

We found that prolonged sitting time watching TV was associated with an increased colorectal cancer risk in women but not in men.

Pines A.
"Sedentary women: sit less, live more!"
Climacteric: The Journal of the International Menopause Society. (2015 December.)

Data on the ill effects of sedentarism keep on increasing, clearly showing a significant adverse impact and increased risk for cardiovascular disease, cancer, fracture and various overweight-related metabolic conditions. The simple fact that prolonged sitting is associated with a shorter life span must be repeatedly discussed with our patients.

4. **President's Council on Fitness, Sports & Nutrition.**
"Facts and Statistics,"
Fitness.gov. (2016, March). Retrieved from http://www.fitness.gov/resource-center/facts-and-statistics/. Accessed June 22, 2016.

5. **Running USA.**
"2014 State of the Sport - Part II: Running Industry Report."
RunningUSA.org. (2014, June 15). Retrieved from http://www.runningusa.org/2014-running-industry-report. Accessed June 22, 2016.

Statistica.
"Number of joggers/runners: Number of people who went jogging or running within the last 12 months in the United States (USA) from spring 2008 to spring 2015 (in millions)." *Statistica.com* (2015). Retrieved from http://www.statista.com/statistics/227423/number-of-joggers-and-runners-usa/. Accessed February 28, 2016.

6. **National Sporting Goods Association.**
"A statistical study of retail purchases in 2013 for representative categories of sporting goods." *NSGA Sorting Goods Market 2014 Edition,* (2014)

7. **Schnohr P, O'Keefe JH, Marott JL, Lange P, Jensen GB.**
"Dose of jogging and long-term mortality: the Copenhagen City Heart Study" *Journal of the American College of Cardiology.* 2015.

Strenuous joggers have a mortality rate not statistically different from that of the sedentary group.

8. **Park A.**
"When Exercise Does More Harm than Good,"
Time Magazine, 2015. Retrieved from http://time.com/3692668/when-exercise-does-more-harm-than-good/ Accessed June 22, 2016.

In a 2015 report published in the Journal of the American College of Cardiology, researchers say that "those who ran at a fast pace more than four hours a week for more than three days a week had about the same risk of dying during the study's 12-year follow up as those who were sedentary and hardly exercised at all. The link held even after the researchers accounted for potentially confounding factors such as age, sex, whether the participants had a history of heart disease or diabetes, or whether they smoked and drank alcohol . . . What [co-author, researcher Jacob] Marrot and his team found was that both too little running and too much running are linked to higher rates of death. The most intense runners ended up with a risk of dying that was similar to that of those who opted to stay on the couch"... That dovetails with the mounting research that so-called micro-workouts—high-intensity but brief workouts that could be as short at 1 minute, according to another recent paper -- may be better for the body than long and continuous workouts.

9. **McGuff D, Little J.**
Body by Science: A Research Based Program for Strength Training, Bodybuilding, *and Complete Fitness in 12 Minutes a Week.* New York: McGraw-Hill, 2009. Print. p. 6.

The scientific literature is filled with data that strongly make the case that long-distance runners are much more likely to develop cardiovascular disease, atrial fibrillation, cancer, liver and gallbladder disorders, muscle damage, kidney dysfunction (renal abnormalities), acute microthrombosis in the vascular system, brain damage, spinal degeneration, and germ-cell cancers than are their less active counterparts.

10. **Patil HR, O'Keefe JH, Lavie CJ, Magalski A, Vogel RA, McCullough PA.**
"Cardiovascular damage resulting from chronic excessive **endurance** exercise." *Modern Medicine.* 2012 July. Review.

Chronic, excessive sustained endurance exercise may cause adverse structural remodeling of the heart and large arteries . . . In veteran extreme endurance athletes, this recurrent myocardial injury and repair may eventually result in patchy myocardial fibrosis, particularly in the atria, interventricular septum and right ventricle, potentially creating a substrate for atrial and ventricular arrhythmias. Furthermore, chronic, excessive, sustained, high-intensity endurance exercise may be associated with diastolic dysfunction, large-artery wall stiffening and coronary artery calcification.

11. **Lavie CJ, O'Keefe JH, Sallis RE.**
"Exercise and the heart--the harm of too little and too much."
Current Sports Medicine Reports. 2015 March. Review.
Very high doses of exercise may be associated with increased risk of atrial fibrillation, coronary artery disease, and malignant ventricular arrhythmias. These acute bouts of excessive exercise may lead to cardiac dilatation, cardiac dysfunction, and release of troponin and brain natriuretic peptide.

12. **Gaudreault V, Tizon-Marcos H, Poirier P, et al.**
"Transient myocardial tissue and function changes during a marathon in less fit marathon runners."
The Canadian Journal of Cardiology. 2013 October. Epub 2013 Jul 30.
Completing a marathon leads to localized myocardial edema, diminished perfusion, and decreased function occurring more extensively in less trained and fit runners. Although reversible, these changes might contribute to the transient increase in cardiac risk reported during sustained vigorous exercise.

13. **Wilson M, O'Hanlon R, Prasad S, Basavarajaiah S, Stephens N, et al.**
"Myocardial fibrosis in an veteran endurance athlete."
Journal of Applied Physiology. 2011.
An unexpectedly high prevalence of myocardial fibrosis (50%) was observed in healthy, asymptomatic, lifelong veteran male [endurance] athletes, compared with zero cases in age-matched veteran controls and young athletes. These data suggest a link between lifelong endurance exercise and myocardial fibrosis that requires further investigation… Cardiovascular MRI demonstrated a pattern of late gadolinium enhancement, which indicated myocardial scarring as a result of previous myocarditis. Myocarditis is a non-ischaemic inflammatory disease of the myocardium associated with cardiac dysfunction and arrhythmogenic substrate. The clinical course of viral myocarditis is mostly insidious with limited cardiac inflammation and dysfunction.

Seidl J, Asplund CA.
"Effects of excessive endurance activity on the heart."
Current Sports Medicine Report. 2014 November.
Excess endurance activity may appear to increase the risk of cardiac abnormalities, which may increase the risk for long-term morbidity or mortality.

Eijsvogels TM, Fernandez AB, Thompson PD.
"Are There Deleterious Cardiac Effects of Acute and Chronic Endurance Exercise?"
Physiology Review. 2016 January. Review.
Recent reports suggest that prodigious amounts of exercise may increase markers for, and even the incidence of, cardiovascular disease. This review examines the

evidence that extremes of endurance exercise may increase cardiovascular disease risk by reviewing the causes and incidence of exercise-related cardiac events, and the acute effects of exercise on cardiovascular function, the effect of exercise on cardiac biomarkers, including "myocardial" creatine kinase, cardiac troponins, and cardiac natriuretic peptides . . . it is possible that prolonged exercise and exercise training can adversely affect cardiac function in some individuals.

Sanchis-Gomar F, Pérez LM, Joyner MJ, Löllgen H, Lucia A.
"Endurance Exercise and the Heart: Friend or Foe?"
Sports Medicine. 2016 Nov 19. [Epub ahead of print]

It has been increasingly suggested that prolonged strenuous endurance exercise could have potential deleterious cardiac effects. In effect, the term "cardiac overuse injury" (or "over-exercise") has been recently reported to group all the possible deleterious cardiac consequences of repeated exposure to strenuous endurance exercise or "over-exercise".

Sanchis-Gomar F, Santos-Lozano A, Garatachea N, et al.
"My patient wants to perform strenuous endurance exercise. What's the right advice?"
International Journal of Cardiology. 2015 Oct 15;197:248-53. Epub 2015 Jun 15. Review.

Prolonged strenuous endurance exercise such as marathon running has recently been associated with potential deleterious cardiac effects, particularly increased risk of atrial fibrillation. This topic is medically important due to the increasing number of participants in strenuous endurance exercise events lasting several hours, including older people.

Doutreleau S, Pistea C, Lonsdorfer E, Charloux A.
"Exercise-induced second-degree atrioventricular block in endurance athletes."
Medicine and Science in Sports and Exercise. 2013 March.

Heart rhythm disorders, such as atrial arrhythmia (including atrial fibrillation and atrial flutter), are a well-established consequence of such long-term endurance practice.

DeMarco VG, Johnson MS, Ma L, et al.
"Overweight female rats selectively bred for low aerobic capacity exhibit increased myocardial fibrosis and diastolic dysfunction."
American Journal of Physiology. Heart Circulatory Physiology. 2012 Apr 15. Epub 2012 Feb 17.

The statistical association between endurance exercise capacity and cardiovascular disease suggests that impaired aerobic metabolism underlies the cardiovascular disease risk in men and women . . . Thus, the combination of risk factors, including female sex, intrinsic low aerobic capacity, and overweightness, promote myocardial stiffness/fibrosis sufficient to induce diastolic dysfunction in the absence of hypertension and left ventricular hypertrophy.

14. **Merghani A, Malhotra A, Sharma S.**
"The U-shaped relationship between exercise and cardiac morbidity."
Trends Cardiovascular Medicine. 2015 Jun 18. [Epub ahead of print] Review.
In the current era, most athletes engage in a volume and intensity of exercise that is at least 5-10-fold greater than the general recommendations for physical activity... Occasionally, however, intense exercise is associated with sudden deaths in athletes harboring quiescent yet potentially sinister cardiac diseases. More recently, there have been an emerging number of reports suggesting that intense [endurance] exercise may have an adverse impact on an otherwise normal heart.

15. **Ozanian, Mike.**
"How *CrossFit* Became A $4 Billion Brand."
Forbes.com / SportsMoney. (2015, February 25).Retrieved from http://www.forbes.com/sites/mikeozanian/2015/02/25/how-*CrossFit*-became-a-4-billion-brand/#2a64742478c1. Accessed February 28, 2016.

16. **Cooperman, Stephanie.**
"Getting Fit, Even if it Kills You."
New York Times | PHYSICAL CULTURE. (2005, December).Retrieved from http://www.nytimes.com/2005/12/22/fashion/thursdaystyles/getting-fit-even-if-it-kills-you.html?_r=0.
After 30 minutes, Mr. Anderson, a 38-year-old member of the [Tacoma, Washington S.W.A.T. team], left the [CrossFit] gym with his muscles sapped and [excruciating back pain] . . .That night he went to the emergency room, where doctors told him he had rhabdomyolysis, which is caused when muscle fiber breaks down and is released into the bloodstream, poisoning the kidneys. He spent six days in intensive care . . . [Greg Glassman], CrossFit's founder, does not discount his regimen's risks, even to those who are in shape and take the time to warm up their bodies before a session. "It can kill you," he said. "I've always been completely honest about that."

17. **Hak PT, Hodzovic E, Hickey B.**
"The nature and prevalence of injury during *CrossFit* training."
Journal of Strength and Conditioning Research. 2013 Nov 22. [Epub ahead of print]
A total of 132 responses were collected with 97 (73.5%) having sustained an injury during CrossFit training. A total of 186 injuries were reported with 9 (7.0%) requiring surgical intervention . . . Injury rates with CrossFit training are similar to that reported in the literature for sports such as Olympic weight-lifting, power-lifting and gymnastics and lower than competitive contact sports such as rugby union and rugby league. Shoulder and spine injuries predominate with no incidences of rhabdomyolysis obtained.

18. Helm B.
"Too Much Pain for *CrossFit* Gains?"
MensJournal.com: Health & Fitness.(2014, March). Retrieved from http://www.mensjournal.com/health-fitness/exercise/too-much-pain-for-*CrossFit*-gains-20140326. Accessed February 28, 2016.

Yuri Feito, a professor of exercise science at Kennesaw State University in Georgia (and a CrossFitter himself), analyzed data from 737 CrossFit participants and found that 51 percent had experienced an injury in the year prior – from minor sprains to muscle tears to broken fingers. Of those, 10 to 15 percent warranted a trip to the hospital.

19. Knapik JJ.
"Extreme Conditioning Programs: Potential Benefits and Potential Risks."
Journal of Special Operations Medicine. 2015, Fall.

Several cases of rhabdomyolysis and cervical carotid artery dissections have been reported during CrossFit training.

20. Glassman, Greg. (Founder of *CrossFit*)
"*CrossFit* Induced Rhabdo"
CrossFit Journal Articles, Issue 38. (2005, October). Retrieved from http://library.*CrossFit*.com/free/pdf/38_05_cf_rhabdo.pdf. Accessed June 27, 2016.

With CrossFit we are dealing with what is known as exertional rhabdomyolysis. It can disable, maim, and even kill. To date we have seen five cases of exertional rhabdo associated with CrossFit workouts. Each case resulted in the hospitalization of the afflicted... The rhabdo we've seen has come from sessions of twenty minutes or less, with mild or low temperature and humidity. The victims were not excessively panting, straining, grunting, or otherwise expressing abnormal discomfort from the workouts. The athletes who came down with rhabdo turned in marginal CrossFit performances and showed no signs of discomfort that were out of the ordinary. They left their workouts seemingly no worse off than anyone else.

21. ESPN and The American Sports Network
"American Muscle: The LifeQuest Triple Crown."
ESPN's American Muscle Magazine. [Video]. YouTube. https://www.youtube.com/watch?v=B842jIVFcMM. Published May 22, 2010. Accessed June 22, 2016.

22. Caparas W.
"Quantum Leap: The Future of Women's Fitness Sports"
Oxygen Magazine. (2000, January)

23. American Heart Association
"Strength and Resistance Training Exercise"
Heart.org: Healthy Living. (2015, March).Retrieved from http://www.heart.org/HEARTORG/HealthyLiving/PhysicalActivity/FitnessBasics/

Strength-and-Resistance-Training-Exercise_UCM_462357_Article.jsp#.WNfz9PkrLcs. Accessed February 28, 2016.

A well-rounded strength-training program provides the following benefits: Increased strength of bones, muscles and connective tissues (tendons and ligaments); Lower risk of injury; Increased muscle mass, which makes it easier for your body to burn calories and thus maintain a healthy weight; Better quality of life.

24. **American Heart Association**
"Tips to Improve Your Workout Routine"
Heart.org. (2016, February). Retrieved from https://www.goredforwomen.org/live-healthy/heart-healthy-exercises/tips-to-improve-your-workout-routine/. Accessed February 28, 2016.

1. Be accountable. 2. Establish a routine. 3. Walk it off. 4. Find a moderate activity you love. 5. Find a vigorous activity you love. 6. Do strength training. 7. Try interval training. 8. Warm up and cool down.

25. **American Heart Association**
"Can Strength Training Help with Blood Pressure?"
Heart.org: Heart Insight Magazine. (2015, Winter). Retrieved from http://heartinsight.heart.org/Winter-2015/Can-Strength-Training-Help-with-Blood-Pressure/. Accessed February 28, 2016.

Studies have reported several benefits of resistance training — or weight training — including strengthening of bones, muscles and connective tissues (tendons and ligaments). Additionally, weight training may lower your risk of injury. And increased muscle mass may make it easier for you to burn calories and maintain a healthy weight. You'll feel better and stronger and want to do more . . . Researchers reported that only four weeks of [strength training] exercises resulted in a 10 percent drop in both blood pressure measures. Aerobic exercise, however, has shown evidence of reducing systolic and diastolic blood pressure by an average of 2 to 5 mm Hg and 1 to 4 mm Hg, respectively.

26. **Gibala MJ, Little JP, van Essen M, et al.**
"Short-term sprint interval versus traditional endurance training: similar initial adaptations in human skeletal muscle and exercise performance."
Journal of Physiology. 2006 September. Epub 2006 Jul 6.

27. **McGuff, Little.** p.15-16. (see note 8 for bibliography)

28. **De Luca CJ, Contessa P.**
"Hierarchical control of motor units in voluntary contractions."
Journal of Neurophysiology. 2012 January. Epub 2011 Oct 5.

This hierarchical control scheme describes a mechanism that provides an effective economy of force generation for the earlier-recruited lower force-twitch motor units, and reduces the fatigue of later-recruited higher force-twitch motor units--both characteristics being well suited for generating and sustaining force during the fight-or-flight response.

29. **Andersen JL, Aagaard P.**
"Effects of strength training on muscle fiber types and size; consequences for athletes training for high-intensity sport."
*Scandinavian Journal of Medicine & Science in Sports.*2010 October. Review.

Further, aerobic exercise may fully or partially blunt the hypertrophic muscle response from concurrent resistance training

30. **Schnohr P, O'Keefe JH, Marott JL, Lange P, Jensen GB.**
"Dose of jogging and long-term mortality: the Copenhagen City Heart Study."
Journal of American College of Cardiology. 2015.

31. **Stacey P.**
"Fast-Twitch, Slow-Twitch: What's The Difference And Does It Matter?"
nasm.org: National Academy of Sports Medicine. (2015, Jan). Retrieved from: http://blog.nasm.org/fitness/fast-twitch-slow-twitch-whats-difference-matter/ Accessed February 28, 2016.

32. **Holt NC, Wakeling JM, Biewener AA.**
"The effect of fast and slow motor unit activation on whole-muscle mechanical performance: the size principle may not pose a mechanical paradox."
Proceedings, Biological Sciences, Royal Society. 2014 April.

The findings presented here suggest that recruitment according to the size principle, where slow motor units are activated first and faster ones recruited as demand increases, may not pose a mechanical paradox, as has been previously suggested.

Sale DG.
"Influence of exercise and training on motor unit activation."
Exercise and Sport Sciences Review. 1987. Review.

The recruitment order of [muscle fiber motor units] according to size is based on the inverse relation between susceptibility to discharge and motoneuron size. Thus, for evenly distributed and increasing excitatory synaptic input to a pool of motoneurons, smaller motoneurons will begin to fire before larger motoneurons. This arrangement ensures, for example, that the small, fatigue-resistant [muscle fiber motor units] will be preferentially activated in prolonged, low-intensity exercise, to which these units are most suited. In brief, intense exercise, the associated greater excitatory input will also recruit the large [muscle fiber motor units], taking advantage of their greater strength and contractile speed. A frequent question is whether rapid, ballistic or explosive contractions and movements are associated with selective or preferential recruitment of large, fast twitch [muscle fiber motor units]. There is evidence of synaptic input systems that preferentially excite large, fast twitch [muscle fiber motor units] and inhibit small twitch [muscle fiber motor units]; however, the majority of evidence from human experiments indicates that the recruitment order is not reversed in ballistic contractions.

33. De Luca CJ, Contessa P.

34. Kesidis N, Metaxas TI, Vrabas IS, et. al.

"Myosin heavy chain isoform distribution in single fibres of bodybuilders."

European Journal of Applied Physiology. 2008 July.

The percentage of fibres expressing [fast twitch and slow/fast twitch] was larger in bodybuilders ($P < 0.05$), while [super fast twitch fibre expression] was completely absent ($P < 0.05$).

35. Nilwik R, Snijders T, Leenders M, et al.

"The decline in skeletal muscle mass with aging is mainly attributed to a reduction in type II muscle fiber size."

Experimental Gerontology. 2013 May.

Reduced muscle mass with aging is mainly attributed to smaller type II [fast and super fast twitch] muscle fiber size . . . the increase in muscle mass following prolonged resistance type exercise training can be attributed entirely to specific type II [fast and super fast twitch] muscle fiber hypertrophy.

Paillard T.

"Neuromuscular system and aging: involutions and implications."

Geriatr. Psychol. and Neuropsychiatr.Vieil. 2013 December. Review. French.

In aged humans, the number of muscle fibers and motor units decreases. The remaining motor units lose their functionality (decrease of the discharge frequency, greater fluctuation of the discharge) particularly those which contain type II [fast and super fast twitch] fibers . . . strength training counteracts the noxious effects mentioned above by generating muscular hypertrophy *thanks to a reactive increase in the production of anabolic hormones.*

36. Pearson SJ, Young A, Macaluso A, et al.

"Muscle function in elite master weightlifters."

Journal of Medicine & Science in Sports & Exercise. 2002 July.

The absolute differences between the weightlifters and [non-trained healthy controls] were such that an 85-yr-old weightlifter was as powerful as a 65-yr-old control subject. This would therefore represent an apparent age advantage of approximately 20 yr for the weightlifters.

37. LeBrasseur NK, Walsh K, Arany Z.

"Metabolic benefits of resistance training and fast glycolytic skeletal muscle."

American Journal of Physiology, Endocrinology and Metabolism. 2011 January. Epub 2010 Nov 2. Review.

Collectively, these data suggest that even modest increases in skeletal muscle mass, the growth of [fast and super fast twitch] glycolytic fibers and modest changes in glycolytic capacity can have remarkable effects on metabolic homeostasis. They also suggest that interventions targeting skeletal muscle may directly or indirectly alter the metabolic profile of other organs affected by insulin resistance and [type 2 diabetes]. It is now evident that skeletal muscle is a key node in the powerful and complex cross-talk between metabolically active tissues . . . In view of the coordinated responses of muscle, liver, adipose tissue [body fat], and the vasculature highlighted in these models, it is likely that 1) increasing skeletal muscle mass will have favorable effects on affected tissues of [type 2 diabetes] and cardiovascular disease; and 2) a network of hormonal communication exists between muscle and other metabolically important organs . . . Although a growing body of experimental evidence suggests that resistance training improves metabolic homeostasis in a manner distinct from endurance training, our understanding of how this precisely occurs is rudimentary.

38. McCaulley GO, McBride JM, Cormie P, et al.
"Acute hormonal and neuromuscular responses to hypertrophy, strength and power type resistance exercise."
European Journal of Applied Physiology. 2009 March. Epub 2008 Dec 9.

These data indicate that significant acute increases in hormone concentrations are limited to hypertrophy *type protocols [i.e. 4 sets of 10 repetitions at 75% of max] independent of the volume of work completed. In addition, it appears the* hypertrophy *protocol also elicits a unique pattern of muscle activity as well. Resistance exercise protocols of varying intensity and rest periods elicit strikingly different acute neuroendocrine responses which indicate a unique physiological stimulus.*

39. Gordon SE, Kraemer WJ, Looney DP, Flanagan SD, Comstock BA, Hymer WC.
"The influence of age and exercise modality on growth hormone bioactivity in women."
Growth Hormone and IGF Research. 2014 April.

The greater [bioactive growth hormone] response to the heavy resistance exercise protocol found in the younger group can be attributed to an unknown serum factor . . . that either potentiated growth hormone bioactivity in response to heavy resistance exercise or inhibited growth hormone bioactivity in response to aerobic exercise.

40. Walker S, Santolamazza F, Kraemer W, Häkkinen K.
"Effects of prolonged hypertrophic resistance training on acute endocrine responses in young and older men."
Journal of Aging and Physical Activity. 2015 April.

The present study investigated changes in acute serum hormone responses to a resistance exercise bout following [twenty weeks] of hypertrophic resistance training in young and older men . . . in general, young men demonstrate greater adaptability within the endocrine system compared with older men. However, adaptability in growth hormone response was associated with larger training-induced gains independent of age.

41. Wahl P, Zinner C, Achtzehn S, Bloch W, Mester J.
"Effect of high- and low-intensity exercise and metabolic acidosis on levels of GH, IGF-I, IGFBP-3 and cortisol."
Journal of the Growth Hormone Research Society. 2010 October. Epub 2010 Aug 30.
Serum cortisol and human growth hormone concentrations were significantly increased 10 min post exercise in High-intensity Training interventions. High-volume Endurance Training showed no significant effects on cortisol, human growth hormone, insulin-like growth factor-1, and Insulin-like growth factor-binding protein-3 levels.

42. Akasaki Y, Ouchi N, Izumiya Y, Bernardo BL, Lebrasseur NK, Walsh K.
'Glycolytic fast-twitch muscle fiber restoration counters adverse age-related changes in body composition and metabolism."
Anatomical Society: Aging Cell. 2014 February.
Aging is associated with the development of insulin resistance, increased adiposity [body fat stores], and accumulation of ectopic lipid deposits in tissues and organs. Starting in mid-life there is a progressive decline in lean muscle mass associated with the preferential loss of glycolytic, fast-twitch [and super fast-twitch] myofibers . . . the loss of lean muscle mass is a significant contributor to the development of age-related metabolic dysfunction and interventions that preserve or restore fast/glycolytic muscle may delay the onset of metabolic disease.

Wang Y, Pessin JE.
"Mechanisms for fiber-type specificity of skeletal muscle atrophy."
Current Opinions in Clinical Nutrition and Metabolic Care. 2013 May. Review.
Fast-twitch glycolytic fibers are more vulnerable than slow-twitch oxidative fibers under a variety of atrophic conditions . . . nutrient-related atrophy such as cancer/aging cachexia, sepsis, and diabetes are more directed to [fast and super fast twitch] glycolytic fiber wasting.

43. Shefer G, Van de Mark DP, Richardson JB, Yablonka-Reuveni Z.
"Satellite-cell pool size does matter: defining the myogenic potency of aging skeletal muscle." *Developmental Biology.* 2006 June. Epub 2006 Mar 22.
The study establishes that abundance of resident satellite cells declines with age in myofibers from both fast- and slow-twitch muscles. Nevertheless, the inherent myogenic potential of satellite cells does not diminish with age . . . Altogether, satellite cell abundance, but not myogenic potential, deteriorates with age.

Bruusgaard JC, Johansen IB, Egner IM, Rana ZA, Gundersen K.
"Myonuclei acquired by overload exercise precede hypertrophy and are not lost on detraining."
The National Academy of Sciences. 2010 August. Epub 2010 Aug 16.
The old and newly acquired nuclei are retained during severe atrophy caused by subsequent denervation lasting for a considerable period of the animal's lifespan. The myonuclei seem to be protected from the high apoptotic activity found in

inactive muscle tissue. A hypertrophy *episode leading to a lasting elevated number of myonuclei retarded disuse atrophy, and the nuclei could serve as a cell biological substrate for such memory. Because the ability to create myonuclei is impaired in the elderly, individuals may benefit from strength training at an early age.*

44. **Relaix F, Zammit PS.**
"Satellite cells are essential for skeletal muscle regeneration: the cell on the edge returns centre stage".
Development. 2012 August. Review.
The clear consensus is that skeletal muscle does not regenerate without satellite cells, confirming their pivotal and non-redundant role.

45. **Gundersen K.**
"Muscle memory and a new cellular model for muscle atrophy and hypertrophy."
Journal of Experimental Biology. 2016 January. Review.
Fibres that have acquired a higher number of myonuclei grow faster when subjected to overload exercise, thus the nuclei represent a functionally important "memory" of previous strength. This memory might be very long lasting in humans, as myonuclei are stable for at least 15 years and might even be permanent. However, myonuclei are harder to recruit in the elderly, and if the long-lasting muscle memory also exists in humans, one should consider early strength training as a public health advice.

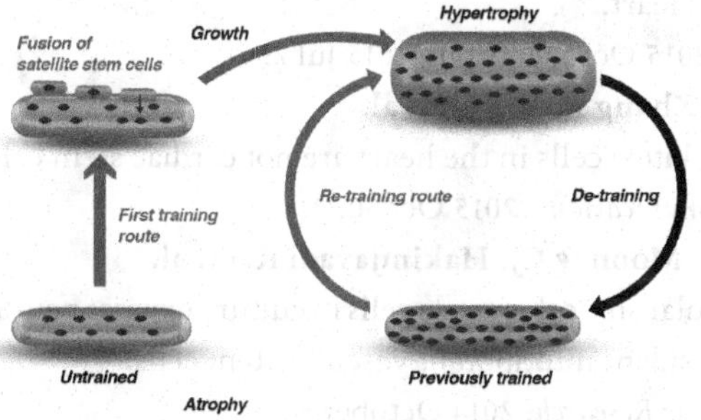

Figure 1: Gundersen's satellite stem cell fusion and muscle memory diagram (reproduction)

46. Ibid.

47. **Verdijk LB, Snijders T, Drost M, Delhaas T, Kadi F, van Loon LJ.**
"Satellite cells in human skeletal muscle; from birth to old age."
Age (Dordr). 2014 April.
Changes in satellite cell content play a key role in regulating skeletal muscle growth and atrophy . . . From birth to adulthood, muscle fiber size increased tremendously

with no major changes in muscle fiber satellite cell content, and no differences between [slow twitch and fast/super fast twitch] fibers. In contrast to [slow twitch] muscle fibers, [fast and super fast twitch] muscle fiber size was substantially smaller with increasing age in adults . . . This was accompanied by an age-related reduction in [fast and super fast twitch] muscle fiber satellite cell content . . . Twelve weeks of resistance-type exercise training significantly increased [fast and super fast twitch] muscle fiber size and satellite cell content. We conclude that [fast and super fast] muscle fiber atrophy with aging is accompanied by a specific decline in [fast and super fast twitch] muscle fiber satellite cell content. Resistance-type exercise training represents an effective strategy to increase satellite cell content and reverse [fast and super fast twitch] muscle fiber atrophy.

48. Ibid.

49. Ibid.

50. **Beltrami AP, Barlucchi L, Torella D, et. al.**
"Adult cardiac stem cells are multipotent and support myocardial regeneration."
Cell. 2003 Sep 19.

51. **Patsch C, Challet-Meylan L, Thoma EC, et.al.**
"Generation of vascular endothelial and smooth muscle cells from human pluripotent stem cells."
Nature Cell Biology. 2015 August. Epub 2015 Jul 27.
Zhang Y, Sivakumaran P, Newcomb AE, et. al.
"Cardiac Repair With a Novel Population of Mesenchymal Stem Cells Resident in the HumanHeart."
Stem Cells. 2015 October. Epub 2015 Jul 29.
Sultana N, Zhang L, Yan J, et. al.
"Resident c-kit(+) cells in the heart are not cardiac stem cells."
Nature Communications. 2015 Oct 30.
Kennedy E, Mooney CJ, Hakimjavadi R, et. al.
"Adult vascular smooth muscle cells in culture express neural stem cell markers typical of resident multipotent vascular stem cells."
Cell and Tissue Research. 2014 October.

52. **Anderson CH.**
"8 Reasons Why [Women] Should Lift Heavier Weights... And no, you will not "bulk up!""
Shape Magazine / Fitness / Workouts. (2012) Retrieved from http://www.shape.com/fitness/workouts/8-reasons-why-you-should-lift-heavier-weights. Accessed February 28, 2016.

You may have been told that cardio is the ultimate fat burner, but that effect stops the minute you hop off the treadmill. Build more muscle and you'll keep your body burning fat all day long. According to one study, adding just two sessions per week of heavy lifting can reduce your body fat by three percent without cutting calories.

Another study from the University of Alabama in Birmingham showed that dieters who lifted heavy weights lost the same amount of weight as dieters who did just card, but all the weight lost by the weight lifters was primarily fat while the cardio queens lost a lot of muscle along with some fat. And more muscle, less fat translated to smaller clothing sizes than their less muscular counterparts.

Hunter GR, Byrne NM, Sirikul B, et al.

"Resistance training conserves fat-free mass and resting energy expenditure following weight loss."

Obesity (Silver Spring). 2008 May. Epub 2008 Mar 6.

Following weight loss in both African American and European American, resistance training conserved fat-free mass, resting energy expenditure, and strength fitness when compared to women who aerobic trained or did not train.

Cullinen K, Caldwell M.

"Weight training increases fat-free mass and strength in untrained young women." *Journal of the American Dietetic Association.* 1998 April. *A moderate-intensity weight training program increased strength and fat-free mass and decreased body fat in normal-weight young women. Favorable changes in body composition were obtained without restricting food intake.*

Opitz D, Lenzen E, Schiffer T, et. al.

"Endurance training alters skeletal muscle MCT contents in T2DM men." *International Journal of Sports Medicine.* 2014 December.

53. Vaara JP, Kokko J, Isoranta M, Kyröläinen H.

"Effects of Added Resistance Training on Physical Fitness, Body Composition, and Serum Hormone Concentrations During Eight Weeks of Special Military Training Period."

Journal of Strength and Conditioning Research. 2015 November.

In conclusion, interference with strength gains might be related to the high-volume of aerobic activities and too low volume of resistance training during strength training. To develop strength characteristics, careful periodization and individualization should be adopted in strength training.

Hagerman FC, Walsh SJ, Staron RS, et al.

"Effects of high-intensity resistance training on untrained older men. I. Strength, cardiovascular, and metabolic responses."

The Journals of Gerontology, Series A, Biological Science and Medical Science. 2000 July.

The results show that skeletal muscle in older, untrained men will respond with significant strength gains accompanied by considerable increases in fiber size and capillary density. Maximal working capacity, VO2max, and serum lipid profiles also benefited from high-intensity resistance training... Older men may not only tolerate very high-intensity workloads but will exhibit intramuscular, cardiovascular, and metabolic changes similar to younger subjects.

54. Fell J.
"Why lifting weights is better than cardio if you're trying to lose fat."
FoxNews.com: Health. (2015, April) Retrieved from http://www.foxnews.com/health/2015/04/21/why-lifting-weights-is-better-than-cardio-if-youre-trying-to-lose-fat.html. Accessed February 28. 2016

It takes about 2,500 calories to build a pound of muscle, whereas you need to burn 3,500 calories to lose a pound of fat. What this means is that for every pound of muscle you build, that's 2,500 calories worth of eating that you didn't have to worry about in terms of your overall energy balance equation for losing fat.

55. Kliszczewicz B, Quindry CJ, Blessing LD, Oliver DG, Esco RM, Taylor JK.
"Acute Exercise and Oxidative Stress: *CrossFit*(™) vs. Treadmill Bout."
Journal of Human Kinetics. 2015. eCollection 2015 Sep 29.

Based on these findings, we interpret the oxidative stress outcomes of the current study to indicate that when closely matched for exercise time and intensity, the CrossFit™ bout "Cindy" produces a similar physiological stress response to a running modality.

56. Goertzen M, Schöppe K, Lange G, Schulitz KP.
"[Injuries and damage caused by excess stress in bodybuilding and powerlifting]."
Sportverletz Sportschaden.1989 March. German.

The upper extremity, particularly the shoulder and elbow joint, showed the highest injury rate. More than 40% of all injuries occurred in this area. The low back region and the knee were other sites of elevated injury occurrences. Muscular injuries (muscle pulls, tendonitis, sprains) were perceived to account for 83.6% of all injury types. Powerlifting showed a twice as high injury rate as bodybuilding, probably of grounds of a more uniform training program.

Sparto PJ, Parnianpour M, Reinsel TE, Simon S.
"The effect of fatigue on multijoint kinematics and load sharing during a repetitive lifting test."
Spine (Phila Pa). 1997.

The significant decrease in postural stability and force generation capability because of the repetitive lifting task indicated a higher risk of injury in the presence of unexpected perturbation.

König M, Biener K.
"Sport-specific injuries in weight lifting."
Schweiz Z Sportmed. 1990 April. German.

From the remaining 68%, 202 instances of injuries related to weight lifting were reported. They affected the knees (25%), scapular girdle (22%), back (21%), wrist (12%) and the elbows (6%). In about 10% of the known cases of knee injury, the rest period without any sports activity lasted more than 28 days. More often than not, it was due to degenerative processes of the joint.

Siewe J, Rudat J, Röllinghoff M, Schlegel UJ, Eysel P, Michael JW.
"Weight training-related injuries in the high school athlete."
American Journal of Sports Medicine. 1982 January.

In 37 of the 80 athletes, it was difficult to pinpoint the cause of injury since the history revealed, in addition to weight training, either a program of running excessive mileage or participation in repetitive lap running in the gymnasium. The injuries of the remaining 43 athletes had a direct causal relationship to the weight training program. Twenty-nine developed lumbosacral pain. Seven of the 29 were hospitalized, and four required surgical treatment. Anterior iliac spine avulsion occurred in six cases, and laceration of the knee meniscus occurred as an initial injury in four athletes who required surgery. Four athletes developed a cervical sprain.

57. **Kesidis N, Metaxas TI, Vrabas IS, et al.**
"Myosin heavy chain isoform distribution in single fibres of bodybuilders."
European Journal of Applied Physiology. 2008 July. Epub 2008 May 7.

The percentage of fibres expressing [fast twitch and slow/fast twitch] was larger in bodybuilders ($P < 0.05$), while [super fast twitch fibre expression] was completely absent ($P < 0.05$).

58. **Cortez-Cooper MY, DeVan AE, Anton MM, et al.**
"Effects of high-intensity resistance training on arterial stiffness and wave reflection in women."
American Journal of Hypertension. 2005 July.

We concluded that a [high-intensity strength and power training program] increases arterial stiffness and wave reflection in young healthy women. Our present interventional results are consistent with the previous cross-sectional studies in men in which [high-intensity strength and power training] is associated with arterial stiffening.

59. **McCaulley GO, McBride JM, Cormie P, et al.**
"Acute hormonal and neuromuscular responses to hypertrophy, strength and power type resistance exercise."
European Journal of Applied Physiology. 2009 March. Epub 2008 Dec 9.

These data indicate that significant acute increases in hormone concentrations are limited to hypertrophy *type protocols [i.e. 4 sets of 10 repetitions at 75% of max] independent of the volume of work completed. In addition, it appears the* hypertrophy *protocol also elicits a unique pattern of muscle activity as well. Resistance exercise protocols of varying intensity and rest periods elicit strikingly different acute neuroendocrine responses which indicate a unique physiological stimulus.*

60. **Wahl P, Mathes S, Köhler K, Achtzehn S, Bloch W, Mester J.**
"Acute metabolic, hormonal, and psychological responses to different endurance training protocols."
Hormone and Metabolic Research. 2013 October. Epub 2013 Jun 21.
In conclusion, the results suggest that High-intensity [Low Volume] Training promotes anabolic processes more than High-volume Endurance Training, due to higher increases of human growth hormone, testosterone, and the testosterone/cortisol ratio. It can be speculated that the acute hormonal increase and the metabolic perturbations might play a positive role in optimizing training adaptation and in eliciting health benefits as it has been shown by previous long term training studies using similar exercise protocols.

61. **Reed ML, Merriam GR, Kargi AY.**
"Adult Growth Hormone Deficiency – Benefits, Side Effects, and Risks of Growth Hormone Replacement."
Frontiers *in Endocrinology* (Lausanne) 2013.Published online 2013 June 4.
Deficiency of growth hormone in adults results in a syndrome characterized by decreased muscle mass and exercise capacity, increased visceral fat, impaired quality of life, unfavorable alterations in lipid profile and markers of cardiovascular risk, decrease in bone mass and integrity, and increased mortality.

62. **Dunstan DW, Daly RM, Owen N, et al.**
"High-intensity resistance training improves glycemic control in older patients with type 2 diabetes."
Diabetes Care. 2002 October.
Karstoft K, Winding K, Knudsen SH, et al.
"Mechanisms behind the superior effects of interval vs continuous training on glycaemic control in individuals with type 2 diabetes: a randomised controlled trial."
Diabetologia. 2014 October.

63. **American Heart Association**
"Sugar 101"
Heart.org. Healthy Living. (2016, July). Retrieved from http://www.heart.org/HEARTORG/HealthyLiving/HealthyEating/Nutrition/Sugar-101_UCM_306024_Article.jsp#.V4UJYbgrLcs

64. **Larsson SC, Giovannucci EL, Wolk A.**
"Sweetened Beverage Consumption and Risk of Biliary Tract and Gallbladder Cancer in a Prospective Study."
Journal of the National Cancer Institute. 2016 Jun 8. Print 2016 October.
Sugar-sweetened beverage consumption raises blood glucose concentration and has been positively associated with weight gain and type 2 diabetes, all of which have been implicated in the development of biliary tract cancer . . . particularly gallbladder cancer.

65. **Melkonian SC, Daniel CR, Ye Y, Pierzynski JA, Roth JA, Wu X.**
"Glycemic Index,_Glycemic Load, and Lung Cancer Risk in Non-Hispanic Whites."
Cancer, Epidemiology, Biomarkers, & Prevention. 2016 March.

Postprandial glucose and insulin responses play a role in carcinogenesis. We evaluated the association between dietary glycemic index and glycemic load, markers of carbohydrate intake and postprandial glucose, and lung cancer risk in non-Hispanic whites . . . This study suggests that dietary glycemic index and other lung cancer risk factors may jointly and independently influence lung cancer etiology.

66. **Jiang Y, Pan Y, Rhea PR, et. al.**
"A Sucrose-Enriched Diet Promotes Tumorigenesis in Mammary Gland in Part through the 12-Lipoxygenase Pathway."
American Association of Cancer Research. 2016 January.

Epidemiologic studies have shown that dietary sugar intake has a significant impact on the development of breast cancer. One proposed mechanism for how sugar impacts cancer development involves inflammation. We determined that fructose derived from the sucrose was responsible for facilitating lung metastasis and 12-HETE production in breast tumors. Overall, our data suggested that dietary sugar induces 12-LOX signaling to increase risks of breast cancer development and metastasis.

67. **McGuff D, Little J.** p.35-40. (see note 8 for bibliography)

68. **Logan GR, Harris N, Duncan S, Plank LD, Merien F, Schofield G.**
"Low-Active Male Adolescents: A Dose Response to High-Intensity Interval Training."
Medicine and Science in Sports and Exercise. 2015 October. [Epub ahead of print]

Low-active adolescent males performing a single HIIT set twice weekly, in addition to one resistance training session, gained meaningful improvements in fitness and body composition. Performing additional HIIT sets provided no additional improvements to those of the lowest dose in this study.

69. **Di Blasio A, Izzicupo P, Tacconi L, et. al.**
"Acute and delayed effects of high-intensity interval resistance training organization on cortisol and testosterone production."
Journal of Sports Medicine and Physical Fitness. 2014 November. [Epub ahead of print]

In order to offer a more complete training, resistance exercises have been added to HIIT (HIIRT [high-intensity interval resistance training]) . . . Even if exercises, load, and number of repetitions were maintained fixed, exercise order, structured recovery and speed of execution determined different acute and prolonged effects.

70. Liou K, Ho S, Fildes J, Ooi SY.
"High-intensity Interval versus Moderate Intensity Continuous Training in Patients with Coronary Artery Disease: A Meta-analysis of Physiological and Clinical Parameters."
Journal of Heart and Lung Circulation. 2016 Feb.

High-intensity interval training improves the mean VO2peak in patients with Coronary Artery Disease more than moderate intensity continuous training

71. McGuff D, Little J. p.17. (see note 8 for bibliography)

Your heart and lungs cannot tell whether you're working your muscles intensely for thirty seconds on a stationary bike or working them intensely on a leg press. The heart and lungs know only about energy requirements, which they dutifully attempt to meet. Four thirty-second intervals of high-intensity muscular exertion is four thirty-second intervals of high-intensity muscular exertion, whether that takes place exclusively in the lower body, as in stationary cycling, or in both the upper and lower body, as in resistance exercise. In either scenario, it is mechanical work by muscles that is the passkey to the aerobic and other metabolic machinery within the body's cells.

72. American Heart Association
"Can Strength Training Help with Blood Pressure?"
Heart.org, Heart Insight Magazine. (2015, Winter). Retrieved from http://heartinsight.heart.org/Winter-2015/Can-Strength-Training-Help-with-Blood-Pressure/. Accessed February 28, 2016.

Studies have reported several benefits of resistance training — or weight training — including strengthening of bones, muscles and connective tissues (tendons and ligaments). Additionally, weight training may lower your risk of injury. And increased muscle mass may make it easier for you to burn calories and maintain a healthy weight. You'll feel better and stronger and want to do more . . . Researchers reported that only four weeks of [strength training] exercises resulted in a 10 percent drop in both blood pressure measures. Aerobic exercise, however, has shown evidence of reducing systolic and diastolic blood pressure by an average of 2 to 5 mm Hg and 1 to 4 mm Hg, respectively.

73. Andersen JL, Aagaard P.
"Effects of strength training on muscle fiber types and size; consequences for athletes training for high-intensity sport."
*Scandinavian Journal of Medicine & Science in Sports.*2010 October. Review.

74. Ibid.

75. Gundersen K.
"Muscle memory and a new cellular model for muscle atrophy and hypertrophy."
Journal of Experimental Biology. 2016 January. Review.

Fibres that have acquired a higher number of myonuclei grow faster when subjected to overload exercise, thus the nuclei represent a functionally important "memory" of previous strength. This memory might be very long lasting in humans, as myonuclei are stable for at least 15 years and might even be permanent. However, myonuclei are harder to recruit in the elderly, and if the long-lasting muscle memory also exists in humans, one should consider early strength training as a public health advice.

76. American Heart Association
"Weight Training After a Stroke"
StrokeAssociation.org. Life After Stroke. (2014, January). Retrieved from http://www.strokeassociation.org/STROKEORG/LifeAfterStroke/RegainingIndependence/PhysicalChallenges/Weight-Training-After-Stroke_UCM_309780_Article.jsp#.VrT6KfkrLcs. Accessed February 28, 2016.
Many healthcare professionals are concerned that resistance training can have a detrimental effect on spastic muscles. A recent review of the professional literature found no scientific evidence to back up that position. In fact, in a recent article in NeuroRehabilitation, investigators determined that targeted strength training in patients with muscle weakness due to strokes significantly increased muscle power without any negative effects on spasticity.

77. O'Connor P, Herring M, Caravalho A.
"Mental Health Benefits of Strength Training in Adults"
American Journal of Lifestyle Medicine (2010, May). Retrieved from http://ajl.sagepub.com/content/4/5/377.abstract, Accessed July 23, 2016.

78. Ramirez A, Kravitz L.
"Resistance Training Improves Mental Health"
University of New Mexico, UNM.edu. (2010) Retrieved from https://www.unm.edu/~lkravitz/Article%20folder/RTandMentalHealth.html. Accessed February 28, 2016.
Silva BA, Cassilhas RC, Attux C, et al.
"A 20-week program of resistance or concurrent exercise improves symptoms of schizophrenia: results of a blind, randomized controlled trial."
Rev Bras Psiquiatr. 2015 December. Epub 2015.

79. Reynolds G.
"Ask Well: Is It Good to Sweat?"
New York Times: Well. (2013, December). Retrieved from http://well.blogs.nytimes.com/2013/12/27/ask-well-is-it-good-to-sweat/?partner=rss&emc=rss Accessed June 23, 2016.

80. Mercola J.
"Is It Good to Sweat?"
Mercola.com, Peak Fitness. (2014, March). Retrieved from
http://fitness.mercola.com/sites/fitness/archive/2014/01/10/sweating-benefits.aspx.

81. Melov S., Tarnopolsky Mark A,Beckman K, Felkey C, Hubbard A.
"Resistance Exercise Reverses Aging in Human Skeletal Muscle"
Public Library of Science. (2007, May). Retrieved from http://journals.plos.org/plosone/article?id=10.1371/journal.pone.0000465. Accessed June 23, 2016.

Following exercise training the transcriptional signature of aging was markedly reversed back to that of younger levels for most genes that were affected by both age and exercise. We conclude that healthy older adults show evidence of mitochondrial impairment and muscle weakness, but that this can be partially reversed at the phenotypic level, and substantially reversed at the transcriptome level, following six months of resistance exercise training.

82. McGuff D, Little J. p.247-248. (see note 8 for bibliography)

When the drug Resveratrol was shown to produce some reversal of aging in mice and worms, it flew off the shelves as an age-reversal agent -- without any proof that it had a similar effect in humans. Now here, after millennia of searching for the "fountain of youth" . . . a clinical study has essentially said, "Look, here it is -- an actual functional reversal of aging at the molecular level!" . . . But it's not surprising to us, nor to anyone who performs the type of training that we advocate . . . Having said this, the most amazing thing that happened after this study came out in 2007 was -- nothing. That news of this magnitude should come out during our lifetimes and not be on the front page of every newspaper and on every evening news program was inexplicable to us. Perhaps it failed to garner much attention because people are more than willing to take a pill, thinking it's going to reverse their aging, and it's only the exceptional individual who would hear such news and say, "I can do something for myself, by the sweat of my brow; by applying my own effort and my own work ethic, I can achieve this for myself!" Perhaps.

83. Centers for Disease Control and Prevention
"Adult Obesity Facts"
CDC.gov, Division of Nutrition, Physical Activity, and Obesity. (2016, April). Retrieved from http://www.cdc.gov/obesity/data/adult.html. Accessed April 28, 2016.

84. Sanchis-Gomar F, Pérez LM, Joyner MJ, Löllgen H, Lucia A.
"Endurance Exercise and the Heart: Friend or Foe?"
Sports Medicine. 2016 April. Epub 2015 November.

It has been increasingly suggested that prolonged strenuous endurance exercise could have potential deleterious cardiac effects. In effect, the term "cardiac overuse injury" (or "over-exercise") has been recently reported to group all the possible deleterious cardiac consequences of repeated exposure to strenuous endurance exercise or "over-exercise.

85. Centers for Disease Control and Prevention.
"Injury Prevention & Control: Traumatic Brain Injury & Concussion" *CDC.gov.* (2016, August). Retrieved from http://www.cdc.gov/traumaticbraininjury/get_the_facts.html

More than half (55%) of traumatic brain injuries among children 0 to 14 years were caused by falls.

86. Kesidis N, Metaxas TI, Vrabas IS, et. al.
"Myosin heavy chain isoform distribution in single fibres of bodybuilders." *European Journal of Applied Physiology.* 2008 July.

The percentage of fibres expressing [fast twitch and lower order fast twitch] was larger in bodybuilders . . . while [super fast twitch fibre expression] was completely absent.

87. Andersen JL, Aagaard P. (see note 71 for bibliography)

[The super fast twitch fiber] percentage in the vastus lateralis muscle of the subjects decreased from 9% to only 2% in a 3 months [heavy] training period, but somewhat more remarkable the [super fast twitch fiber] percentage subsequently increased to 17% after an additional period of 3 months of detraining

88. Ibid.

89. De Souza RW, Aguiar AF, Carani FR, Campos GE, Padovani CR, Silva MD.
"High-intensity resistance training with insufficient recovery time between bouts induce atrophy and alterations in myosin heavy chain content in rat skeletal muscle."
Anatomical Record, (Hoboken). 2011 August.

Change in muscle fiber-type frequency was supported by a significant decrease in [slow twitch] and [lower order fast twitch fibers] accompanied by a significant increase in [super fast twitch fiber] content . . . These data show that high-intensity resistance training with insufficient recovery time between bouts promoted muscle atrophy...

90. Andersen JL, Aagaard P. (see note 71 for bibliography)

91. Unhjem RJ, Nygård M, van den Hoven LT, Sidhu SK, Hoff J, Wang E.
"Lifelong strength training mitigates the age-related decline in efferent drive."
Journal of Applied Physiology. 2016 June.

These observations suggest that lifelong strength training has a protective effect against age-related attenuation of efferent drive. In contrast, no beneficial effect seems to derive from habitual recreational activity, indicating that strength training may be particularly beneficial for counteracting age-related loss of neuromuscular function.

Di Rienzo F, Blache Y, Kanthack TF, Monteil K, Collet C, Guillot A.
"Short-term effects of integrated motor imagery practice on muscle activation and force performance."
Neuroscience. 2015 October.

The effect of motor imagery practice on isometric force development is well-documented . . . priming effects of motor imagery practice [yields] higher muscle activation and force performance.

92. **Folland JP, Williams AG.**
"The adaptations to strength training : morphological and neurological contributions to increased strength."
Sports Medicine. 2007. Review.

The gains in strength with high resistance strength training are undoubtedly due to a wide combination of neurological and morphological factors. Whilst the neurological factors may make their greatest contribution during the early stages of a training programme, hypertrophic processes also commence at the onset of training.

93. **Calatayud J, Vinstrup J, Jakobsen MD, Sundstrup et. al.**
"Importance of mind-muscle connection during progressive resistance training."
European Journal Applied Physiology. 2016 March. . Epub 2015 Dec 23.

This study evaluates whether focusing on using specific muscles during bench press can selectively activate these muscles . . . In both [pectorals and triceps] muscles, focusing on using the respective muscles increased muscle activity . . . Resistance-trained individuals can increase [triceps] or [pectorals] muscle activity during the bench press when focusing on using the specific muscle at intensities up to 60 % of [one repetition maximum].

94. **Even-Esh Z, Shwarzenegger.com**
"The Most Powerful Training Tool"
Shwarzenegger.com, 2012 September. Retrieved from http://www.schwarzenegger.com/fitness/post/the-most-powerful-training-tool.

The Body Is Very Important, But The Mind Is MORE Important Than The Body

95. **Bunno Y, Suzuki T, Iwatsuki H.**
"Motor imagery muscle contraction strength influences spinal motor neuron excitability and cardiac sympathetic nerve activity."
Journal of Physical Therapy Science. 2015 December.

Motor imagery can increase the spinal motor neuron excitability and cardiac sympathetic nerve activity . . . These results might account for priming effects of motor imagery practice yielding to higher muscle activation and force performance. Present findings may be of interest for applications in sports training and neurologic rehabilitation.

Lebon F, Collet C, Guillot A.
"Benefits of motor imagery training on muscle strength."
Journal of Strength and Conditioning Research. 2010 June.

It is well established that motor imagery (MI) improves motor performance and motor learning efficiently. Previous studies provided evidence that muscle strength may benefit from MI training, mainly when movements are under the control of large cortical areas in the primary motor cortex.

Yue G, Cole KJ.
"Strength increases from the motor program: comparison of training with maximal voluntary and imagined muscle contractions."
Journal of Neurophysiology. 1992 May.

Strength increases can be achieved without repeated muscle activation. These force gains appear to result from practice effects on central motor programming/ planning. The results of these experiments add to existing evidence for the neural origin of strength increases that occur before muscle hypertrophy.

96. Ingram TG, Kraeutner SN, Solomon JP, Westwood DA, Boe SG.
"Skill acquisition via motor imagery relies on both motor and perceptual learning."
Behavioral Neuroscience. 2016 April. Epub 2016 Feb 8.

Motor imagery, the mental rehearsal of movement, is an effective means for acquiring a novel skill, even in the absence of physical practice . . . Generally, physical practice-based training led to lower response times compared with motor imagery-based training for implicit and random sequences . . . Our results suggest that motor imaging-based training relies on both perceptual and motor learning . . . These results reveal details regarding the mechanisms underlying motor imagery, and inform its use as a modality for skill acquisition.

97. Calatayud J, Vinstrup J, Jakobsen MD, Sundstrup et. al. (see note 90 for bibliography)

98. Schuenke MD, Herman JR, Gliders RM, et. al.
"Early-phase muscular adaptations in response to slow-speed versus traditional resistance-training regimens."
European Journal of Applied Physiology. 2012 October.

[The cross-sectional area of slow, fast, and super fast twitch fibers] increased in [traditional strength training]. In [super slow training], only the [cross-sectional area of fast and super fast twitch] fibers increased . . . slow-speed strength training induced a greater adaptive response compared to training with a similar resistance at "normal" speed

99. Westcott WL, Winett RA, Anderson ES, et. al.
"Effects of regular and slow speed resistance training on muscle strength."
Journal of Sports Medicine & Physical Fitness. 2001 June.

Slower repetition speed may effectively increase intensity throughout the lifting phase while decreasing momentum. Super-Slow training is an effective method for middle-aged and older adults to increase strength. Although studies still need to be done with at-risk populations, repetition speed should be considered when prescribing resistance training.

100. Gabriel DA, Kamen G, Frost G.
"Neural adaptations to resistive exercise: mechanisms and recommendations for training practices."
Sports Medicine. 2006. Review.

There are several lines of evidence for central [brain] control of training-related adaptation to resistive exercise. Mental practice using imagined contractions has been shown to increase the excitability of the cortical areas involved in movement and motion planning. However, training using imagined contractions is unlikely to be as effective as physical training, and it may be more applicable to rehabilitation. Retention of strength gains after dissipation of physiological effects demonstrates a strong practice effect . . . A reduction in antagonist co-activation would allow increased expression of agonist muscle force, while an increase in antagonist co-activation is important for maintaining the integrity of the joint… Motor learning theory and imagined contractions should be incorporated into strength-training practice… Submaximal eccentric contractions should be used when there are issues of muscle pain, detraining or limb immobilisation.

101. Goto K, Ishii N, Kizuka T, Takamatsu K.
"The impact of metabolic stress on hormonal responses and muscular adaptations."
Medicine and Science in Sports and Exercise. 2005 June.

The [no rest between reps within sets] regimen induced strong lactate, growth hormone, epinephrine, and norepinephrine responses, whereas the [rest between reps within sets] regimen did not . . . These results suggest that exercise-induced metabolic stress is associated with acute Growth Hormone, Epinephrine, and Norepinephrine responses and chronic muscular adaptations following resistance training.

102. Gabriel DA, Kamen G, Frost G. (see note 97 for bibliography)

103. McGuff D, Little J., pg. 53 (see note 8 for bibliography)

Physiologists R.N. Carpinelli and R.M. Otto conducted a study out of Adelphi University that surveyed all of the known scientific literature [up to 1998] concerning single-set versus multiple-set resistance training. They found that, on the whole, performing multiple sets brought absolutely no additional increase in results compared with single-set training. The literature came down overwhelmingly in favor of a single set of exercise as being sufficient; only two out of the forty seven studies surveyed showed any benefit (and a marginal improvement at that) to be had from the performance of multiple sets.

Starkey DB, Pollock ML, Ishida Y, et. al.

"Effect of resistance training volume on strength and muscle thickness."

Medicine and Science in Sports and Exercise. 1996 October.

> *In conclusion, one set of high-intensity resistance training was as effective as three sets for increasing [knee extension] and [knee flexion] isometric torque and muscle thickness in previously untrained adults.*

104. Kemmler WK, Lauber-D, Engelke K, Weineck J.

"Effects of single- vs. multiple-set resistance training on maximum strength and body composition in trained postmenopausal women."

Journal of Strength & Conditioning Research. 2004 November.

> *Multiple-set training resulted in significant increases (3.5-5.5%) for all 4 strength measurements, whereas single-set training resulted in significant decreases (-1.1 to -2.0%). Body mass and body composition did not change during the study. The results show that, in pretrained subjects, multiple-set protocols are superior to single-set protocols in increasing maximum strength.*

Rønnestad BR, Egeland W, Kvamme NH, Refsnes PE, Kadi F, Raastad T.

"Dissimilar effects of one- and three-set strength training on strength and muscle mass gains in upper and lower body in untrained subjects."

Journal of Strength and Conditioning Research. 2007 Feb.

> *The results demonstrate that 3-set strength training is superior to 1-set strength training with regard to strength and muscle mass gains in the leg muscles, while no difference exists between 1- and 3-set training in upper-body muscles in untrained men.*

105. Fröhlich M, Emrich E, Schmidtbleicher D.

"Outcome effects of single-set versus multiple-set training--an advanced replication study."

Research in Sports Medicine. 2010 July.

> *On the basis of 72 primary studies, the meta-analysis dealt with the problem of single-set vs. multiple-set training . . . Generally speaking, it can be stated that multiple-set training, depending on factors like age, training experience, duration of the study, etc., offers several advantages over single-set regimes, especially when combined with periodization strategies, and it can be applied very successfully for increasing maximal strength in long-time effects. Therefore, the outcome effects of both methods are the same in short-time interventions. For longer-time interventions and for advanced subjects with the goal of optimizing their strength gain, however, multiple-set strategies are superior.*

106. Verdijk LB, Snijders T, Drost M, Delhaas T, Kadi F, van Loon LJ. (see note 45 for bibliography)

107. Lebon F, Collet C, Guillot A.

"Benefits of motor imagery training on muscle strength."

Journal of Strength and Conditioning Research. 2010 June.

It is well established that motor imagery (MI) improves motor performance and motor learning efficiently. Previous studies provided evidence that muscle strength may benefit from MI training, mainly when movements are under the control of large cortical areas in the primary motor cortex.

Calatayud J, Vinstrup J, Jakobsen MD, Sundstrup et. al. (see note 90 for bibliography)

Yue G, Cole KJ.

"Strength increases from the motor program: comparison of training with maximal voluntary and imagined muscle contractions."

Journal of Neurophysiology. 1992 May.

Strength increases can be achieved without repeated muscle activation. These force gains appear to result from practice effects on central motor programming/planning. The results of these experiments add to existing evidence for the neural origin of strength increases that occur before muscle hypertrophy.

108. De Luca CJ, Contessa P.

"Hierarchical control of motor units in voluntary contractions."

Journal of Neurophysiology. 2012 January. Epub 2011 Oct 5.

This hierarchical control scheme describes a mechanism that provides an effective economy of force generation for the earlier-recruited lower force-twitch motor units, and reduces the fatigue of later-recruited higher force-twitch motor units-both characteristics being well suited for generating and sustaining force during the fight-or-flight response.

109. Ahtiainen JP, Pakarinen A, Kraemer WJ, Häkkinen K.

"Acute hormonal responses to heavy resistance exercise in strength athletes versus nonathletes."

Canadian Journal of Applied Physiology. 2004 October.

These data suggest that, at least in experienced strength athletes, the forced-repetition protocol is a viable alternative to the more traditional maximum-repetition protocol and may even be a superior approach.

110. Anderson JL, Aagaard P. (see note 71 for bibliography)

111. Schoenfeld BJ, Pope ZK, Benik FM, et. al.

"Longer Interset Rest Periods Enhance Muscle Strength and Hypertrophy in Resistance-Trained Men."

Journal of Strength and Conditioning. Research. 2016 July.

This study provides evidence that longer rest periods promote greater increases in muscle strength and hypertrophy *in young resistance-trained men.*

112. McKendry J, Pérez-López A, McLeod M, et. al.
"Short inter-set rest blunts resistance exercise-induced increases in myofibrillar protein synthesis and intracellular signaling in young males."
Experimental Physiology. 2016 July. Epub 2016 Jun 2.

We demonstrate that short rest (1 min) between sets of moderate-intensity, high-volume resistance exercise blunts the acute muscle anabolic response compared with a longer rest period (5 min), despite a superior circulating hormonal milieu. These data have important implications for the development of training regimens to maximize muscle hypertrophy. *Manipulating the rest-recovery interval between sets of resistance exercise may influence training-induced muscle remodeling.*

113. Scudese E, Simão R, Senna G, et. al.
"Long Rest Interval Promotes Durable Testosterone Responses in High-intensity Bench Press."
Journal of Strength and Conditioning Research. 2015 Oct 6. [Epub ahead of print]

In conclusion, although both short and long rest periods [between sets] enhanced acute testosterone values, the longer rest promoted a longer lasting elevation for both total testosterone and free testosterone.

114. Bain J, Chang l.
"New Ideas on Proper Stretching Techniques"
WebMD.com, Fitness & Exercise. 2010 October. Retrieved from http://www.webmd.com/fitness-exercise/new-ideas-on-proper-stretching-techniques?page=1

[According to Dr. Bill Holcomb, professor of athletic training at UNLV] you should never stretch a cold muscle in any way. And doing static stretches -- meaning the kind where you hold the stretch before a workout or competition -- may decrease your strength, power, and performance . . . After warming up [one should perform] dynamic (not static) stretches. Dynamic stretching means slow, controlled movements rather than remaining still and holding a stretch. They may include simple movements like arm circles and hip rotations, flowing movements as in yoga or walking . . . increasing numbers of experts agree that dynamic stretching is the best stretching routine before a workout or competition.

115. Andersen JL, Aagaard P. (see note 71 for bibliography)

116. Heavens KR, Szivak TK, Hooper DR, et. al.
"The effects of high-intensity short rest resistance exercise on muscle damage markers in men and women."
Journal of Strength and Conditioning Research. 2014 April.

Overall, [when following the short rest protocol] women demonstrated a faster inflammatory response with increased acute damage, whereas men demonstrated a greater prolonged damage response. Therefore, strength and conditioning professionals need to be aware of the level of stress imposed on individuals when creating such volitional high-intensity metabolic type workouts and allow for adequate progression and recovery from such workouts.

117. Gentil P, Fischer B, Martorelli AS, Lima RM, Bottaro M.
"Effects of equal-volume resistance training performed one or two times a week in upper body muscle size and strength of untrained young men."
The Journal of Sports Medicine and Physical Fitness. 2015 March. Epub 2014 Apr 14.
The results from the present study suggest that untrained men experience similar gains in muscle mass and strength with equal volume resistance training [whether] performed one or two days per week.

118. Andersen JL, Aagaard P. (see note 71 for bibliography)

119. Kesidis N, Metaxas TI, Vrabas IS, et. al.
"Myosin heavy chain isoform distribution in single fibres of bodybuilders."
European Journal of Applied Physiology. 2008 July.
The percentage of fibres expressing [fast twitch and slow/fast twitch] was larger in bodybuilders ($P < 0.05$), while [super fast twitch fibre expression] was completely absent ($P < 0.05$).

120. Andersen JL, Aagaard P. (see note 71 for bibliography)

121. Glassman G. (Founder of *CrossFit*) (see note 19 for bibliography)

122. Kesidis N, Metaxas TI, Vrabas IS, et. al. (see note 117 for bibliography)

123. Wilson J.
"Ask the Muscle Prof: How Do I Target Fast-Twitch Muscle Fibers?"
Bodybuilding.com. (2016, April). Retrieved from http://www.bodybuilding.com/fun/ask-the-muscle-prof-how-do-i-target-fast-twitch-muscle-fibers.html
Fast-twitch muscle fibers are indeed the largest and most powerful muscular movers in your body. Unfortunately, they're also neglected in most bodybuilders' programs. It's time to change this! . . . Studies show that individuals who neglect training in a heavier range will not program their nervous system to effectively recruit their largest [super] fast-twitch fibers. Along with intensity, fatigue is the second surefire way to increase fast-twitch muscle fiber recruitment. Your body's first impulse is to recruit slow-twitch fibers, but once you fatigue those fibers, it has to recruit fast-twitch fibers to do what is being asked of it.

124. Trappe S, Creer A, Slivka D, Minchev K, Trappe T.
"Single muscle fiber function with concurrent exercise or nutrition countermeasures during 60 days of bed rest in women."
Journal of Applied Physiology. 2007 October.
In [the exercise group] conditions, [muscle fiber] size and contractile function were preserved during bed rest. These data show that the concurrent exercise program preserved the myocellular profile of the vastus lateralis muscle during 60-day bed rest. To combat muscle atrophy and function with long-term unloading, the exercise prescription program used in this study should be considered as a viable training program for the upper leg muscles, whereas the nutritional intervention used cannot be recommended as a countermeasure for skeletal muscle.

125. Merriam-Webster.com
"Scientific method"
Merriam-Webster Dictionary, (2016, July). Retrieved from http://www.merriam-webster.com/dictionary/scientific%20method. Accessed on July 20, 2016.

126. Easter M.
"4 Muscle Myths Debunked"
Men's Health, MensHealth.com, Fitness. (2013 January). Retrieved from http://www.menshealth.com/fitness/common-exercise-mistakes

You don't have to constantly add new moves and workouts to your routine to prevent your body from adapting. Actually, you want adaptation—this is how muscles grow. Sustain it with small weekly tweaks: Alter your grip, pace, or rest. That can help your muscles adapt over time, preventing plateaus, says Nick Tumminello, C.P.T., owner of Performance University in Fort Lauderdale.

Smith C.
"The Muscle Confusion Controversy -- Fact or Myth?
Fierce Strength, fiercestrength.com. (2014 October). Retrieved from http://www.fiercestrength.com/muscle-confusion/

When you search for information regarding the muscle confusion principle and whether it's a fact or a myth, most "experts" will tell you that there's absolutely no truth to it and that anyone who thinks it's a fact is dumber than a bag of rocks. They claim that the best results come from using progressive overload and sticking to a strict routine.

127. Bain J, Chang L. (see note 112 for bibliography)

128. Bodybuilding.com Contributing Writer
"Stretching for Weight Training!"
Bodybuilding.com, Stretching. 2014 September. Retrieved from http://www.bodybuilding.com/fun/donald1.htm

Dynamic stretching . . . involves moving parts of your body and gradually increasing reach, speed of movement, or both . . . Do not confuse dynamic stretching with ballistic stretching! Dynamic stretching consists of controlled leg and arm swings that take you (gently!) to the limits of your range of motion. Ballistic stretches involve trying to force a part of the body beyond its range of motion. In dynamic stretches, there are no bounces or "jerky" movements. An example of dynamic stretching would be slow, controlled leg swings, arm swings, or torso twists.

129. Kokkonen J, Nelson AG, Tarawhiti T, Buckingham P, Winchester JB.
"Early-phase resistance training strength gains in novice lifters are enhanced by doing static stretching."
Journal of Strength and Conditioning Research. 2010 Feb.

Based on results of this study, it is recommended that to maximize strength gains in the early phase of training, novice lifters should include static stretching exercises to their resistance training programs.

130. Di Rienzo F, Blache Y, Kanthack TF, Monteil K, Collet C, Guillot A (see note 88(2) for bibliography)

131. Lam LC, Chau RC, Wong BM, et. al.
"A 1-year randomized controlled trial comparing mind body exercise (Tai Chi) with stretching and toning exercise on cognitive function in older Chinese adults at risk of cognitive decline."
Journal of the American Medical Directors Association. 2012 July.

132. Fields LL.
"The Fitness-Driven Church"
ChristianityToday.com, Cultural Trends. (2013, June). Retrieved from http://www.christianitytoday.com/ct/2013/june/fitness-driven-church.html?start=2.

133. Centers for Disease Control and Prevention
"Childhood Obesity Facts"
CDC.gov, Overweight and Obesity. (2016) Retrieved from http://www.cdc.gov/healthyschools/obesity/facts.htm. Accessed February 28. 2016.

134. Hazell TJ, Islam H, Townsend LK, Schmale MS, Copeland JL.
"Effects of exercise intensity on plasma concentrations of appetite-regulating hormones: Potential mechanisms." *ScienceDirect, Appetite.* 2016. Epub 2015 Dec 22. Review.

> *Overall, changes in appetite-regulating hormones following acute exercise appear to be intensity-dependent, with increasing intensity leading to a greater suppression of orexigenic [appetite-stimulating] signals and greater stimulation of anorexigenic [appetite-inhibiting] signals.*

135. Mayo Clinic.
"Water: How much should you drink every day?"
MayoClinic.com, Healthy Lifestyle, Nutrition and healthy eating, (2016). Retrieved from http://www.mayoclinic.org/healthy-lifestyle/nutrition-and-healthy-eating/in-depth/water/art-20044256. Accessed June 23, 2016.

136. Jacobsen MT, WebMD staff
"Protein: Are You Getting Enough?"
WebMD.com. 2014, September. Retrieved from http://www.webmd.com/food-recipes/protein.

137. Mercola J.
"Vitamin D--One of the Simplest Solutions to Wide-Ranging Health Problems"
Mercola.com. 2013, December. Retrieved from http://articles.mercola.com/sites/articles/archive/2013/12/22/dr-holick-vitamin-d-benefits.aspx.

Mercola J.
"7 Signs You May Have a Vitamin D Deficiency"
Mercola.com. 2014, May. http://articles.mercola.com/sites/articles/archive/2014/05/28/vitamin-d-deficiency-signs-symptoms.aspx

Jacobsen MT, WebMD staff
"Vitamin D Deficiency"
WebMD.com. (2016, May) Retrieved from http://www.webmd.com/diet/guide/vitamin-d-deficiency

138. **University of Maryland Medical Center**
"Turmeric"
UMM.edu. 2016. Retrieved from https://umm.edu/health/medical/altmed/herb/turmeric. Accessed June 23, 2016.

139. **Zuckerman D, Gallo A, Levin M; Chen C.**
"Can eating fish be dangerous? The facts about methylmercury" *Center4Research.org, National Center for Health Research,* (2014). Retrieved from http://center4research.org/healthy-living-prevention/diet-weight-control-and-food-safety/can-eating-fish-be-dangerous-the-facts-about-methylmercury/. Accessed June 23, 2016.

140. **Consumer Reports**
How safe is your shrimp?"
Consumer Reports, Special Report: Shrimp Safety. (2015, April). Retrieved from http://www.consumerreports.org/cro/magazine/2015/06/shrimp-safety/index.htm.

141. **Gammon C.**
"Weed-Whacking Herbicide Proves Deadly to Human Cells"
Scientific American, Environmental Health News. (2009, June) Retrieved from http://www.scientificamerican.com/article/weed-whacking-herbicide-p/. Accessed June 23, 2016.

142. **Hyman M.**
"Milk is Dangerous for your Health"
DrHyman.com. (2016).
Retrieved from http://drhyman.com/blog/2013/10/28/milk-dangerous-health/. Accessed June 23, 2016.

143. **National Sleep Foundation**
"How Much Sleep Do We Really Need?"
SleepFoundation.org, How Sleep Works. (2016). Retrieved from https://sleepfoundation.org/how-sleep-works/how-much-sleep-do-we-really-need. Accessed June 23, 2016.

APPENDIX II

Categorized Research with Excerpts for Further Reading

In this section of the Appendix, you will find fourteen categories that I believe will be of highest interest to specific audiences of large populations who want to drill deeper into the research. In each category, you will find the sources grouped according to subject matter, and sequenced in order of highest relevance to the average reader. While many of these sources can also be found in the *Notated Bibliography with Citations*, you will also find with additional sources—many with yet unseen citations—that I believe will be useful as further reading. While I will cite the full source bibliography for each, not all sources in each category will include an excerpt (which, where they occur, were taken directly from the full study *or* the published abstract). Each source and citation will be recorded in every category to which it applies, so you can expect to see several sources in multiple categories.

Dangers of Running, Aerobics, and Other Endurance Exercise

Lavie CJ, O'Keefe JH, Sallis RE.
"Exercise and the heart--the harm of too little and too much."
Current Sports Medicine Reports. 2015 March. Review.

> *Very high doses of exercise may be associated with increased risk of atrial fibrillation, coronary artery disease, and malignant ventricular arrhythmias. These acute bouts of excessive exercise may lead to cardiac dilatation, cardiac dysfunction, and release of troponin and brain natriuretic peptide.*

Sanchis-Gomar F, Pérez LM, Joyner MJ, Löllgen H, Lucia A.
"Endurance Exercise and the Heart: Friend or Foe?"
Sports Medicine. 2016 April. Epub 2015 November.

> *It has been increasingly suggested that prolonged strenuous endurance exercise could have potential deleterious cardiac effects. In effect, the term "cardiac overuse injury" (or*

"over-exercise") has been recently reported to group all the possible deleterious cardiac consequences of repeated exposure to strenuous endurance exercise or "over-exercise."

Seidl J, Asplund CA. "Effects of excessive endurance activity on the heart." *Current Sports Medicine Report*. 2014 November.

Excess endurance activity may appear to increase the risk of cardiac abnormalities, which may increase the risk for long-term morbidity or mortality.

Park, Alice.
"When Exercise Does More Harm than Good"
Time Magazine, 2015. Retrieved from http://time.com/3692668/when-exercise-does-more-harm-than-good/ Accessed June 22, 2016.

In a 2015 report published in the Journal of the American College of Cardiology, researchers say that "those who ran at a fast pace more than four hours a week for more than three days a week had about the same risk of dying during the study's 12-year follow up as those who were sedentary and hardly exercised at all. The link held even after the researchers accounted for potentially confounding factors such as age, sex, whether the participants had a history of heart disease or diabetes, or whether they smoked and drank alcohol" . . . What [co-author, researcher Jacob] Marrot and his team found was that both too little running and too much running are linked to higher rates of death. The most intense runners ended up with a risk of dying that was similar to that of those who opted to stay on the couch... That dovetails with the mounting research that so-called micro-workouts—high-intensity but brief workouts that could be as short at 1 minute, according to another recent paper -- may be better for the body than long and continuous workouts.

Eijsvogels TM, Fernandez AB, Thompson PD.
"Are There Deleterious Cardiac Effects of Acute and Chronic Endurance Exercise?"
Physiology Review. 2016 January. Review.

Recent reports suggest that prodigious amounts of exercise may increase markers for, and even the incidence of, cardiovascular disease. This review examines the evidence that extremes of endurance exercise may increase cardiovascular disease risk by reviewing the causes and incidence of exercise-related cardiac events, and the acute effects of exercise on cardiovascular function, the effect of exercise on cardiac biomarkers, including "myocardial" creatine kinase, cardiac troponins, and cardiac natriuretic peptides . . . it is possible that prolonged exercise and exercise training can adversely affect cardiac function in some individuals.

Patil HR, O'Keefe JH, Lavie CJ, Magalski A, Vogel RA, McCullough PA.
"Cardiovascular damage resulting from chronic excessive endurance exercise."
Modern Medicine. 2012 July. Review.

Chronic, excessive sustained endurance exercise may cause adverse structural remodeling of the heart and large arteries . . . In veteran extreme endurance athletes, this recurrent myocardial injury and repair may eventually result in patchy myocardial fibrosis, particularly in the atria, interventricular septum and right ventricle, potentially creating a substrate for atrial and ventricular arrhythmias. Furthermore, chronic, excessive, sustained, high-intensity endurance exercise may be associated with diastolic dysfunction, large-artery wall stiffening and coronary artery calcification.

Gaudreault V, Tizon-Marcos H, Poirier P, et al.

"Transient myocardial tissue and function changes during a marathon in less fit marathon runners."

The Canadian Journal of Cardiology. 2013 October.

Completing a marathon leads to localized myocardial edema, diminished perfusion, and decreased function occurring more extensively in less trained and fit runners. Although reversible, these changes might contribute to the transient increase in cardiac risk reported during sustained vigorous exercise.

Wilson M, O'Hanlon R, Prasad S, Basavarajaiah S, Stephens N, et al.

"Myocardial fibrosis in an veteran endurance athlete."

Journal of Applied Physiology. 2011.

An unexpectedly high prevalence of myocardial fibrosis (50%) was observed in healthy, asymptomatic, lifelong veteran male [endurance] athletes, compared with zero cases in age-matched veteran controls and young athletes. These data suggest a link between lifelong endurance exercise and myocardial fibrosis that requires further investigation... Cardiovascular MRI demonstrated a pattern of late gadolinium enhancement, which indicated myocardial scarring as a result of previous myocarditis. Myocarditis is a non-ischaemic inflammatory disease of the myocardium associated with cardiac dysfunction and arrhythmogenic substrate. The clinical course of viral myocarditis is mostly insidious with limited cardiac inflammation and dysfunction.

Sanchis-Gomar F, Santos-Lozano A, Garatachea N, et al.

"My patient wants to perform strenuous endurance exercise. What's the right advice?" *International Journal of Cardiology.* 2015 Oct 15;197:248-53. Epub 2015 Jun 15. Review.

Prolonged strenuous endurance exercise such as marathon running has recently been associated with potential deleterious cardiac effects, particularly increased risk of atrial fibrillation. This topic is medically important due to the increasing number of participants in strenuous endurance exercise events lasting several hours, including older people.

Doutreleau S, Pistea C, Lonsdorfer E, Charloux A.

"Exercise-induced second-degree atrioventricular block in endurance athletes."

Medicine and Science in Sports and Exercise. 2013 March.

Heart rhythm disorders, such as atrial arrhythmia (including atrial fibrillation and atrial flutter), are a well-established consequence of such long-term endurance practice.

Izquierdo M, Ibáñez J, Häkkinen K, Kraemer WJ, Ruesta M, Gorostiaga EM. "Maximal strength and power, muscle mass, endurance and serum hormones in weightlifters and road cyclists."

Journal of Sports Sciences. 2004 May.

> *Basal serum total testosterone and free testosterone concentrations were lower in elite amateur cyclists than in age-matched weightlifters or untrained individuals . . . in cycling, long-term endurance training may interfere more with the development of muscle power than with the development of maximal strength, probably mediated by long-term cycling-related impairment in anabolic hormonal status.*

Gordon SE, Kraemer WJ, Looney DP, Flanagan SD, Comstock BA, Hymer WC. "The influence of age and exercise modality on growth hormone bioactivity in women."

Growth Hormone and IGF Research. 2014 April.

> *The greater [bioactive growth hormone] response to the heavy resistance exercise protocol found in the younger group can be attributed to an unknown serum factor . . . that either potentiated growth hormone bioactivity in response to heavy resistance exercise or* ***inhibited growth hormone bioactivity in response to aerobic exercise.***

Seeger JP, Lenting CJ, Schreuder TH, et. al.

"Interval exercise, but not endurance exercise, prevents endothelial ischemia-reperfusion injury in healthy subjects."

The American Journal of Physiology, Heart and Circulatory Physiology. 2015 February. Epub 2014 Nov 21.

> *In conclusion, a single bout of lower limb interval exercise, but not moderate-intensity endurance exercise, effectively prevents [brachial artery injury]. This indicates the presence of a remote preconditioning effect of exercise, which is selectively present after short-term interval but not continuous exercise in healthy young subjects.*

Widrick JJ, Trappe SW, Costill DL, Fitts RH.

"Force-velocity and force-power properties of single muscle fibers from elite master runners and sedentary men."

American Journal of Physiology, Cell Physiology. 1996 August.

> *[Super fast twitch] fibers produced twice as much peak power as [fast twitch] fibers, whereas [fast twitch] fibers produced about five times more peak power than [slow twitch] fibers . . . Endurance-trained master runners' slow twitch and fast twitch] fibers were smaller in diameter and produced less peak force than [middle-aged sedentary men's slow twitch and fast twitch fibers]. The absolute peak power output of [the runners' slow twitch and fast twitch] fibers was 13% and 27% less, respectively, than peak power of similarly typed [sedentary men's] fibers.*

Vaara JP, Kokko J, Isoranta M, Kyröläinen H.
"Effects of Added Resistance Training on Physical Fitness, Body Composition, and Serum Hormone Concentrations During Eight Weeks of Special Military Training Period."
Journal of Strength and Conditioning Research. 2015 November.

In conclusion, interference with strength gains might be related to the high-volume of aerobic activities and too low volume of resistance training during strength training. To develop strength characteristics, careful periodization and individualization should be adopted in strength training.

Farup J, Sørensen H, Kjølhede T.
"Similar changes in muscle fiber phenotype with differentiated consequences for rate of force development: endurance versus resistance training."
Human Movement Science. 2014 April.

Resistance Training significantly increased eccentric, concentric and isometric strength for both knee extensors and flexors, whereas Endurance Training did not. In conclusion, resistance training may be very important for maintaining the rate of force development, whereas endurance training may negatively impact rate of force development.

Howden EJ, Perhonen M, Peshock RM, et. al.
"Females have a blunted cardiovascular response to one year of intensive supervised endurance training."
Journal of Applied Physiology. 2015 July.

We demonstrate for the first time clear sex differences in response to 1 yr of matched endurance training, such that the development of ventricular hypertrophy *and increase in Vo2max in females is markedly blunted compared with males.*

Luke AC, Stehling C, Stahl R, et. al.
"High-field magnetic resonance imaging assessment of articular cartilage before and after marathon running: does long-distance running lead to cartilage damage?"
American Journal of Sports Medicine. 2010 November.

Runners showed elevated T1ρ and T2 values after a marathon, suggesting biochemical changes in articular cartilage, T1ρ values remain elevated after 3 months of reduced activity. The patellofemoral joint and medial compartment of the knee show the highest signal changes, suggesting they are at higher risk for degeneration.

Fitts RH, Widrick JJ.
"Muscle mechanics: adaptations with exercise-training."
Exercise and Sport Sciences Reviews. 1996. Review.

Regular endurance exercise training had no effect on fiber size, but with prolonged durations of daily training it depressed peak force and peak power. When the training is maintained over prolonged periods, it may even induce atrophy of the slow [twitch] and fast [twitch] fibers.

Burt D, Lamb K, Nicholas C, Twist C.
"Lower-volume muscle-damaging exercise protects against high-volume muscle-damaging exercise and the detrimental effects on endurance performance."
European Journal of Applied Physiology. 2015 July.

This study demonstrates that the protective effect of lower-volume exercise-induced muscle damage [EIMD] on subsequent high-volume EIMD is transferable to endurance running.

Sato K, Iemitsu M, Katayama K, Ishida K, Kanao Y, Saito M.
"Responses of sex steroid hormones to different intensities of exercise in endurance athletes."
Experimental Physiology. 2016 January. Epub 2015 Dec 9.

These results indicate that in endurance athletes, serum sex steroid hormone concentrations, especially serum DHEA and 5α-dihydrotestosterone concentrations, increased only with high-intensity exercise, suggesting that different responses of sex steroid hormone secretion are induced by different exercise intensities in individuals with low and high levels of physical fitness. In athletes, therefore, high-intensity exercise may be required to increase circulating sex steroid hormone concentrations.

Wang Y, Pessin JE.
"Mechanisms for fiber-type specificity of skeletal muscle atrophy."
Current Opinions in Clinical Nutrition and Metabolic Care. 2013 May. Review.

Fast-twitch glycolytic fibers are more vulnerable than slow-twitch oxidative fibers under a variety of atrophic conditions . . . nutrient-related atrophy such as cancer/aging cachexia, sepsis, and diabetes are more directed to [fast and super fast twitch] glycolytic fiber wasting.

Tong TK, Lin H, Lippi G, Nie J, Tian Y.
"Serum oxidant and antioxidant status in adolescents undergoing professional endurance sports training."
Oxidative Medicine and Cellular Longevity. 2012.

Schnohr P, O'Keefe JH, Marott JL, Lange P, Jensen GB.
"Dose of jogging and long-term mortality: the Copenhagen City Heart Study."
Journal of American College of Cardiology. 2015.

Siebelt M, Groen HC, Koelewijn SJ, et. al.
"Increased physical activity severely induces osteoarthritic changes in knee joints with papain induced sulfate-glycosaminoglycan depleted cartilage."
Arthritis Research and Therapy. 2014 January.

Arbab-Zadeh A, Perhonen M, Howden E, et. al.
"Cardiac remodeling in response to 1 year of intensive endurance training."
Circulation. 2014 December.

Dangers of CrossFit Type Strength Training

Drum SN, Bellovary B, Jensen R, Moore M, Donath L.
"Perceived demands and post-exercise physical dysfunction in *CrossFit®* compared to an acsm based training session.»
Journal of Sports Medicine and Physical Fitness. 2016 Feb 12. [Epub ahead of print]

CrossFit® is considered an intense and extreme conditioning program that can cause overtraining and injury. Exertional Rhabdomyolysis - breakdown of muscle tissue - after *[CrossFit] has been reported . . . CrossFit®* leads to «very hard» perceived exertion causing detrimental post-exercise effects on muscle and ventilatory function in experienced athletes. Improved training progression with adequate *recovery schedules are needed to prevent severe muscle injury, such as Exertional Rhabdomyolysis.*

Knapik JJ.
"Extreme Conditioning Programs: Potential Benefits and Potential Risks."
Journal of Special Operations Medicine. 2015 Fall.

Several cases of rhabdomyolysis and cervical carotid artery dissections [both potentially deadly] have been reported during CrossFit training.

Cooperman, Stephanie.
"Getting Fit, Even if it Kills You"
New York Times | PHYSICAL CULTURE. (2005, December).Retrieved from http://www.nytimes.com/2005/12/22/fashion/thursdaystyles/getting-fit-even-if-it-kills-you.html?_r=0. Accessed February 28, 2016.

After 30 minutes, Mr. Anderson, a 38-year-old member of the {Tacoma, Washington S.W.A.T. team], left the [CrossFit] gym with his muscles sapped and [excruciating back pain] . . .That night he went to the emergency room, where doctors told him he had rhabdomyolysis, which is caused when muscle fiber breaks down and is released into the bloodstream, poisoning the kidneys. He spent six days in intensive care . . . [Greg Glassman], CrossFit's founder, does not discount his regimen's risks, even to those who are in shape and take the time to warm up their bodies before a session. "It can kill you," he said. 'I've always been completely honest about that.

Glassman, Greg. (Founder of *CrossFit*)
"*CrossFit* Induced Rhabdo"
CrossFit Journal Articles, Issue 38. (2005, October). Retrieved from http://library.CrossFit.com/free/pdf/38_05_cf_rhabdo.pdf. Accessed June 27, 2016.

With CrossFit we are dealing with what is known as exertional rhabdomyolysis. It can disable, maim, and even kill. To date we have seen five cases of exertional rhabdo associated with CrossFit workouts. Each case resulted in the hospitalization of the afflicted,.. The rhabdo we've seen has come from sessions of twenty minutes or less, with mild or low temperature and humidity. The victims were not excessively panting, straining, grunting, or otherwise expressing abnormal discomfort from the workouts. The athletes who came down with rhabdo turned in marginal CrossFit performances and showed no signs of discomfort that were out of the ordinary. They left their workouts seemingly no worse off than anyone else.

New York Post, News.com.au

"Can *CrossFit* Kill You?"

NYPost.com, New York Post/Living, (2013, September).Retrieved from http://nypost.com/2013/09/22/can-*CrossFit*-kill-you/. Accessed June 28, 2016.

Still entrenched in the CrossFit culture of deplete, endure, repeat, [a physical therapist and regular CrossFit-goer] quieted the alarms and stoically pressed on to go to work. It didn't take long to realise she not only couldn't bend her arms, they also had no strength . . . By that evening, her slender arms had continued to swell into plump hot dogs of ache and regret, and she was starting to come to the realisation that the morning's danger alarms were legitimate. The woman was diagnosed with acute rhabdomyolysis, and hospitalised for over a week . . . While in the hospital, she called to cancel her CrossFit membership. As is standard when something is cancelled, the CrossFit coach asked the reason for her decision. She replied, "I'm in the hospital." The instructor quickly asked, "Is it rhabdo?"

Robertson, Eric.

"*CrossFit*'s Dirty Little Secret"

Medium.com. (2013, September). Retrieved from https://medium.com/@ericrobertson/*CrossFits*-dirty-little-secret-97bcce70356d#.dqkkb2lhu.

[Potentially deadly] Rhabdomyolysis isn't a common condition, yet it's so commonly encountered in CrossFit that they have a cartoon about it, nonchalantly casting humor on something that should never happen.

Hak PT, Hodzovic E, Hickey B.

"The nature and prevalence of injury during *CrossFit* training."

Journal of Strength and Conditioning Research. 2013 Nov 22. [Epub ahead of print]

A total of 132 responses were collected with 97 (73.5%) having sustained an injury during CrossFit training. A total of 186 injuries were reported with 9 (7.0%) requiring surgical intervention.

Helm, Burt.

"Too Much Pain for *CrossFit* Gains?"

Men's Journal. Health & Fitness. (2014, March). Retrieved from http://www.mensjournal.com/health-fitness/exercise/too-much-pain-for-*CrossFit*-gains-20140326

Yuri Feito, a professor of exercise science at Kennesaw State University in Georgia (and a CrossFitter himself), analyzed data from 737 CrossFit participants and found that 51 percent had experienced an injury in the year prior – from minor sprains to muscle tears to broken fingers. Of those, 10 to 15 percent warranted a trip to the hospital.

Fell, James S.
"Is It Time To Admit That *CrossFit*'s Just Too Dangerous?"
The Good Men Project, goodmenproject.com. (2015, January). Retrieved from http://goodmenproject.com/featured-content/is-it-time-to-admit-that-*CrossFits*-just-too-dangerous-hesaid/. Accessed February 28 2016.

My main criticism of CrossFit in regards to injury is that it takes an activity — resistance training — that has an excellent safety record, and sometimes seems to relish making it unsafe.

Kliszczewicz B, Quindry CJ, Blessing LD, Oliver DG, Esco RM, Taylor JK.
"Acute Exercise and Oxidative Stress: *CrossFit*(™) vs. Treadmill Bout."
Journal of Human Kinetics. 2015 October.

Based on these findings, we interpret the oxidative stress outcomes of the current study to indicate that when closely matched for exercise time and intensity, the CrossFit™ bout "Cindy" produces a similar physiological stress response to a running modality.

Diamond D.
"Is *CrossFit* Safe? What '60 Minutes' Didn't Tell You"
Forbes / Pharma & Healthcare. (2015, May) Retrieved from http://www.forbes.com/sites/dandiamond/2015/05/11/is-*CrossFit*-good-for-you-what-60-minutes-didnt-say/#4d8ef1593845. Accessed June 27, 2016.

Writing at the New Yorker, cardiologist Lisa Rosenbaum last year examined the evidence into whether intense workouts are linked to risk of heart attack and stroke. She notes that one of the biggest truisms in health and diet is that too much of anything can ultimately backfire, and that some scientists believe moderate exercise is the best approach."Moderate" doesn't fit with the CrossFit mentality, though. One challenge, which 60 Minutes didn't mention at all, is a condition called rhabdomyolysis. It's generally rare, but involves muscle fibers being pushed to the point that they break down, enter the bloodstream, and lead to life-threatening kidney damage. And there have been a number of anecdotal examples tied to CrossFit, Kent Sepkowitz writes at the Daily Beast.

Easter M.
"4 Muscle Myths Debunked"
Men's Health, MensHealth.com, Fitness. (2013 January). Retrieved from http://www.menshealth.com/fitness/common-exercise-mistakes

You don't have to constantly add new moves and workouts to your routine to prevent your body from adapting. Actually, you want adaptation—this is how muscles grow. Sustain it with small weekly tweaks: Alter your grip, pace, or rest. That can help your muscles adapt over time, preventing plateaus, says Nick Tumminello, C.P.T., owner of Performance University in Fort Lauderdale.

Smith C.
"The Muscle Confusion Controversy -- Fact or Myth?
Fierce Strength, fiercestrength.com. (2014 October). Retrieved from http://www.fiercestrength.com/muscle-confusion/

When you search for information regarding the muscle confusion principle and whether it's a fact or a myth, most "experts" will tell you that there's absolutely no truth to it and that anyone who thinks it's a fact is dumber than a bag of rocks. They claim that the best results come from using progressive overload and sticking to a strict routine.

Joondeph SA, Joondeph BC.
"Retinal Detachment due to *CrossFit* Training Injury."
Case Reports in Ophthalmological Medicine. 2013.

Weisenthal BM, Beck CA, Maloney MD, DeHaven KE, Giordano BD.
"Injury Rate and Patterns Among *CrossFit* Athletes."
Orthopedic Journal of Sports Medicine. 2014 April.

Ozanian, Mike.
"How *CrossFit* Became A $4 Billion Brand"
Forbes / SportsMoney. Forbes.com. (2015, February 25). Retrieved from http://www.forbes.com/sites/mikeozanian/2015/02/25/how-*CrossFit*-became-a-4-billion-brand/#2a64742478c1. Accessed February 28, 2016.

Dangers of other High-Volume, High-Variability Strength Training Programs

Greco CC, Oliveira AS, Pereira MP, et. al.

"Improvements in metabolic and neuromuscular fitness after 12-week bodypump® training."

Journal of Strength and Conditioning Research. 2011 December.

> *No significant improvements in running aerobic fitness nor in body mass and body fat were observed.*

Borawski BJ.

"BodyPump Group Exercise: Does It Work or Not?"

BreakingMuscle.com. (2016, February). Retrieved from http://breakingmuscle.com/strength-conditioning/bodypump-group-exercise-does-it-work-or-not.

Casey DP, Beck DT, Braith RW.

"Progressive resistance training without volume increases does not alter arterial stiffness and aortic wave reflection."

Experimental Biology and Medicine (Maywood). 2007 October.

> *High-intensity, high-volume resistance training has been shown to increase arterial stiffness in young adults… These results suggest that a resistance training protocol consisting of progressively higher intensity without concurrent increases in training volume does not increase central or peripheral arterial stiffness or alter aortic pressure wave characteristics in young subjects.*

Cortez-Cooper MY, DeVan AE, Anton MM, et. al.

"Effects of high-intensity resistance training on arterial stiffness and wave reflection in women."

American Journal of Hypertension. 2005 July.

> *We concluded that a [high-intensity, high-volume strength and power training program] increases arterial stiffness and wave reflection in young healthy women. Our present interventional results are consistent with the previous cross-sectional studies in men in which [high-intensity strength and power training] is associated with arterial stiffening.*

Casey DP, Pierce GL, Howe KS, Mering MC, Braith RW.

"Effect of resistance training on arterial wave reflection and brachial artery reactivity in normotensive postmenopausal women."

European Journal of Applied Physiology. 2007 July.

> *This prospective, randomized study demonstrated that moderate intensity whole body resistance training in previously sedentary, normotensive postmenopausal women does not alter central aortic pressure wave reflection.*

Sparto PJ, Parnianpour M, Reinsel TE, Simon S

"The effect of fatigue on multijoint kinematics and load sharing during a repetitive lifting test.".

Spine (Phila Pa). 1997 November.

The significant decrease in postural stability and force generation capability because of the repetitive lifting task indicated a higher risk of injury in the presence of unexpected perturbation.

Goertzen M, Schöppe K, Lange G, Schulitz KP.

"[Injuries and damage caused by excess stress in bodybuilding and powerlifting]."

Sportverletz Sportschaden. 1989 March. German.

Powerlifting showed a twice as high injury rate as bodybuilding, probably of grounds of a more uniform training program.

Siewe J, Rudat J, Röllinghoff M, Schlegel UJ, Eysel P, Michael JW.

"Injuries and overuse syndromes in powerlifting."

International Journal of Sports Medicine. 2011 September.

Most commonly injured body regions were the shoulder, lower back and the knee. The use of weight belts increased the injury rate of the lumbar spine. Rate of injury to the upper extremities was significantly increased based on age >40 years and female gender.

Brady TA, Cahill BR, Bodnar LM.

"Weight training-related injuries in the high school athlete."

*American Journal Sports Medicine.*1982 January.

In 37 of the 80 athletes, it was difficult to pinpoint the cause of injury since the history revealed, in addition to weight training, either a program of running excessive mileage or participation in repetitive lap running in the gymnasium. The injuries of the remaining 43 athletes had a direct causal relationship to the weight training program. Twenty-nine developed lumbosacral pain. Seven of the 29 were hospitalized, and four required surgical treatment. Anterior iliac spine avulsion occurred in six cases, and laceration of the knee meniscus occurred as an initial injury in four athletes who required surgery. Four athletes developed a cervical sprain.

König M, Biener K.

"Sport-specific injuries in weightlifting."

Schweiz Z Sportmed. 1990 Apr;38(1):25-30. German.

202 instances of injuries related to weight lifting were reported. They affected the knees (25%), scapular girdle (22%), back (21%), wrist (12%) and the elbows (6%). In about 10% of the known cases of knee injury, the rest period without any sports activity lasted more than 28 days. More often than not, it was due to degenerative processes of the joint.

Kesidis N, Metaxas TI, Vrabas IS, et. al.

"Myosin heavy chain isoform distribution in single fibres of bodybuilders."

European Journal of Applied Physiology. 2008 July.

The percentage of fibres expressing [fast twitch and lower order fast twitch] was larger in bodybuilders . . . while [super fast twitch fibre expression] was completely absent.

Yoshizawa M, Maeda S, Miyaki A, et. al.
"Effect of 12 weeks of moderate-intensity resistance training on arterial stiffness: a randomised controlled trial in women aged 32-59 years."
British Journal of Sports Medicine. 2009 August.

This study found that moderate-intensity resistance training did not increase arterial stiffness in middle-aged women, which may have great importance for health promotion with resistance training.

Pansarasa O, Rinaldi C, Parente V, Miotti D, Capodaglio P, Bottinelli R.
"Resistance training of long-duration modulates force and unloaded shortening velocity of single muscle fibres of young women."
Journal of Electromyography and Kinesiology. 2009 October.

No muscle fibre hypertrophy *and no shift in [muscle fibre type] content was observed.*

Harber MP, Fry AC, Rubin MR, Smith JC, Weiss LW.
"Skeletal muscle and hormonal adaptations to circuit weight training in untrained men."
Scandinavian Journal of Medicine & Science in Sports. 2004 June.

[Circuit weight training] of the type used resulted in improved muscular strength and a tendency toward increased lean mass. Compared with other types of weight training, fewer adaptations of the muscle fibers were evident. This is likely due in part to the relatively low loads used with this type of resistance exercise.

Crewther BT, Cronin J, Keogh JW.
"The contribution of volume, technique, and load to single-repetition and total-repetition kinematics and kinetics in response to three loading schemes."
Journal of Strength and Conditioning Research. 2008 November.

The interaction of load, volume, and technique plays an important role in determining the mechanical responses (stimuli) afforded by these workouts. These findings may explain disparities cited within research, regarding the effectiveness of different loading strategies for hypertrophy, *maximal strength, and power adaptation.*

Greco CC, Oliveira AS, Pereira MP, et. al.
"Improvements in metabolic and neuromuscular fitness after 12-week bodypump® training."
Journal of Strength and Conditioning Research. 2011 December.

No significant improvements in running aerobic fitness nor in body mass and body fat were observed.

Brown EW, Kimball RG.
"Medical history associated with adolescent powerlifting."
*Pediatrics.*1983 November.

Fast Twitch and Super Fast Twitch Muscle Fibers

De Luca CJ, Contessa P.
"Hierarchical control of motor units in voluntary contractions."
Journal of Neurophysiology. 2012 January. Epub 2011 Oct 5.

This hierarchical control scheme describes a mechanism that provides an effective economy of force generation for the earlier-recruited lower force-twitch motor units [slow twitch fibers], and reduces the fatigue of later-recruited higher force-twitch motor units [fast and super fast twitch fibers] -- both characteristics being well suited for generating and sustaining force during the fight-or-flight response.

LeBrasseur NK, Walsh K, Arany Z.
"Metabolic benefits of resistance training and fast glycolytic skeletal muscle."
American Journal of Physiology, Endocrinology, and Metabolism. 2011 January. Review.

Recent work has shown that interventions such as resistance training, genetic alterations and pharmacological strategies that increase muscle mass and glycolytic capacity, and not necessarily oxidative competence, can improve body composition and systemic metabolism . . . In view of the coordinated responses of muscle, liver, [fat] tissue, and the vasculature highlighted in these models, it is likely that 1) increasing skeletal muscle mass will have favorable effects on affected tissues of [type 2 diabetes] and cardiovascular disease; and 2) a network of hormonal communication (e.g., myokines) exists between muscle and other metabolically important organs.

Akasaki Y, Ouchi N, Izumiya Y, Bernardo BL, Lebrasseur NK, Walsh K.
'Glycolytic fast-twitch muscle fiber restoration counters adverse age-related changes in body composition and metabolism."
Anatomical Society: Aging Cell. 2014 February.

Aging is associated with the development of insulin resistance, increased adiposity [body fat stores], and accumulation of ectopic lipid deposits in tissues and organs. Starting in mid-life there is a progressive decline in lean muscle mass associated with the preferential loss of glycolytic, fast-twitch [and super fast-twitch] myofibers . . . the loss of lean muscle mass is a significant contributor to the development of age-related metabolic dysfunction and interventions that preserve or restore fast/glycolytic muscle may delay the onset of metabolic disease.

Wang Y, Pessin JE.
"Mechanisms for fiber-type specificity of skeletal muscle atrophy."
Current Opinions in Clinical Nutrition and Metabolic Care. 2013 May. Review.

Fast-twitch glycolytic fibers are more vulnerable than slow-twitch oxidative fibers under a variety of atrophic conditions . . . nutrient-related atrophy such as cancer/aging cachexia, sepsis, and diabetes are more directed to [fast and super fast twitch] glycolytic fiber wasting.

Wilson J.
"Ask the Muscle Prof: How Do I Target Fast-Twitch Muscle Fibers?"
Bodybuilding.com. (2016, April). Retrieved from http://www.bodybuilding.com/fun/ask-the-muscle-prof-how-do-i-target-fast-twitch-muscle-fibers.html

Fast-twitch muscle fibers are indeed the largest and most powerful muscular movers in your body. Unfortunately, they're also neglected in most bodybuilders' programs. It's time to change this! . . . Studies show that individuals who neglect training in a heavier range will not program their nervous system to effectively recruit their largest [super] fast-twitch fibers. Along with intensity, fatigue is the second surefire way to increase fast-twitch muscle fiber recruitment. Your body's first impulse is to recruit slow-twitch fibers, but once you fatigue those fibers, it has to recruit fast-twitch fibers to do what is being asked of it.

Cannon J, Marino FE.
"Early-phase neuromuscular adaptations to high- and low-volume resistance training in untrained young and older women."
Journal of Sports Science. 2010 December.

These findings may have practical applications for the prescription of short-duration resistance training programmes to enhance muscle strength and achieve hypertrophic and non-hypertrophic adaptations in untrained women.

Schuenke MD, Herman JR, Gliders RM, et. al.
"Early-phase muscular adaptations in response to slow-speed versus traditional resistance-training regimens."
European Journal of Applied Physiology. 2012 October.

[The cross-sectional area] of fiber types I, IIA, and IIX [slow, fast and super fast twitch] increased in [traditional strength training]. In [super slow training], only the [cross-sectional area] of IIA and IIX [fast and super fast twitch] fibers increased . . . slow-speed strength training induced a greater adaptive response compared to training with a similar resistance at "normal" speed.

Westcott WL, Winett RA, Anderson ES, et. al.
"Effects of regular and slow speed resistance training on muscle strength."
Journal of Sports Medicine & Physcal Fitness. 2001 June.

Slower repetition speed may effectively increase intensity throughout the lifting phase while decreasing momentum. Super-Slow training is an effective method for middle-aged and older adults to increase strength. Although studies still need to be done with at-risk populations, repetition speed should be considered when prescribing resistance training.

Campos GE, Luecke TJ, Wendeln HK, et. al.
"Muscular adaptations in response to three different resistance-training regimens: specificity of repetition maximum training zones."
European Journal of Applied Physiology. 2002 November.

The low to intermediate repetition resistance-training programs induced a greater hypertrophic effect compared to the high repetition regimen . . . these data demonstrate that both physical performance and the associated physiological adaptations are linked to the intensity and number of repetitions performed, and thus lend support to the "strength-endurance continuum".

D'Antona G, Lanfranconi F, Pellegrino MA, et al.
"Skeletal muscle hypertrophy and structure and function of skeletal muscle fibres in male bodybuilders."
The Journal of Physiology. 2006 February.

In [bodybuilders] a preferential hypertrophy *of [fast twitch] and especially type 2X [super fast twitch] fibres was observed...[specific force per cross-sectional area] was significantly lower in [slow twitch] fibres from [bodybuilders] than in [slow twitch] fibres from [active untrained males] whereas both [fast twitch] and [super fast twitch] fibres were significantly stronger in [bodybuilders than in [active untrained males].*

Ahtiainen JP, Pakarinen A, Kraemer WJ, Häkkinen K.
"Acute hormonal responses to heavy resistance exercise in strength athletes versus non-athletes."
Canadian Journal of Applied Physiology. 2004 October.

These data suggest that, at least in experienced strength athletes, the forced-repetition protocol is a viable alternative to the more traditional maximum-repetition protocol and may even be a superior approach.

Goto K, Ishii N, Kizuka T, Takamatsu K.
"The impact of metabolic stress on hormonal responses and muscular adaptations."
Medicine and Science in Sports and Exercise. 2005 June.

The [no rest between reps within sets] regimen induced strong lactate, growth hormone, epinephrine, and norepinephrine responses, whereas the [rest between reps within sets] regimen did not . . . These results suggest that exercise-induced metabolic stress is associated with acute Growth Hormone, Epinephrine, and Norepinephrine responses and chronic muscular adaptations following resistance training.

Fry AC.
"The role of resistance exercise intensity on muscle fibre adaptations."
Sports Medicine. 2004. Review.

When competitive lifters were compared, those typically utilising the heaviest loads (> or =90% [1 rep maximum]), that is weightlifters and powerlifters, exhibited a preferential hypertrophy *of [fast and super fast twitch] fibres when compared with bodybuilders who appear to equally* hypertrophy *both [slow twitch] and [fast twitch] fibres. These data suggest that maximal* hypertrophy *occurs with loads from 80-95% [of the 1 rep maximum].*

Gasier HG, Riechman SE, Wiggs MP, Buentello A, Previs SF, Fluckey JD.
"Cumulative responses of muscle protein synthesis are augmented with chronic resistance exercise training."
Acta Physiologica (Oxf). 2011 March.

The present study demonstrates that anabolic responses to [high-intensity low volume resistance exercise] are still evident after chronic [training], primarily in muscle composed of fast-twitch fibres.

Pearson SJ, Young A, Macaluso A, et al.
"Muscle function in elite master weightlifters."
Journal of Medicine & Science in Sports & Exercise. 2002 July.

The absolute differences between the weightlifters and [non-trained healthy controls] were such that an 85-yr-old weightlifter was as powerful as a 65-yr-old control subject. This would therefore represent an apparent age advantage of approximately 20 yr for the weightlifters.

Nilwik R, Snijders T, Leenders M, et al.
"The decline in skeletal muscle mass with aging is mainly attributed to a reduction in type II muscle fiber size."
Experimental Gerontology. 2013 May.

Reduced muscle mass with aging is mainly attributed to smaller type II [fast and super fast twitch] muscle fiber size . . . the increase in muscle mass following prolonged resistance type exercise training can be attributed entirely to specific type II [fast and super fast twitch] muscle fiber hypertrophy.

Mangine GT, Hoffman JR, Gonzalez AM, et. al.
"The effect of training volume and intensity on improvements in muscular strength and size in resistance-trained men."
Physiological Reports. 2015 August.

This investigation compared the effect of high-volume versus high-intensity resistance training on stimulating changes in muscle size and strength in resistance-trained men… It appears that high-intensity resistance training stimulates greater improvements in some measures of strength and hypertrophy *in resistance-trained men during a short-term training period.*

Bickel CS et al.
"Time course of molecular responses of human skeletal muscle to acute bouts of resistance exercise."
Journal of Applied Physiology. (2005).

These results, along with a number of other published observations, indicate that the mechanisms that regulate the adaptation of skeletal muscle to increased loading respond on a relatively short time scale and that these responses may be useful in evaluating [resistance exercise] training variables with high temporal resolution.

Holt NC, Wakeling JM, Biewener AA.
"The effect of fast and slow motor unit activation on whole-muscle mechanical performance: the size principle may not pose a mechanical paradox."
Proceedings, Biological Sciences, Royal Society. 2014 April.

The findings presented here suggest that recruitment according to the size principle, where slow motor units are activated first and faster ones recruited as demand increases, may not pose a mechanical paradox, as has been previously suggested.

Sale DG.
"Influence of exercise and training on motor unit activation."
Exercise and Sport Sciences Review. 1987. Review.

The recruitment order of [muscle fiber motor units] according to size is based on the inverse relation between susceptibility to discharge and motoneuron size. Thus, for evenly distributed and increasing excitatory synaptic input to a pool of motoneurons, smaller motoneurons will begin to fire before larger motoneurons. This arrangement ensures, for example, that the small, fatigue-resistant [muscle fiber motor units] will be preferentially activated in prolonged, low-intensity exercise, to which these units are most suited. In brief, intense exercise, the associated greater excitatory input will also recruit the large [muscle fiber motor units], taking advantage of their greater strength and contractile speed. A frequent question is whether rapid, ballistic or explosive contractions and movements are associated with selective or preferential recruitment of large, fast twitch [muscle fiber motor units]. There is evidence of synaptic input systems that preferentially excite large, fast twitch [muscle fiber motor units] and inhibit small twitch [muscle fiber motor units]; however, the majority of evidence from human experiments indicates that the recruitment order is not reversed in ballistic contractions.

Sokoloff AJ, Siegel SG, Cope TC.
"Recruitment order among motoneurons from different motor nuclei."
Journal of Neurophysiology. 1999 May.

These findings demonstrate for the first time, that the size principle can extend beyond the boundaries of a single muscle but does not coordinate all coactive muscles in a limb.

Cope TC, Sokoloff AJ.
"Orderly recruitment among motoneurons supplying different muscles."
Journal of Physiology, Paris. 1999 January.

The principle acting to organize the recruitment of motor units within muscles is the size principle, whereby the first motor units to be recruited have the smallest values for axonal conduction velocity and contractile force, and are the slowest to contract and fatigue. Here we consider the possibility that the size principle applies in the recruitment of motor units across muscles, i.e., that regardless of their muscles of origin, active motor units are recruited in rank order, for example, from low to high conduction velocity.

Logan GR, Harris N, Duncan S, Plank LD, Merien F, Schofield G.
"Low-Active Male Adolescents: A Dose Response to High-Intensity Interval Training."
Medicine and Science in Sports and Exercise. 2015 October. [Epub ahead of print]
Low-active adolescent males performing a single HIIT set twice weekly, in addition to one resistance training session, gained meaningful improvements in fitness and body composition. Performing additional HIIT sets provided no additional improvements to those of the lowest dose in this study.
Di Blasio A, Izzicupo P, Tacconi L, et. al.
"Acute and delayed effects of high-intensity interval resistance training organization on cortisol and testosterone production."
Journal of Sports Medicine and Physical Fitness. 2014 November. [Epub ahead of print]
In order to offer a more complete training, resistance exercises have been added to HIIT (HIIRT [high-intensity interval resistance training]) . . . Even if exercises, load, and number of repetitions were maintained fixed, exercise order, structured recovery and speed of execution determined different acute and prolonged effects.
Koutedakis Y, Sharp NC.
"Thigh-muscles strength training, dance exercise, dynamometry, and anthropometry in professional ballerinas."
Journal of Strength and Conditioning Research. 2004 November.
These results suggest that supplementary strength training for hamstring and quadriceps muscles is beneficial to professional ballerinas and their dancing; weaker individuals are more likely to benefit from such regimens than their stronger counterparts, whereas increases in thigh-muscle strength do not alter selected aesthetic components.
Bandy WD, Lovelace-Chandler V, McKitrick-Bandy B.
"Adaptation of skeletal muscle to resistance training."
Journal of Orthopedic and Sports Physical Therapy. 1990.
Changes in nervous system input resulting from resistance training include recruitment of an increased number and firing rate of motor units, increased reflex potentiation, and improved synchronization.
Unhjem RJ, Nygård M, van den Hoven LT, Sidhu SK, Hoff J, Wang E.
"Lifelong strength training mitigates the age-related decline in efferent drive."
Journal of Applied Physiology. 2016 June.
These observations suggest that lifelong strength training has a protective effect against age-related attenuation of efferent drive. In contrast, no beneficial effect seems to derive from habitual recreational activity, indicating that strength training may be particularly beneficial for counteracting age-related loss of neuromuscular function.
Pincivero DM, Campy RM, Karunakara RG.
"The effects of rest interval and resistance training on quadriceps femoris muscle. Part II: EMG and perceived exertion."
The Journal of Sports Medicine and Physical Fitness. 2004 September.

Milner-Brown HS, Stein RB, Yemm R.
"The orderly recruitment of human motor units during voluntary isometric contractions."
Journal of Physiology. 1973 April.
Contessa P, De Luca CJ.
"Neural control of muscle force: indications from a simulation model."
Journal of Neurophysiology. 2013 March.
Rana SR, Chleboun GS, Gilders RM, et. al.
"Comparison of early phase adaptations for traditional strength and endurance, and low velocity resistance training programs in college-aged women."
Journal of Strength and Conditioning Research. 2008 January.
Gentil P, Oliveira E, de Araújo Rocha Júnior V, do Carmo J, Bottaro M
Effects of exercise order on upper-body muscle activation and exercise performance.
Journal of Strength and Conditioning Research. 2007 November.

Fat Burning, Metabolism, and Insulin Sensitivity

Akasaki Y, Ouchi N, Izumiya Y, Bernardo BL, LeBrasseur NK, Walsh K.
'Glycolytic fast-twitch muscle fiber restoration counters adverse age-related changes in body composition and metabolism."
Anatomical Society: Aging Cell. 2014 February.

Aging is associated with the development of insulin resistance, increased adiposity [body fat stores], and accumulation of ectopic lipid deposits in tissues and organs. Starting in mid-life there is a progressive decline in lean muscle mass associated with the preferential loss of glycolytic, fast-twitch [and super fast-twitch] myofibers . . . the loss of lean muscle mass is a significant contributor to the development of age-related metabolic dysfunction and interventions that preserve or restore fast/glycolytic muscle may delay the onset of metabolic disease.

LeBrasseur NK, Walsh K, Arany Z.
"Metabolic benefits of resistance training and fast glycolytic skeletal muscle."
American Journal of Physiology, Endocrinology and Metabolism. 2011 January. Review.

Skeletal muscle exhibits remarkable plasticity with respect to its metabolic properties. Recent work has shown that interventions such as resistance training, genetic alterations and pharmacological strategies that increase muscle mass and glycolytic capacity, and not necessarily oxidative [aerobic] competence, can improve body composition and systemic metabolism . . . Collectively, these data suggest that even modest increases in skeletal muscle mass, the growth of [fast and super fast twitch] glycolytic fibers, and modest changes in glycolytic capacity can have remarkable effects on metabolic homeostasis. They also suggest that interventions targeting skeletal muscle may directly or indirectly alter the metabolic profile of other organs affected by insulin resistance and [type 2 diabetes mellitus]. It is now evident that skeletal muscle is a key node in the powerful and complex cross-talk between metabolically active tissues . . . In view of the coordinated responses of muscle, liver, adipose tissue [fat], and the vasculature highlighted in these models, it is likely that 1) increasing skeletal muscle mass will have favorable effects on affected tissues of [type 2 diabetes mellitus] and cardiovascular disease; and 2) a network of hormonal communication exists between muscle and other metabolically important organs . . . It is now recommended that resistance training be incorporated into the exercise regimen of patients with [type 2 diabetes mellitus]. Similarly, complementary resistance training is also recommended for patients with cardiovascular disease. Although a growing body of experimental evidence suggests that resistance training improves metabolic homeostasis in a manner distinct from endurance training, our understanding of how this precisely occurs is rudimentary.

Tibana RA, Navalta J, Bottaro M, et al.
"Effects of eight weeks of resistance training on the risk factors of metabolic syndrome in overweight /obese women - "A Pilot Study"."
Diabetology and Metabolic Syndrome. 2013 February.

A [resistance training] program without caloric restriction promotes an increase on muscle thickness and strength, with no effects on risk factors of [metabolic syndrome] in overweight/obese women.

Hunter GR, Byrne NM, Sirikul B, et al.

"Resistance training conserves fat-free mass and resting energy expenditure following weight loss."

Obesity (Silver Spring). 2008 May.

Following weight loss in both African American and European American, resistance training conserved fat-free mass, resting energy expenditure, and strength fitness when compared to women who aerobic trained or did not train.

Cullinen K, Caldwell M.

"Weight training increases fat-free mass and strength in untrained young women."

Journal of the American Dietetic Association. 1998 April.

A moderate-intensity weight training program increased strength and fat-free mass and decreased body fat in normal-weight young women. Favorable changes in body composition were obtained without restricting food intake.

Abernethy PJ, Jürimäe J, Logan PA, Taylor AW, Thayer RE.

"Acute and chronic response of skeletal muscle to resistance exercise."

Journal of Sports Medicine. 1994 January. Review.

Lipid metabolism may be of some significance in bodybuilding type activity. Thus, not surprisingly, oxidative enzyme adaptations appear to be affected by the structure and perhaps the modality of resistance training. The dilution of mitochondrial volume and endogenous lipid densities appears mainly because of fibre hypertrophy.

Burt DG, Lamb K, Nicholas C, Twist C.

"Effects of exercise-induced muscle damage on resting metabolic rate, sub-maximal running and post-exercise oxygen consumption."

European Journal of Sports Science. 2014.

Exercise-induced muscle damage (EIMD), described as the acute weakness of the musculature after unaccustomed eccentric exercise, increases oxidative metabolism at rest and during endurance exercise.

Hazell TJ, Islam H, Townsend LK, Schmale MS, Copeland JL.

"Effects of exercise intensity on plasma concentrations of appetite-regulating hormones: Potential mechanisms."

ScienceDirect, Appetite. 2016 March. Epub 2015 Dec 22. Review.

Overall, changes in appetite-regulating hormones following acute exercise appear to be intensity-dependent, with increasing intensity leading to a greater suppression of orexigenic [appetite-stimulating] signals and greater stimulation of anorexigenic [appetite-inhibiting] signals.

Schofield KL, Rehrer NJ, Perry TL, Ross A, Andersen JL, Osborne H.
"Insulin and fiber type in the offspring of T2DM subjects with resistance training and detraining." *Medicine and Science in Sports and Exercise.* 2012 December.

Resistance training has a significant effect on insulin responses and may reduce future risk of type 2 diabetes mellitus among [familial insulin resistant individuals].

Schwarz NA, Rigby BR, La Bounty P, Shelmadine B, Bowden RG.
"A review of weight control strategies and their effects on the regulation of hormonal balance." *Journal of Nutrition and Metabolism.* 2011.

Karstoft K, Winding K, Knudsen SH, et al.
"Mechanisms behind the superior effects of interval vs continuous training on glycaemic control in individuals with type 2 diabetes: a randomised controlled trial."
Diabetologia. 2014 October.

Dunstan DW, Daly RM, Owen N, et al.
"High-intensity resistance training improves glycemic control in older patients with type 2 diabetes."
Diabetes Care. 2002 October.

Ivy JL.
"Role of exercise training in the prevention and treatment of insulin resistance and non-insulin-dependent diabetes mellitus."
Journal of Sports Medicine. 1997 November. Review.

Christ-Roberts CY, Pratipanawatr T, Pratipanawatr W, et. al.
"Exercise training increases glycogen synthase activity and GLUT4 expression but not insulin signaling in overweight nondiabetic and type 2 diabetic subjects."
Metabolism. 2004 September.

Opitz D, Lenzen E, Schiffer T, et. al.
"Endurance training alters skeletal muscle MCT contents in T2DM men."
International Journal of Sports Medicine. 2014 December.

Ishiguro H, Kodama S, Horikawa C, et al.
"In Search of the Ideal Resistance Training Program to Improve Glycemic Control and its Indication for Patients with Type 2 Diabetes Mellitus: A Systematic Review and Meta-Analysis." *Journal of Sports Medicine.* 2016 January.

American Diabetes Association staff
"Statistics About Diabetes"
Diabetes.org. (2014, June). Retrieved from http://www.diabetes.org/diabetes-basics/statistics/

Heart and Cardiovascular Health

Speretta GF, Silva AA, Vendramini RC, et. al.

"Resistance training prevents the cardiovascular changes caused by high-fat diet."

Life Science. 2016 Jan 8. [Epub ahead of print]

> *Resistance training prevented the cardiovascular and inflammatory responses (increases in tumoral necrosis factor-α and interleukin-1β) . . . Resistance training prevented obesity-induced cardiovascular disorders simultaneously with reduced inflammatory responses and modifications.*

de Freitas Brito A, Brasileiro-Santos Mdo S, Coutinho de Oliveira CV, et. al.

"High-Intensity Resistance Exercise Promotes Postexercise Hypotension Greater than Moderate Intensity and Affects Cardiac Autonomic Responses in Women Who Are Hypertensive."

Journal of Strength and Conditioning Research. 2015 December.

> *These results suggest that resistance exercise of higher intensity promoted greater postexercise hypotension accompanied by greater increases in forearm blood flow, vasodilator response, heart rate, and cardiac sympathovagal balance.*

McGuff D, Little J.

"*Body by Science: A Research Based Program for Strength Training,* Bodybuilding, *and Complete Fitness in 12 Minutes a Week.*" New York: McGraw-Hill, 2009. Print. (p.35-36)

> *Strength training is actually the best way to train the cardiovascular system precisely because, unlike what we refer to as "aerobics," strength training actually involves and stimulates all of the components of metabolism . . . This includes the metabolism that goes on in the cytosol (the liquid portion of the cell and in the absence of oxygen) and the metabolism that occurs in the mitochondria (i.e., in the presence of oxygen).*

Storey A, Smith HK.

"Unique aspects of competitive weightlifting: performance, training and physiology."

Sports Medicine. 2012 September. Review.

> *Weightlifting training and competition has been shown to induce significant structural and functional adaptations of the cardiovascular system. The collective evidence shows that these adaptations are physiological as opposed to pathological. Finally, the acute exercise-induced testosterone, cortisol and growth hormone responses of weightlifters have similarities to that of following conventional strength and* hypertrophy *protocols involving large muscle mass exercises.*

Pollock ML, Franklin BA, Balady GJ, et. al.

"AHA Science Advisory. Resistance exercise in individuals with and without cardiovascular disease: benefits, rationale, safety, and prescription: An advisory from the Committee on Exercise, Rehabilitation, and Prevention, Council on

Clinical Cardiology, American Heart Association; Position paper endorsed by the American College of Sports Medicine."

American Heart Association: *Circulation*. 2000 February. Review.

*Although resistance training has long been accepted as a means for developing and maintaining muscular strength, endurance, power, and muscle mass (*hypertrophy*), its beneficial relationship to health factors and chronic disease has been recognized only recently. Prior to 1990, resistance training was not a part of the recommended guidelines for exercise training and rehabilitation for either the* American Heart Association *or the American College of Sports Medicine (ACSM).*

Morra EA, Zaniqueli D, Rodrigues SL, et. al.

"Long-term intense resistance training in men is associated with preserved cardiac structure/function, decreased aortic stiffness, and lower central augmentation pressure."

Journal of Hypertension. 2014 Feb.

There have been contradictory reports regarding resistance exercise and central arterial compliance. The American Heart Association *has recommended its [long term resistance training] use in preventing/treating cardiovascular diseases . . . Long-term resistance training in men is associated with preserved cardiac structure/function, decreased aortic stiffness, and lower cAP [central augmentation index].*

American Heart Association

"Can Strength Training Help with Blood Pressure?"

Heart.org: Heart Insight Magazine. (2015, Winter). Retrieved from http://heartinsight.heart.org/Winter-2015/Can-Strength-Training-Help-with-Blood-Pressure/.

Studies have reported several benefits of resistance training — or weight training — including strengthening of bones, muscles and connective tissues (tendons and ligaments). Additionally, weight training may lower your risk of injury. And increased muscle mass may make it easier for you to burn calories and maintain a healthy weight. You'll feel better and stronger and want to do more . . . Researchers reported that only four weeks of [strength training] exercises resulted in a 10 percent drop in both blood pressure measures. Aerobic exercise, however, has shown evidence of reducing systolic and diastolic blood pressure by an average of 2 to 5 mm Hg and 1 to 4 mm Hg, respectively.

Burgomaster KA, Hughes SC, Heigenhauser GJ, Bradwell SN, Gibala MJ.

"Six sessions of sprint interval training increases muscle oxidative potential and cycle endurance capacity in humans."

Journal of Applied Physiology. 2005 June.

Sprint training dramatically improves endurance capacity during a fixed-workload test in which the majority of cellular energy is derived from aerobic metabolism. These data demonstrate that brief repeated bouts of very intense exercise can rapidly stimulate improvements in muscle oxidative potential that are comparable to or higher than previously reported aerobic-based training studies of similar duration.

McGuff D, Little J. (p.17) (see note 8 for bibliography)

Your heart and lungs cannot tell whether you're working your muscles intensely for thirty seconds on a stationary bike or working them intensely on a leg press. The heart and lungs know only about energy requirements, which they dutifully attempt to meet. Four thirty second intervals of high-intensity muscular exertion is four thirty-second intervals of high-intensity muscular exertion, whether that takes place exclusively in the lower body, as in stationary cycling, or in both the upper and lower body, as in resistance exercise. In either scenario, it is mechanical work by muscles that is the passkey to the aerobic and other metabolic machinery within the body's cells.

Moradi F.

"Changes of Serum Adiponectin and Testosterone Concentrations Following Twelve Weeks Resistance Training in Obese Young Men."

Asian Journal of Sports Medicine. 2015 December.

It is recommended that obese young men do resistance training to benefit useful decreasing/preventive effects of this type of training against the risks of cardiovascular diseases and diabetes.

American Heart Association

"Weight Training After a Stroke"

StrokeAssociation.org. Life After Stroke. (2014, January). Retrieved from http://www.strokeassociation.org/STROKEORG/LifeAfterStroke/RegainingIndependence/PhysicalChallenges/Weight-Training-After-Stroke_UCM_309780_Article.jsp#.VrT6KfkrLcs.

Many healthcare professionals are concerned that resistance training can have a detrimental effect on spastic muscles. A recent review of the professional literature found no scientific evidence to back up that position. In fact, in a recent article in NeuroRehabilitation, investigators determined that targeted strength training in patients with muscle weakness due to strokes significantly increased muscle power without any negative effects on spasticity.

Badics E, Whitmann A, Rupp M, Stabauer B, Zifko UA.

"Systematic muscle building exercises in the rehabilitation of stroke patients"

Neurorehabilitation. (2002). vol. 17, no. 3, pp. 211-214. Retrieved from http://content.iospress.com/articles/neurorehabilitation/nre00143. Accessed February, 28, 2016.

The results of this study showed that targeted strength training significantly increased muscle power in patients with muscle weakness of central origin without any negative effects on spasticity.

Hagerman FC, Walsh SJ, Staron RS, et al.

"Effects of high-intensity resistance training on untrained older men. I. Strength, cardiovascular, and metabolic responses."

The Journals of Gerontology, 2000, July.

The results show that skeletal muscle in older, untrained men will respond with significant strength gains accompanied by considerable increases in fiber size and capillary density. Maximal working capacity, VO2max, and serum lipid profiles also benefited from high-intensity resistance training... Older men may not only tolerate very high-intensity workloads but will exhibit intramuscular, cardiovascular, and metabolic changes similar to younger subjects.

Liou K, Ho S, Fildes J, Ooi SY.

"High-intensity Interval versus Moderate Intensity Continuous Training in Patients with Coronary Artery Disease: A Meta-analysis of Physiological and Clinical Parameters."

Heart and Lung Circulation. 2016 February. Epub 2015 Jul 22.

High-intensity interval training improves the mean VO2peak in patients with Coronary Artery Disease more than moderate intensity continuous training

Gibala MJ, Little JP, van Essen M, et. al.

"Short-term sprint interval versus traditional endurance training: similar initial adaptations in human skeletal muscle and exercise performance."

Journal of Physiology. 2006 September.

These data demonstrate that [sprint interval training] is a time-efficient strategy to induce rapid adaptations in skeletal muscle and exercise performance that are comparable to [high-intensity low volume resistance exercise] in young active men.

Ferketich AK, Kirby TE, Alway SE.

"Cardiovascular and muscular adaptations to combined endurance and strength training in elderly women."

Acta Physiologica Scandanavica. 1998 November.

Greater improvements in sub-maximal time to fatigue and strength is achieved when resistance training is added to an aerobic training programme in healthy elderly women.

Burgomaster KA, Heigenhauser GJ, Gibala MJ.

"Effect of short-term sprint interval training on human skeletal muscle carbohydrate metabolism during exercise and time-trial performance."

Journal of Applied Physiology. 2006 June.

The present data confirm the novel results from our laboratory's recent study (above) that showed skeletal muscle oxidative capacity can be enhanced by a brief 2-wk period of sprint training, equivalent to only 16 min of very intense exercise spread over a total time commitment of ~2.5 h.

Little JP, Safdar A, Wilkin GP, Tarnopolsky MA, Gibala MJ.

"A practical model of low-volume high-intensity interval training induces mitochondrial biogenesis in human skeletal muscle: potential mechanisms."

Journal of Physiology. 2010 March.

A practical model of low volume high-intensity training is a potent stimulus for increasing skeletal muscle mitochondrial capacity and improving exercise performance.

Burgomaster KA, Howarth KR, Phillips SM, et. al.
"Similar metabolic adaptations during exercise after low volume sprint interval and traditional endurance training in humans."
Journal of Physiology. 2008 January.

Data suggest that high-intensity interval training is a time-efficient strategy to increase skeletal muscle oxidative capacity and induce specific metabolic adaptations during exercise that are comparable to traditional endurance training.

Sedano S, Marín PJ, Cuadrado G, Redondo JC.
"Concurrent training in elite male runners: the influence of strength versus muscular endurance training on performance outcomes."
Journal of Strength and Conditioning Research. 2013 September.

We can conclude that concurrent training for both [the high-intensity strength training] and [the low-intensity strength training] groups [both of which continued endurance training] led to improved maximal strength, running economy, and peak velocity with no significant effects on the VO2 kinetics pattern. The [high-intensity strength training group] also seems to show improvements in 3-km time trial tests.

Aagaard P, Andersen JL.
"Effects of strength training on endurance capacity in top-level endurance athletes."
Scandinavian Journal of Medicine and Science in Sports. 2010 October. Review.

It is concluded that strength training can lead to enhanced long-term (>30 min) and short-term (<15 min) endurance capacity both in well-trained individuals and highly trained top-level endurance athletes...

Prista A, Macucule CF, Queiroz AC, et. al.
"A bout of resistance exercise following the 2007 AHA guidelines decreases asleep blood pressure in Mozambican men."
Journal of Strength and Conditioning Research. 2013 March.

Ricci-Vitor AL, Bonfim R, Fosco LC, et. al.
"Influence of the resistance training on heart rate variability, functional capacity and muscle strength in the chronic obstructive pulmonary disease."
European Journal of Physical and Rehabilitation Medicine. 2013 December.

Mathes S, Mester J, Bloch W, Wahl P.
"Impact of high-intensity and high-volume exercise on short-term perturbations in the circulating fraction of different cell types."
Journal of Sports Medicine and Physical Fitness. 2015 Nov 26. [Epub ahead of print]

Toth MJ, Miller MS, VanBuren P et. al.
"Resistance training alters skeletal muscle structure and function in human heart failure: effects at the tissue, cellular and molecular levels."
Journal of Physiology. 2012 March.

Ramos JS, Dalleck LC, Tjonna AE, Beetham KS, Coombes JS.
"The impact of high-intensity interval training versus moderate-intensity continuous training on vascular function: a systematic review and meta-analysis."

Sports Medicine. 2015 May. Review.

Little JP, Jung ME, Wright AE, Wright W, Manders RJ.

"Effects of high-intensity interval exercise versus continuous moderate-intensity exercise on postprandial glycemic control assessed by continuous glucose monitoring in obese adults." *Applied Physiology Nutrition and Metabolism*. 2014 July. Epub 2014 Feb 18.

Ahmadizad S, Avansar AS, Ebrahim K, Avandi M, Ghasemikaram M.

"The effects of short-term high-intensity interval training vs. moderate-intensity continuous training on plasma levels of nesfatin-1 and inflammatory markers."

Hormone Molecular Biology and Clinical Investigation. 2015 March.

Bonsu B, Terblanche E.

"The training and detraining effect of high-intensity interval training on post-exercise hypotension in young overweight/obese women."

European Journal of Applied Physiology. 2016 January. Epub 2015 Aug 21.

Duffell LD, Rowlerson AM, Donaldson Nde N, Harridge SD, Newham DJ.

"Effects of endurance and strength-directed electrical stimulation training on the performance and histological properties of paralyzed human muscle: a pilot study."

Muscle & Nerve. 2010 November.

Aagaard P, Andersen JL, Bennekou M, et. al.

"Effects of resistance training on endurance capacity and muscle fiber composition in young top-level cyclists."

Scandinavian Journal of Medicine and Science in Sports. 2011 December.

Hickson RC, Dvorak BA, Gorostiaga EM, Kurowski TT, Foster C.

'Potential for strength and endurance training to amplify endurance performance."

Journal of Applied Physiology. 1988 November.

Hormone and Anti-Aging Research

Herbert P, Grace FM, Sculthorpe NF.
"Exercising caution: prolonged recovery from a single session of high-intensity interval training in older men."
Journal of the American Geriatrics Society. 2015 April.

Extremely short-duration high-intensity training substantially improves the physical function and self-reported health status of elderly adults.

Walker S, Santolamazza F, Kraemer W, Häkkinen K.
"Effects of prolonged hypertrophic resistance training on acute endocrine responses in young and older men."
Journal of Aging and Physical Activity. 2015 April.

The present study investigated changes in acute serum hormone responses to a resistance exercise bout following [twenty weeks] of hypertrophic resistance training in young and older men . . . in general, young men demonstrate greater adaptability within the endocrine system compared with older men. However, adaptability in growth hormone response was associated with larger training-induced gains independent of age.

Paillard T.
"Neuromuscular system and aging: involutions and implications."
Geriatr. Psychol. and Neuropsychiatr.Vieil. 2013 December. Review. French.

In aged humans, the number of muscle fibers and motor units decreases. The remaining motor units lose their functionality (decrease of the discharge frequency, greater fluctuation of the discharge) particularly those which contain type II [fast and super fast twitch] fibers . . . strength training counteracts the noxious effects mentioned above by generating muscular hypertrophy *thanks to a reactive increase in the production of anabolic hormones.*

Häkkinen K, Pakarinen A, Kraemer WJ, Häkkinen A, Valkeinen H, Alen M.
"Selective muscle hypertrophy, changes in EMG and force, and serum hormones during strength training in older women."
Journal of Applied Physiology. 2001 August.

The magnitude and time duration of the acute growth hormone response [to strength training protocols] may be important physiological indicators of anabolic adaptations during strength training even in older women.

Wahl P, Mathes S, Köhler K, Achtzehn S, Bloch W, Mester J.
"Acute metabolic, hormonal, and psychological responses to different endurance training protocols."
Hormone and Metabolic Research. 2013 October.

In conclusion, the results suggest that High-intensity [Low Volume] Training promotes anabolic processes more than High-volume Endurance Training, due to higher increases of human growth hormone, testosterone, and the testosterone/cortisol ratio. It can be speculated that the acute hormonal increase and the metabolic perturbations might play a positive role in optimizing training adaptation and in eliciting health benefits as it has been shown by previous long term training studies using similar exercise protocols.

American Heart Association

"Health Benefits of Weight Training for Women"

GoRedForWomen.org. (2016, February). Retrieved from https://www.goredforwomen.org/live-healthy/heart-healthy-exercises/health-benefits-of-weight-training-for-women/. Accessed April 28, 2016.

The main hormone that contributes to increasing muscle size is testosterone, which is typically associated with the male body, but isn't generally as abundant in females. In order for a woman to develop "bodybuilder" muscles, it would be necessary to exceed the recommended amount of strength training, take hormones and focus intensely on increasing muscle mass. However, the average woman who lifts moderate weights will not experience that type of muscle growth.

Rubin DA, Pham HN, Adams ES, et. al.

"Endocrine response to acute resistance exercise in obese versus lean physically active men." *European Journal of Applied Physiology.* 2015, June.

These findings suggest that [obesity] does not appear to negatively affect the immediate Growth Hormone and Testosterone responses to Resistance Training in active males...

Chia-Liang T, Chun-Hao W, Chien-Yu P, Fu-Chen C.

"The effects of long-term resistance exercise on the relationship between neurocognitive performance and GH, IGF-1, and homocysteine levels in the elderly." *Frontiers in Behavioral Neuroscience.* 2015.

In conclusion, increasing the level of physical activity via high-intensity [low volume] resistance exercise could assist in lowering the rate of age-related neurocognitive decreases in healthy elderly males. In addition, increases in basal Insulin-like Growth Factor-1 levels achieved via such an exercise protocol could have positive effects on both neuropsychological (i.e., resistance training) and neuroelectric (i.e., P3b amplitude) performance in the elderly. This study's findings imply that healthy elderly individuals who regularly engage in resistance exercise might delay the onset of age-related decline in executive functions, and that this protective effect may be modulated by the growth factor-IGF-1.

Luk HY, Kraemer WJ, Szivak TK, et al.

"Acute resistance exercise stimulates sex-specific dimeric immunoreactive growth hormone responses."

Growth Hormone and IGF Research. 2015, June.

Heavy resistance exercise increases immunoreactive growth hormone concentrations in men and women, with larger increases in women and more sustained response in men. The physiological significance of a sexually dimorphic growth hormone response adds to the growing literature on aggregate growth hormone and may be explained by differences in sex hormones and the structure of the growth hormone cell network.

McCaulley GO, McBride JM, Cormie P, et al.

"Acute hormonal and neuromuscular responses to hypertrophy, strength and power type resistance exercise."

European Journal of Applied Physiology. 2009 March. Epub 2008 Dec 9.

These data indicate that significant acute increases in hormone concentrations are limited to hypertrophy *type protocols [i.e. 4 sets of 10 repetitions at 75% of max] independent of the volume of work completed. In addition, it appears the* hypertrophy *protocol also elicits a unique pattern of muscle activity as well. Resistance exercise protocols of varying intensity and rest periods elicit strikingly different acute neuroendocrine responses which indicate a unique physiological stimulus.*

Wahl P, Zinner C, Achtzehn S, Bloch W, Mester J.

"Effect of high- and low-intensity exercise and metabolic acidosis on levels of GH, IGF-I, IGFBP-3 and cortisol."

Journal of the Growth Hormone Research Society. 2010 October.

Serum cortisol and human growth hormone concentrations were significantly increased 10 min post exercise in High-intensity Training interventions. High-volume Endurance Training showed no significant effects on cortisol, human growth hormone, insulin-like growth factor-1, and Insulin-like growth factor-binding protein-3 levels.

Ahtiainen JP, Pakarinen A, Kraemer WJ, Häkkinen K.

"Acute hormonal and neuromuscular responses and recovery to forced vs maximum repetitions multiple resistance exercises."

International Journal of Sports Medicine. 2003 August.

Both [resistance training] protocols led to the great acute increases in serum testosterone, free testosterone, cortisol and growth hormone concentrations. However, the responses in cortisol and growth hormone were larger in the forced repetitions group than in the maximum repetitions group . . . The data indicate that the forced repetition exercise system induced greater acute hormonal and neuromuscular responses than a traditional maximum repetition exercise system and therefore it may be used to manipulate acute resistance exercise variables in athletes.

Häkkinen K, Pakarinen A, Hannonen P, et al

"Effects of strength training on muscle strength, cross-sectional area, maximal electromyographic activity, and serum hormones in premenopausal women with fibromyalgia." *Journal of Rheumatology.* 2002 June.

Observations recorded during the acute loading conditions might be considered an indication of the training induced adaptation of the endocrine system, showing that the acute growth hormone response may become systematic after strength training in both women with fibromyalgia and [those who are healthy].

Goto K, Ishii N, Kizuka T, Takamatsu K.
"The impact of metabolic stress on hormonal responses and muscular adaptations."
Medicine and Science in Sports and Exercise. 2005 June.

The [no rest between reps within sets] regimen induced strong lactate, growth hormone, epinephrine, and norepinephrine responses, whereas the [rest within sets] regimen did not . . . These results suggest that exercise-induced metabolic stress is associated with acute Growth Hormone, Epinephrine, and Norepinephrine responses and chronic muscular adaptations following resistance training.

Godfrey RJ, Madgwick Z, Whyte GP.
"The exercise-induced growth hormone response in athletes."
Journal of Sports Medicine. 2003. Review.

A growing body of evidence suggests that higher intensity [lower volume] exercise is effective in eliciting beneficial health, well-being and training outcomes. In a great many cases, the impact of some of the deleterious effects of ageing could be reduced if exercise focused on promoting the exercise-induced growth hormone response [EIGR]. This review examines the current knowledge and proposed mechanisms for the EIGR, the physiological consequences of endurance, strength and power training on the EIGR and its potential effects in elderly populations, including the aged athlete.

Ahtiainen JP, Pakarinen A, Alen M, Kraemer WJ, Häkkinen K.
"Short vs. long rest period between the sets in hypertrophic resistance training: influence on muscle strength, size, and hormonal adaptations in trained men."
Strength and Conditioning Research. 2005 August.

Both protocols before the experimental training period (month 0) led to large acute increases in serum Testosterone, Free Testosterone, Cortisol, and Growth Hormone concentrations . . . The present study indicated that, within typical hypertrophic strength-training protocols used in the present study, the length of the recovery times between the sets (2 vs. 5 minutes) did not have an influence on the magnitude of acute hormonal and neuromuscular responses or long-term training adaptations in muscle strength and mass in previously strength-trained men.

Gordon SE, Kraemer WJ, Looney DP, Flanagan SD, Comstock BA, Hymer WC.
"The influence of age and exercise modality on growth hormone bioactivity in women."
Growth Hormone and IGF Research. 2014 April.

The greater [bioactive growth hormone] response to the heavy resistance exercise protocol found in the younger group can be attributed to an unknown serum factor . . . that either potentiated growth hormone bioactivity in response to heavy resistance exercise or inhibited growth hormone bioactivity in response to aerobic exercise.

West DW, Phillips SM.

"Associations of exercise-induced hormone profiles and gains in strength and hypertrophy in a large cohort after weight training."

European Journal of Applied Physiology. 2012 July. Epub 2011 Nov 22.

> *The purpose of this study was to investigate associations between acute exercise-induced hormone responses and adaptations to high-intensity resistance training in a large cohort (n = 56) of young men . . . We report that the acute exercise-induced systemic hormonal responses of cortisol and Growth Hormone are weakly correlated with resistance training-induced changes in fibre cross-sectional area and lean body mass(cortisol only), but not with changes in strength.*

Häkkinen K, Pakarinen A, Kraemer WJ, Newton RU, Alen M.

"Basal concentrations and acute responses of serum hormones and strength development during heavy resistance training in middle-aged and elderly men and women."

Journal of Gerontology Series A. 2000 Feb.

> *The single exercise session both before and after the training resulted in significant responses in serum total and free testosterone concentrations in both male groups, but not in the female groups, as well as in serum growth hormone levels in all groups except in [the elderly women group]. In summary, the present strength training led to great increases in maximal strength not only in middle-aged but also in elderly men and women. The strength gains were accompanied by large increases in the maximal voluntary activation of the trained muscles.*

Eliakim A, Nemet D, Most G, Rakover N, Pantanowitz M, Meckel Y.

"Effect of gender on the GH-IGF-I response to anaerobic exercise in young adults."

The Journal of Strength and Conditioning Research. 2014 December.

> *In summary, supramaximal anaerobic exercise was associated with a greater and earlier postexercise GH peak in women compared with men. All together, the results suggest anaerobic exercise-related anabolic-type hormonal response.*

Taipale R, Häkkinen K.

"Acute Hormonal and Force Responses to Combined Strength and Endurance Loadings in Men and Women: The "Order Effect""

Public Library of Science, One. 2013.

> *These observed differences in hormonal responses despite similarities in neuromuscular fatigue in men indicate the presence of an order effect as the body was not fully recovered at 48 h following [strength training followed by endurance training]. These findings may be applicable in training prescription in order to optimize specific training adaptations . . . The present study does, however, demonstrate an order effect in hormone responses, particularly in testosterone of men that indicated that the body may not have been fully recovered 24 h and 48 h following [strength training followed by endurance training when compared to the reverse order].*

Oöpik V, Timpmann S, Kreegipuu K, Unt E, Tamm M.
"Heat acclimation decreases the growth hormone response to acute constant-load exercise in the heat."
Growth Hormone and IGF Research. 2014 February. Epub 2013 Oct 17.

Heat acclimation decreases the GH response to moderate intensity exhausting exercise in the heat.

Calixto R, Verlengia R, Crisp A, et al.
"Acute effects of movement velocity on blood lactate and growth hormone responses after eccentric bench press exercise in resistance-trained men."
Biology of Sports. 2014 December.

In conclusion, the velocity of eccentric muscle action influences acute responses following bench press exercises performed by resistance-trained men using a slow velocity resulting in a greater metabolic stress and hormone response.

Shaner AA, Vingren JL, Hatfield DL, Budnar RG Jr, Duplanty AA, Hill DW.
"The acute hormonal response to free weight and machine weight resistance exercise."
Journal of Strength Conditioning Research. 2014 April.

Free weight exercises seem to induce greater hormonal responses to resistance exercise than machine weight exercises using similar lower-body multijoint movements and primary movers.

Gupta V.
"Adult growth hormone deficiency."
Indian Journal of Endocrinology and Metabolism. 2011 September.

Adult growth hormone deficiency is being recognized increasingly and has been thought to be associated with premature mortality. Pituitary tumors are the commonest cause for Adult growth hormone deficiency. Growth hormone deficiency has been associated with neuropsychiatric-cognitive, cardiovascular, neuromuscular, metabolic, and skeletal abnormalities.

Tritos NA.
"Skeletal health in adult growth hormone deficiency."
Endocrine. 2016 January.

These data affirm and extend previous observations on the effects of GH on the adult skeleton. Indeed, several retrospective studies have reported an increased risk of fracture (vertebral or all sites combined) among GH-deficient adults in comparison with either the general population or hypopituitary patients without GH deficiency.

Bove RM, White CC, Gerweck AV, et al.
"Effect of growth hormone on cognitive function in young women with abdominal obesity."
Clinical Endocrinology. (Oxf). 2015 Dec 10.

The hormonal milieu of obesity, including relative growth hormone deficiency and resultant relative insulin-like growth factor-1 deficiency, may mediate the emerging association between midlife adiposity and longitudinal cognitive decline.

Wang Y, Pessin JE.
"Mechanisms for fiber-type specificity of skeletal muscle atrophy."
Current Opinions in Clinical Nutrition and Metabolic Care. 2013 May. Review.

Fast-twitch glycolytic fibers are more vulnerable than slow-twitch oxidative fibers under a variety of atrophic conditions . . . nutrient-related atrophy such as cancer/aging cachexia, sepsis, and diabetes are more directed to [fast and super fast twitch] glycolytic fiber wasting.

Rosa C, Vilaça-Alves J, Fernandes HM, Saavedra FJ, Pinto RS, dos Reis VM.
"Order effects of combined strength and endurance training on testosterone, cortisol, growth hormone, and IGF-1 binding protein 3 in concurrently trained men."
Journal of Strength and Conditioning Research. 2015 January.

Smilios I, Pilianidis T, Karamouzis M, Tokmakidis SP.
"Hormonal responses after various resistance exercise protocols."
Medical Science in Sports Exercise. 2003 April.

Ahtiainen JP, Pakarinen A, Alen M, Kraemer WJ, Häkkinen K.
"Muscle hypertrophy, hormonal adaptations and strength development during strength training in strength-trained and untrained men."
European Journal of Applied Physiology. 2003 August.

Vendelbo MH, Christensen B, Grønbæk SB, et. al.
"GH signaling in human adipose and muscle tissue during "feast and famine": amplification of exercise stimulation following fasting compared to glucose administration."
European Journal of Endocrinology. 2015 September.

Padilla Colon CJ, Sanchez Collado P, Cuevas MJ.
"[Benefits of strength training for the prevention and treatment of sarcopenia]."
Nutricion Hospitalaria. 2014 May. Review. Spanish.

Nascimento Dda C, Tibana RA, Benik FM, et al.
"Sustained effect of resistance training on blood pressure and hand grip strength following a detraining period in elderly hypertensive women: a pilot study."
Clinical Interventions in Aging. 2014 January.

Gonzalez AM, Hoffman JR, Stout JR, Fukuda DH, Willoughby DS.
"Intramuscular Anabolic Signaling and Endocrine Response Following Resistance Exercise: Implications for Muscle Hypertrophy".
Journal of Sports Medicine. 2015 Dec 14.

Muscle Psychology, Motor Imagery, and Neural Adaptations in Strength Training

Calatayud J, Vinstrup J, Jakobsen MD, Sundstrup et. al.
"Importance of mind-muscle connection during progressive resistance training."
European Journal Applied Physiology. 2016 March. . Epub 2015 Dec 23.

This study evaluates whether focusing on using specific muscles during bench press can selectively activate these muscles . . . In both [pectorals and triceps] muscles, focusing on using the respective muscles increased muscle activity . . . Resistance-trained individuals can increase [triceps] or [pectorals] muscle activity during the bench press when focusing on using the specific muscle at intensities up to 60 % of [one repetition maximum].

Gabriel DA, Kamen G, Frost G.
"Neural adaptations to resistive exercise: mechanisms and recommendations for training practices."
Sports Medicine. 2006. Review.

There are several lines of evidence for central [brain] control of training-related adaptation to resistive exercise. Mental practice using imagined contractions has been shown to increase the excitability of the cortical areas involved in movement and motion planning. However, training using imagined contractions is unlikely to be as effective as physical training, and it may be more applicable to rehabilitation. Retention of strength gains after dissipation of physiological effects demonstrates a strong practice effect . . . A reduction in antagonist co-activation would allow increased expression of agonist muscle force, while an increase in antagonist co-activation is important for maintaining the integrity of the joint... Motor learning theory and imagined contractions should be incorporated into strength-training practice... Submaximal eccentric contractions should be used when there are issues of muscle pain, detraining or limb immobilisation.

Martin K, Thompson KG, Keegan R, Ball N, Rattray B
"Mental fatigue does not affect maximal anaerobic exercise performance."
European Journal of Applied Physiology. 2015 April. Epub 2014 Nov 26.

Whereas mental fatigue can negatively impact submaximal endurance exercise, it appears that explosive power, voluntary maximal strength and anaerobic work capacity are unaffected.

Ingram TG, Kraeutner SN, Solomon JP, Westwood DA, Boe SG.
"Skill acquisition via motor imagery relies on both motor and perceptual learning."
Behavioral Neuroscience. 2016 April. Epub 2016 Feb 8.

Motor imagery, the mental rehearsal of movement, is an effective means for acquiring a novel skill, even in the absence of physical practice . . . Generally, physical practice-based training led to lower response times compared with motor imagery-based training for implicit and random sequences . . . Our results suggest that motor imaging-based training relies on both perceptual and motor learning . . . These results reveal details regarding the mechanisms underlying motor imagery, and inform its use as a modality for skill acquisition.

Lebon F, Collet C, Guillot A.

"Benefits of motor imagery training on muscle strength."

Journal of Strength and Conditioning Research. 2010 June.

It is well established that motor imagery (MI) improves motor performance and motor learning efficiently. Previous studies provided evidence that muscle strength may benefit from MI training, mainly when movements are under the control of large cortical areas in the primary motor cortex.

Di Rienzo F, Blache Y, Kanthack TF, Monteil K, Collet C, Guillot A.

"Short-term effects of integrated motor imagery practice on muscle activation and force performance."

Neuroscience. 2015 October.

The effect of motor imagery (MI) practice on isometric force development is well-documented.

Kumar VK, Chakrapani M, Kedambadi R.

"Motor Imagery Training on Muscle Strength and Gait Performance in Ambulant Stroke Subjects-A Randomized Clinical Trial."

Journal of Clinical and Diagnostic Research. 2016 March.

Motor imagery (MI) is an active process during which a specific action is reproduced within working memory without any actual movements. MI training enhances motor learning, neural reorganization and cortical activation . . . Additional task specific MI training improves paretic muscle strength and gait performance in ambulant stroke patients.

Lee M, Carroll TJ.

"Cross education: possible mechanisms for the contralateral effects of unilateral resistance training."

Sports Medicine. 2007. Review.

One piece of indirect evidence to indicate that neural adaptations accompany resistance training comes from the phenomenon of "cross education", which describes the strength gain in the opposite, untrained limb following unilateral resistance training. Since its discovery in 1894, subsequent studies have confirmed the existence of cross education in contexts involving voluntary, imagined and electrically stimulated contractions. The cross-education effect is specific to the contralateral homologous muscle but not restricted to particular muscle groups, ages or genders. A recent meta-analysis determined that the magnitude of cross education is approximately equal to 7.8% of the initial strength of the untrained limb... unilateral resistance training may activate neural circuits that chronically modify the efficacy of motor pathways that project to the opposite untrained limb. This may subsequently lead to an increased capacity to drive the untrained muscles and thus result in increased strength. A number of spinal and cortical circuits that exhibit the potential for this type of adaptation are considered. The second hypothesis suggests that unilateral resistance training induces adaptations in motor areas that are primarily involved in the control of movements of the trained limb. The opposite untrained limb may access these modified neural circuits during maximal voluntary contractions in ways that are analogous to motor learning.

Farthing JP, Borowsky R, Chilibeck PD, Binsted G, Sarty GE.
"Neuro-physiological adaptations associated with cross-education of strength."
Brain Topography. 2007 Winter.

These results suggest that cross-education of strength may be partly controlled by adaptations within sensorimotor cortex, consistent with previous studies of motor learning. However, this research demonstrates the involvement of temporal lobe regions that subserve semantic memory for movement, which has not been previously studied in this context. We argue that temporal lobe regions might play a significant role in the cross-education of strength.

Yue G, Cole KJ.
"Strength increases from the motor program: comparison of training with maximal voluntary and imagined muscle contractions."
Journal of Neurophysiology. 1992 May.

Strength increases can be achieved without repeated muscle activation. These force gains appear to result from practice effects on central motor programming/planning. The results of these experiments add to existing evidence for the neural origin of strength increases that occur before muscle hypertrophy.

Folland JP, Williams AG.
"The adaptations to strength training : morphological and neurological contributions to increased strength."
Sports Medicine. 2007. Review.

The gains in strength with high resistance strength training are undoubtedly due to a wide combination of neurological and morphological factors. Whilst the neurological factors may make their greatest contribution during the early stages of a training programme, hypertrophic processes also commence at the onset of training.

Enoka RM.
"Neural adaptations with chronic physical activity."
Journal of Biomechanics. 1997 May. Review.

Behm DG, Sale DG.
"Velocity specificity of resistance training."
Sports Medicine. 1993 June. Review.

Sale DG.
"Neural adaptation to resistance training."
Medicine and Science in Sports and Exercise. 1988 October. Review.

Other Healing Effects of BioLogic Strength Training

Unhjem RJ, Nygård M, van den Hoven LT, Sidhu SK, Hoff J, Wang E.
"Lifelong strength training mitigates the age-related decline in efferent drive."
Journal of Applied Physiology. 2016 June.

These observations suggest that lifelong strength training has a protective effect against age-related attenuation of efferent drive. In contrast, no beneficial effect seems to derive from habitual recreational activity, indicating that strength training may be particularly beneficial for counteracting age-related loss of neuromuscular function.

Wang Y, Pessin JE.
"Mechanisms for fiber-type specificity of skeletal muscle atrophy."
Current Opinions in Clinical Nutrition and Metabolic Care. 2013 May. Review.

Fast-twitch glycolytic fibers are more vulnerable than slow-twitch oxidative fibers under a variety of atrophic conditions . . . nutrient-related atrophy such as cancer/aging cachexia, sepsis, and diabetes are more directed to [fast and super fast twitch] glycolytic fiber wasting.

Winters-Stone KM, Dobek JC, Bennett JA, Dieckmann et. al.
"Resistance training reduces disability in prostate cancer survivors on androgen deprivation therapy: evidence from a randomized controlled trial."
Archives of Physical Medicine and Rehabilitation. 2015 January.

Findings from this study contribute to the mounting evidence that [resistance training] exercise should become a routine part of clinical care in older men with advanced prostate cancer.

Hagstrom AD, Marshall PW, Lonsdale C, et. al.
"Resistance training improves fatigue and quality of life in previously sedentary breast cancer survivors: a randomised controlled trial."
European Journal of Cancer Care. (Engl). 2015 November. [Epub ahead of print]

We demonstrated both statistically and clinically important improvements in fatigue and quality of life in response to resistance training in breast cancer survivors.

Shaw G, Reviewed by Nazario B.
"Women and Weight Training for Osteoporosis"
WebMD Feature Article. (2009, January). Retrieved from http://www.webmd.com/osteoporosis/living-with-osteoporosis-7/weight-training

Studies show that strength training over a period of time can help prevent bone loss -- and may even help build new bone. In one study, postmenopausal women who participated in a strength training program for a year saw significant increases in their bone density in the spine and hips, areas affected most by osteoporosis in older women.

Gillies EM, Putman CT, Bell GJ.
"The effect of varying the time of concentric and eccentric muscle actions during resistance training on skeletal muscle adaptations in women."
European Journal of Applied Physiology. 2006 July.

[Long concentric] resistance training was more effective than [long eccentric] for increasing both [slow twitch and fast twitch] fibre area and cortisol when time under tension and intensity of muscle actions were matched between the two modes of resistance training in young healthy women.

Coughlin SS, Yoo W, Whitehead MS, Smith SA.
"Advancing breast cancer survivorship among African-American women."
Breast Cancer Research and Treatment. 2015 September.

For addressing physical and mental health concerns, a variety of interventions have been evaluated, including exercise and weight training, dietary interventions, yoga and mindfulness-based stress reduction, and support groups or group therapy. Obesity has been associated with breast cancer recurrence and poorer survival. Relative to white survivors, African-American breast cancer survivors are more likely to be obese and less likely to engage in physical activity, although exercise improves overall quality of life and cancer-related fatigue.

Stephen PM, Shannon LM, Daniel PB, et. al.
"Strength Training for Arthritis Trial (START): design and rationale"
BioMed Central, Musculoskeletal Disorders. 2013.

Muscle loss and fat gain contribute to the disability, pain, and morbidity associated with knee osteoarthritis, and thigh muscle weakness is an independent, modifiable risk factor. While treatment guidelines recommend strengthening exercise to combat sarcopenia in knee osteoarthritis patients, the appropriate intensities or loads (defined as percent of one repetition maximum, or %1RM) recommended are unclear.

Seeger JP, Lenting CJ, Schreuder TH, et. al.
"Interval exercise, but not endurance exercise, prevents endothelial ischemia-reperfusion injury in healthy subjects."
The American Journal of Physiology, Heart and Circulatory Physiology. 2015 February. Epub 2014 Nov 21.

In conclusion, a single bout of lower limb interval exercise, but not moderate-intensity endurance exercise, effectively prevents [brachial artery injury]. This indicates the presence of a remote preconditioning effect of exercise, which is selectively present after short-term interval but not continuous exercise in healthy young subjects.

Farup J, Sørensen H, Kjølhede T.
"Similar changes in muscle fiber phenotype with differentiated consequences for rate of force development: endurance versus resistance training."
Human Movement Science. 2014 April.

Resistance Training significantly increased eccentric, concentric and isometric strength for both knee extensors and flexors, whereas Endurance Training did not. In conclusion, resistance training may be very important for maintaining the rate of force development, whereas endurance training may negatively impact rate of force development.

Häkkinen K, Pakarinen A, Hannonen P, et. al.

"Effects of strength training on muscle strength, cross-sectional area, maximal electromyographic activity, and serum hormones in premenopausal women with fibromyalgia."

Journal of Rheumatology. 2002 June.

Both the magnitude and time course of adaptations of the neuromuscular system to resistance training in [women with fibromyalgia] were completely comparable to those taking place in healthy women. Basal levels of the anabolic hormones seem to be similar in women with [fibromyalgia] compared to age matched healthy women. Observations recorded during the acute loading conditions might be considered an indication of the training induced adaptation of the endocrine system, showing that the acute growth hormone response may become systematic after strength training in both women with fibromyalgia and [those who are healthy].

Correa CS, Teixeira BC, Cobos RC, et. al.

"High-volume resistance training reduces postprandial lipaemia in postmenopausal women."

Journal of Sports Science. 2015.

The results of this investigation suggest that [high-volume resistance training] reduces PPL in postmenopausal women.

American Heart Association

'Weight Training After a Stroke"

StrokeAssociation.org, Life After Stroke. American Heart Association. (2014, January). Retrieved from http://www.strokeassociation.org/STROKEORG/LifeAfterStroke/RegainingIndependence/PhysicalChallenges/Weight-Training-After-Stroke_UCM_309780_Article.jsp#.VrT6KfkrLcs

Many healthcare professionals are concerned that resistance training can have a detrimental effect on spastic muscles. A recent review of the professional literature found no scientific evidence to back up that position. Tom Wisenbaker, as special needs fitness trainer, has been using strength training with stroke survivors for 15 years. According to Wisenbaker: "I get people after everyone else has given up on them, and they've been going downhill a long time. So many doctors and therapists who assess stroke survivors give only a few tests to decide if someone has plateaued. What we have found is that plateauing in one area doesn't mean they've plateaued in every area. We have not seen someone who doesn't continue to improve. We had a lady from Denmark who was more than 20 years post-stroke, and she got her gait back after limping for all those years. People actually develop new muscle on their affected side. The experts didn't think that was possible, but we clearly see it. One of my clients was talking to his neurologist, who was impressed with how much improvement he had made. He asked the patient if we had planned that improvement because he didn't believe that you could target areas and have them improve. The big thing I've learned is how amazingly adaptable and capable we are. The medical community is so external and passive and unwilling for us to look inside. When are they going to realize that the head is part of the body, that the brain cells are attached to the body, so our thoughts and desires are part of our body? It's amazing what we can accomplish when we stop focusing on our limitations."

American Heart Association

"Safe Workouts Post-Heart Attack"

GoRedForWomen.com, American Heart Association. (2016. February). Retrieved from https://www.goredforwomen.org/live-healthy/heart-healthy-exercises/safe-workouts-post-heart-attack/

After a heart attack, some resistance exercises are beneficial. You can start with bicep curls without weight. Start small and work your way up to eight or 12 of those as a set. Do two or three sets and when that gets easy, grab a can of soup to start doing it with a little weight.

Recovery, Recuperation, & Rest: Mission Critical

Heavens KR, Szivak TK, Hooper DR, et. al.
"The effects of high-intensity short rest resistance exercise on muscle damage markers in men and women."
Journal of Strength and Conditioning Research. 2014 April.

Overall, [when following the short rest protocol] women demonstrated a faster inflammatory response with increased acute damage, whereas men demonstrated a greater prolonged damage response. Therefore, strength and conditioning professionals need to be aware of the level of stress imposed on individuals when creating such volitional high-intensity metabolic type workouts and allow for adequate progression and recovery from such workouts.

Andersen JL, Aagaard P.
"Effects of strength training on muscle fiber types and size; consequences for athletes training for high-intensity sport."
*Scandinavian Journal of Medicine & Science in Sports.*2010 October. Review.

Data from our lab indicate that heavy resistance training followed by detraining can evoke a boosting in proportions of the [super fast twitch fiber] isoform....[the super fast twitch fiber] percentage in the vastus lateralis muscle of the subjects decreased from 9% to only 2% in a 3 months training period, but somewhat more remarkable the [super fast twitch fiber] percentage subsequently increased to 17% after an additional period of 3 months of detraining . . . The fact is that muscle fibers containing predominantly [super fast twitch cells] are also fibers that rely on a metabolism that enables them to produce very high amounts of energy in short time (i.e. exerting very high power), but only over a very limited period of time (seconds). Consequently, the [super fast twitch] fibers need to rest to avoid exhaustion . . . However, if the intention is to produce a very fast [sprinter] . . . avoid training involving hours of continuous work at a moderate aerobic level, as this type of exercise may lead to an increased number of fibers expressing [as slow twitch fibers] . . . Further, aerobic exercise may fully or partially blunt the hypertrophic muscle response from concurrent resistance training . . . Two of the major processes evidentially leading to hypertrophy *are (i) increase in muscle protein synthesis and (ii) myogenic satellite cell proliferation. The increase in protein synthesis is the immediate response of the muscle fibers to the training stimulus received, whereas the activation (proliferation) of satellite cells are trailing somewhat behind, as if the muscle fibers are "waiting" to see if this stimulus are withheld over a longer period, before the costly affair of incorporating new nuclei into the fibers are implemented.*

De Souza RW, Aguiar AF, Carani FR, Campos GE, Padovani CR, Silva MD.
"High-intensity resistance training with insufficient recovery time between bouts induce atrophy and alterations in myosin heavy chain content in rat skeletal muscle."
Anatomical Record, (Hoboken). 2011 August.

Change in muscle fiber-type frequency was supported by a significant decrease in [slow twitch] and [lower order fast twitch fibers] accompanied by a significant increase in [super fast twitch fiber] content . . . These data show that high-intensity resistance training with insufficient recovery time between bouts promoted muscle atrophy.

Gentil P, Fischer B, Martorelli AS, Lima RM, Bottaro M.
"Effects of equal-volume resistance training performed one or two times a week in upper body muscle size and strength of untrained young men."
The Journal of Sports Medicine and Physical Fitness. 2015 March. Epub 2014 Apr 14.

The results from the present study suggest that untrained men experience similar gains in muscle mass and strength with equal volume resistance training [whether] performed one or two days per week.

Schoenfeld BJ, Pope ZK, Benik FM, et. al.
"Longer Interset Rest Periods Enhance Muscle Strength and Hypertrophy in Resistance-Trained Men."
Journal of Strength and Conditioning. Research. 2016 July.

This study provides evidence that longer rest periods promote greater increases in muscle strength and hypertrophy *in young resistance-trained men.*

McKendry J, Pérez-López A, McLeod M, et. al.
"Short inter-set rest blunts resistance exercise-induced increases in myofibrillar protein synthesis and intracellular signaling in young males."
Experimental Physiology. 2016 July. Epub 2016 Jun 2.

We demonstrate that short rest (1 min) between sets of moderate-intensity, high-volume resistance exercise blunts the acute muscle anabolic response compared with a longer rest period (5 min), despite a superior circulating hormonal milieu. These data have important implications for the development of training regimens to maximize muscle hypertrophy. *Manipulating the rest-recovery interval between sets of resistance exercise may influence training-induced muscle remodeling.*

Scudese E, Simão R, Senna G, et. al.
"Long Rest Interval Promotes Durable Testosterone Responses in High-intensity Bench Press."
Journal of Strength and Conditioning Research. 2015 Oct 6. [Epub ahead of print]

In conclusion, although both short and long rest periods [between sets] enhanced acute testosterone values, the longer rest promoted a longer lasting elevation for both total testosterone and free testosterone.

Miranda H, Simão R, Moreira LM, et. al.
"Effect of rest interval length on the volume completed during upper body resistance exercise."
Journal of Sports Science and Medicine. 2009 September.

The results of the current study indicate that during a resistance exercise session, if sufficient time is available, resting 3 minutes between sets and exercises allows greater workout volume for the upper body exercises examined.

Pincivero DM, Lephart SM, Karunakara RG.
"Effects of rest interval on isokinetic strength and functional performance after short-term high-intensity training."
British Journal of Sports Medicine. 1997 September.

The findings indicate that a relatively longer intrasession rest period resulted in a greater improvement in hamstring muscle strength during short term high-intensity training.

Häkkinen K, Kallinen M.
"Distribution of strength training volume into one or two daily sessions and neuromuscular adaptations in female athletes."
Electromyography and Clinical Neurophysiology. 1994 March.

The present results with female athletes suggest that the distribution of the volume of intensive strength training into smaller units, such as two daily sessions, may create more optimal conditions not only for muscular hypertrophy *but by producing effective training stimuli especially for the nervous system. These kinds of training conditions may lead to further strength development in athletes being greater than obtained during "normal" strength training of the same [total] duration.*

Martorelli A, Bottaro M, Vieira A, et. al.
"Neuromuscular and blood lactate responses to squat power training with different rest intervals between sets."
Journal of Sports Science & Medicine. 2015 May.

From a practical point of view, the results suggest that 1 to 2 minute of rest interval between sets during squat exercise may be sufficient to recover power output in a designed power training protocol. However, if training duration is malleable, we recommend 2 min of rest interval for optimal recovery and power output maintenance during the subsequent exercise sets.

Theou O, Gareth JR, Brown LE
"Effect of rest interval on strength recovery in young and old women.".
Journal of Strength and Conditioning Research. 2008 November.

Old women required only a 1:1 exercise-to-rest ratio for knee flexor recovery, whereas younger women required a longer 1:2 exercise-to-rest ratio. Practitioners should consider age and gender when prescribing rest intervals between sets.

Hartman MJ, Clark B, Bembens DA, Kilgore JL, Bemben MG.
"Comparisons between twice-daily and once-daily training sessions in male weight lifters."
International Journal of Sports Physiology Performance. 2007 June.

The increase in [isometric strength] and [neuromuscular] activity for the twice-daily group might provide some rationale for dividing training load in an attempt to reduce the risk of overtraining.

Rønnestad BR, Egeland W, Kvamme NH, Refsnes PE, Kadi F, Raastad T.
"Dissimilar effects of one- and three-set strength training on strength and muscle mass gains in upper and lower body in untrained subjects."
Journal of Strength and Conditioning Research. 2007 Feb.

The results demonstrate that 3-set strength training is superior to 1-set strength training with regard to strength and muscle mass gains in the leg muscles, while no difference exists between 1- and 3-set training in upper-body muscles in untrained men." (supports the 3-F progression)

Trappe S, Creer A, Slivka D, Minchev K, Trappe T.
"Single muscle fiber function with concurrent exercise or nutrition countermeasures during 60 days of bed rest in women."
Journal of Applied Physiology. 2007 October.

In [the exercise group] conditions, [muscle fiber] size and contractile function were preserved during bed rest. These data show that the concurrent exercise program preserved the myocellular profile of the vastus lateralis muscle during 60-day bed rest. To combat muscle atrophy and function with long-term unloading, the exercise prescription program used in this study should be considered as a viable training program for the upper leg muscles, whereas the nutritional intervention used cannot be recommended as a countermeasure for skeletal muscle.

Häkkinen K, Alen M, Kraemer WJ, et. al.
"Neuromuscular adaptations during concurrent strength and endurance training versus strength training."
European Journal of Applied Physiology. 2003 March.

The mean fibre areas of [the various muscle fiber types] increased after the training both in [strength training only] and [strength plus endurance training] ($p<0.05$ and $p<0.01$ respectively). [Strength training only] showed an increase in rate of force development ($p<0.01$), while no change occurred in [strength plus endurance training]."

Fröhlich M, Emrich E, Schmidtbleicher D.
"Outcome effects of single-set versus multiple-set training--an advanced replication study."
Research in Sports Medicine. 2010 July.

On the basis of 72 primary studies, the meta-analysis dealt with the problem of single-set vs. multiple-set training . . . Generally speaking, it can be stated that multiple-set training, depending on factors like age, training experience, duration of the study, etc., offers several advantages over single-set regimes, especially when combined with periodization strategies, and it can be applied very successfully for increasing maximal strength in long-time effects. Therefore, the outcome effects of both methods are the same in short-time interventions. For longer-time interventions and for advanced subjects with the goal of optimizing their strength gain, however, multiple-set strategies are superior.

McGuff D, Little J., pg. 53

Physiologists R.N. Carpinelli and R.M. Otto conducted a study out of Adelphi University that surveyed all of the known scientific literature [up through 1998] concerning single-set versus multiple-set resistance training. They found that, on the whole, performing multiple sets brought absolutely no additional increase in results compared with single-set training. The literature came down overwhelmingly in favor of a single set of exercise as being sufficient; only two out of the forty seven studies surveyed showed any benefit (and a marginal improvement at that) to be had from the performance of multiple sets.

Kemmler WK, Lauber-D, Engelke K, Weineck J.

"Effects of single- vs. multiple-set resistance training on maximum strength and body composition in trained postmenopausal women."

Journal of Strength & Conditioning Research. 2004 November.

Multiple-set training resulted in significant increases (3.5-5.5%) for all 4 strength measurements, whereas single-set training resulted in significant decreases (-1.1 to -2.0%). Body mass and body composition did not change during the study. The results show that, in pretrained subjects, multiple-set protocols are superior to single-set protocols in increasing maximum strength.

Radaelli R, Wilhelm EN, Botton CE, et al.

"Effects of single vs. multiple-set short-term strength training in elderly women."

Age (Dordr). 2014.

These results suggest that during the initial stages of strength training, single- and multiple-set training demonstrate similar capacity for increasing dynamic strength, [muscle thickness], and [muscle quality] of the knee extensors in elderly women.

Starkey DB, Pollock ML, Ishida Y, et. al.

"Effect of resistance training volume on strength and muscle thickness."

Medicine and Science in Sports and Exercise. 1996 October.

In conclusion, one set of high-intensity resistance training was as effective as three sets for increasing [knee extension] and [knee flexion] isometric torque and muscle thickness in previously untrained adults.

Buresh R, Berg K, French J.

"The effect of resistive exercise rest interval on hormonal response, strength, and hypertrophy with training."

Journal of Strength and Conditioning Research. 2009 January.

These results show that in healthy, recently untrained males, strength training with 1 minute of rest between sets elicits a greater hormonal response than 2.5-minute rest intervals in the first week of training, but these differences diminish by week 5 and disappear by week 10 of training. Furthermore, the hormonal response is highly variable and may not necessarily be predictive of strength and lean tissue gains in a 10-week training program.

Simão R, de Salles BF, Figueiredo T, Dias I, Willardson JM.
"Exercise order in resistance training."
Sports Medicine. 2012 March.

> *In terms of chronic adaptations, greater strength increases were evident by untrained subjects for the first exercise of a given sequence, while strength increases were inhibited for the last exercise of a given sequence. Additionally, based on strength and* hypertrophy *(i.e. muscle thickness and volume) effect-size data, the research suggests that exercises be ordered based on priority of importance as dictated by the training goal of a programme, irrespective of whether the exercise involves a relatively large or small muscle group.*

Simão R, Spineti J, de Salles BF, et. al.
"Influence of exercise order on maximum strength and muscle thickness in untrained men."
Journal of Sports Science & Medicine. 2010 March.

> *If an exercise is important for the training goals of a program, then it should be placed at the beginning of the training session, whether or not it is a large or a small muscle group exercise.*

Ahtiainen JP, Pakarinen A, Alen M, Kraemer WJ, Häkkinen K.
"Short vs. long rest period between the sets in hypertrophic resistance training: influence on muscle strength, size, and hormonal adaptations in trained men."
Journal of Strength and Conditioning Research. 2005 August.

Resting Movements and Stretching

Zakaria AA, Kiningham RB, Sen A.
"Effects of Static and Dynamic Stretching on Injury Prevention in High School Soccer Athletes: A Randomized Trial."
Journal of Sport Rehabilitation. 2015 August.

Static stretching does not provide any added benefit to dynamic stretching in the prevention of injury in this population before exercise.

Haddad M, Dridi A, Chtara M, et. al.
"Static stretching can impair explosive performance for at least 24 hours."
Journal of Strength and Conditioning Research. 2014 January.

The static stretching of the lower limbs and hip muscles had a negative effect on explosive performances up to 24 hours post stretching with no major effects on the repeated sprint ability. Conversely, the dynamic stretching of the same muscle groups are highly recommended 24 hours before performing sprint and long-jump performances. In conclusion, the positive effects of DS on explosive performances seem to persist for 24 hours.

Bain J, Chang L.
"New Ideas on Proper Stretching Techniques"
WebMD.com, Fitness & Exercise. 2010 October. Retrieved from http://www.webmd.com/fitness-exercise/new-ideas-on-proper-stretching-techniques?page=1

[According to Dr. Bill Holcomb, professor of athletic training at UNLV] you should never stretch a cold muscle in any way. And doing static stretches -- meaning the kind where you hold the stretch before a workout or competition -- may decrease your strength, power, and performance . . . After warming up [one should perform] dynamic (not static) stretches. Dynamic stretching means slow, controlled movements rather than remaining still and holding a stretch. They may include simple movements like arm circles and hip rotations, flowing movements as in yoga or walking . . . increasing numbers of experts agree that dynamic stretching is the best stretching routine before a workout or competition."

Bodybuilding.com Contributing Writer.
"Stretching for Weight Training!"
Bodybuilding.com, Stretching. 2014 September. Retrieved from http://www.bodybuilding.com/fun/donald1.htm

Dynamic stretching . . . involves moving parts of your body and gradually increasing reach, speed of movement, or both . . . Do not confuse dynamic stretching with ballistic stretching! Dynamic stretching consists of controlled leg and arm swings that take you (gently!) to the limits of your range of motion. Ballistic stretches involve trying to force a part of the body beyond its range of motion. In dynamic stretches, there are no bounces or "jerky" movements. An example of dynamic stretching would be slow, controlled leg swings, arm swings, or torso twists.

Kay AD, Blazevich AJ.

"Effect of acute static stretch on maximal muscle performance: a systematic review."

Medicine and Science in Sports and Exercise. 2012 January. Review.

The detrimental effects of static stretch are mainly limited to longer durations (≥60s) . . . Shorter durations of stretch (<60s) can be performed in a pre-exercise routine without compromising maximal muscle performance.

Kokkonen J, Nelson AG, Tarawhiti T, Buckingham P, Winchester JB.

"Early-phase resistance training strength gains in novice lifters are enhanced by doing static stretching."

Journal of Strength and Conditioning Research. 2010 February.

Based on results of this study, it is recommended that to maximize strength gains in the early phase of training, novice lifters should include static stretching exercises to their resistance training programs.

Lam LC, Chau RC, Wong BM, et. al.

"A 1-year randomized controlled trial comparing mind body exercise (Tai Chi) with stretching and toning exercise on cognitive function in older Chinese adults at risk of cognitive decline."

Journal of the American Medical Directors Association. 2012 July.

Regular exercise, especially mind-body exercise with integrated cognitive and motor coordination, may help with preservation of global ability in elders at risk of cognitive decline.

Monteiro WD, Simão R, Polito MD, et. al.

"Influence of strength training on adult women's flexibility."

Journal of Strength and Conditioning Research. 2008 May.

In conclusion, weight training can increase flexibility in previously sedentary middle-aged women in some, but not all joint movements.

Aquino CF, Fonseca ST, Gonçalves GG, Silva PL, Ocarino JM, Mancini MC.

"Stretching versus strength training in lengthened position in subjects with tight hamstring muscles: a randomized controlled trial."

Manual Therapy. 2010 Feb.

Stretching is used to modify muscle length. However, its effects seem to be temporary. There is evidence in animal models that strengthening in a lengthened position may induce long lasting changes in muscle length... The results demonstrated that strengthening in a lengthened position produced a shift of the torque-angle curve, which suggests an increase in muscle length. Conversely, stretching did not produce modification of torque-angle curve and flexibility; its effects appear restricted to increases in stretch tolerance.

Black JD, Stevens ED.
"Passive stretching does not protect against acute contraction-induced injury in mouse EDL muscle."
Journal of Muscle Research and Cell Motility. 2001.
Brooks SV, Zerba E, Faulkner JA.
"Injury to muscle fibres after single stretches of passive and maximally stimulated muscles in mice."
Journal of Physiology. 1995 October.

Risks of Prolonged Sitting and a Sedentary Living

Younger AM, Pettitt RW, Sexton PJ, Maass WJ, Pettitt CD.
"Acute moderate exercise does not attenuate cardiometabolic function associated with a bout of prolonged sitting."
Journal of Sports Science. 2016 April. Epub 2015 Jul 17.
Epidemiological studies suggest that prolonged sitting increases all-cause mortality; yet, physiological causes underpinning prolonged sitting remain elusive . . . We conclude prolonged sitting may be related to decreased posterior tibial artery blood velocity. Moreover, an acute bout of moderate exercise does not seem to attenuate cardiometabolic function during prolonged sitting in healthy, young adults.
Pines A.
"Sedentary women: sit less, live more!"
Climacteric. 2015 December. Epub 2015 Apr 14.

> *Data on the ill effects of sedentarism keep on increasing, clearly showing a significant adverse impact and increased risk for cardiovascular disease, cancer, fracture and various overweight-related metabolic conditions. The simple fact that prolonged sitting is associated with a shorter life span must be repeatedly discussed with our patients.*

Koehne K.
"A New Threat to the Nursing Workforce: Take a Stand!"
Creative Nursing. 2015.

> *The consequences of a sedentary lifestyle have been extensively studied, and the findings have been broadly reported in scientific journals as well as all forms of media. The development of cancer, cardiovascular disease, metabolic syndrome, venous thromboembolism, and extensive musculoskeletal strain can all result from prolonged immobility and repetitive computer use.*

Keum N, Cao Y, Oh H, et. al.
"Sedentary behaviors and light-intensity activities in relation to colorectal **cancer** risk."
International Journal of Cancer. 2015 December. [Epub ahead of print]
We found that prolonged sitting time watching TV was associated with an increased colorectal cancer risk in women but not in men.
Gao Y, Cronin NJ, Pesola AJ, Finni T.
"Muscle activity patterns and spinal shrinkage in office workers using a sit-stand workstation versus a sit workstation."
Ergonomics. 2016 February. [Epub ahead of print]

> *This cross-sectional study compared the effects of using a sit-stand workstation to a sit workstation on muscle activity patterns and spinal shrinkage in office workers. It provides evidence that working with a sit-stand workstation can promote more light muscle activity time and less inactivity without negative effects on spinal shrinkage.*

Bailey DP, Locke CD.
"Breaking up prolonged sitting with light-intensity walking improves postprandial glycemia, but breaking up sitting with standing does not."
Journal of Science and Medicine in Sports. 2015 May.

> *This study suggests that interrupting sitting time with frequent brief bouts of light-intensity activity, but not standing, imparts beneficial postprandial responses that may enhance cardiometabolic health.*

Restaino RM, Holwerda SW, Credeur DP, Fadel PJ, Padilla J.
"Impact of prolonged sitting on lower and upper limb micro- and macrovascular dilator function."
Experimental Physiology. 2015 July.

> *Collectively, these data suggest that prolonged sitting markedly reduces lower leg micro- and macrovascular dilator function, but these impairments can be fully normalized with a short bout of walking. In contrast, upper arm microvascular reactivity is selectively impaired with prolonged sitting, and walking does not influence this effect.*

Satellite Muscle Stem Cells

Verdijk LB, Snijders T, Drost M, Delhaas T, Kadi F, van Loon LJ.
"Satellite cells in human skeletal muscle; from birth to old age."
Age (Dordr). 2014 April.

Changes in satellite cell content play a key role in regulating skeletal muscle growth and atrophy . . . From birth to adulthood, muscle fiber size increased tremendously with no major changes in muscle fiber satellite cell content, and no differences between [slow twitch and fast/super fast twitch] fibers. In contrast to [slow twitch] muscle fibers, [fast and super fast twitch] muscle fiber size was substantially smaller with increasing age in adults . . . This was accompanied by an age-related reduction in [fast and super fast twitch] muscle fiber satellite cell content . . . Twelve weeks of resistance-type exercise training significantly increased [fast and super fast twitch] muscle fiber size and satellite cell content. We conclude that [fast and super fast] muscle fiber atrophy with aging is accompanied by a specific decline in [fast and super fast twitch] muscle fiber satellite cell content. Resistance-type exercise training represents an effective strategy to increase satellite cell content and reverse [fast and super fast twitch] muscle fiber atrophy.

Relaix F, Zammit PS.
"Satellite cells are essential for skeletal muscle regeneration: the cell on the edge returns centre stage".
Development. 2012 August. Review.

The clear consensus is that skeletal muscle does not regenerate without satellite cells, confirming their pivotal and non-redundant role.

Wang YX, Dumont NA, Rudnicki MA.
"Muscle stem cells at a glance."
Journal of Cell Science. 2014 November.

Muscle stem cells facilitate the long-term regenerative capacity of skeletal muscle. This self-renewing population of satellite cells has only recently been defined through genetic and transplantation experiments. Although muscle stem cells remain in a dormant quiescent state in uninjured muscle, they are poised to activate and produce committed progeny. Unlike committed myogenic progenitor cells, the self-renewal capacity gives muscle stem cells the ability to engraft as satellite cells and capitulate long-term regeneration.

Gundersen K.
"Muscle memory and a new cellular model for muscle atrophy and hypertrophy."
Journal of Experimental Biology. 2016 January. Review.

Fibres that have acquired a higher number of myonuclei grow faster when subjected to overload exercise, thus the nuclei represent a functionally important "memory" of previous strength. This memory might be very long lasting in humans, as myonuclei are stable for at least 15 years and might even be permanent. However, myonuclei are harder to recruit in the elderly, and if the long-lasting muscle memory also exists in humans, one should consider early strength training as a public health advice.

Dumont NA, Wang YX, Rudnicki MA

"Intrinsic and extrinsic mechanisms regulating satellite cell function.". *Development.* 2015 May. Review.

Satellite cells are the protagonists of muscle regeneration. To appropriately fulfill their functions, they must maintain a dynamic balance between their different cell states, namely quiescence, commitment, differentiation and self-renewal. As we have highlighted above, many intrinsic mechanisms are required to regulate the cell cycle and cell fate determination in satellite cells, and dysregulation of these mechanisms results in the loss of regeneration in degenerative conditions, including aging . . . These discoveries could represent a cornerstone in the treatment of pathologies such as sarcopenia, an irreversible loss of muscle mass induced by aging that causes serious health issues and currently has no therapy. It is likely that intrinsic perturbations in satellite cell regulatory mechanisms are present in other pathologies, including muscular dystrophies, and further studies are needed to explore these possibilities and to aid our understanding of muscle development, regeneration and degeneration.

Shefer G, Van de Mark DP, Richardson JB, Yablonka-Reuveni Z.

"Satellite-cell pool size does matter: defining the myogenic potency of aging skeletal muscle." *Developmental Biology.* 2006 June.

The study establishes that abundance of resident satellite cells declines with age in myofibers from both fast- and slow-twitch muscles. Nevertheless, the inherent myogenic potential of satellite cells does not diminish with age… Altogether, satellite cell abundance, but not myogenic potential, deteriorates with age.

Cermak NM, Snijders T, McKay BR, et. al.

"Eccentric exercise increases satellite cell content in type II muscle fibers." *Medicine and Science in Sports and Exercise.* 2013 Feb.

A single bout of high-force eccentric exercise increases muscle fiber [satellite cell] content and activation status in [fast and super fast twitch] but not [slow twitch] muscle fibers.

Ono Y, Masuda S, Nam HS, Benezra R, Miyagoe-Suzuki Y, Takeda S.

"Slow-dividing satellite cells retain long-term self-renewal ability in adult muscle." *Journal of Cellular Science.* 2012 March.

Our results indicate that undifferentiated slow-dividing satellite cells retain stemness for generating progeny capable of long-term self-renewal, and so might be essential for muscle homeostasis throughout life.

Day K, Shefer G, Richardson JB, Enikolopov G, Yablonka-Reuveni Z.
"Nestin-GFP reporter expression defines the quiescent state of skeletal muscle satellite cells."
Developmental Biology. 2007 April.

Repair of adult skeletal muscle depends on satellite cells, quiescent myogenic stem cells located beneath the myofiber basal lamina. Satellite cell numbers and performance decline with age and disease...

Shigemoto T, Kuroda Y, Wakao S, Dezawa M.
"A novel approach to collecting satellite cells from adult skeletal muscles on the basis of their stress tolerance."
Stem Cells Translational Medicine. 2013 July.

Satellite cells, which are skeletal muscle stem cells, have the ability to regenerate damaged muscles and are expected to be applicable for treatment of muscle degeneration.

Bruusgaard JC, Johansen IB, Egner IM, Rana ZA, Gundersen K.
"Myonuclei acquired by overload exercise precede hypertrophy and are not lost on detraining."
The National Academy of Sciences. 2010 August.

The old and newly acquired nuclei are retained during severe atrophy caused by subsequent denervation lasting for a considerable period of the animal's lifespan. The myonuclei seem to be protected from the high apoptotic activity found in inactive muscle tissue. A hypertrophy *episode leading to a lasting elevated number of myonuclei retarded disuse atrophy, and the nuclei could serve as a cell biological substrate for such memory. Because the ability to create myonuclei is impaired in the elderly, individuals may benefit from strength training at an early age.*

Fry CS, Lee JD, Jackson JR, et. al.
"Regulation of the muscle fiber microenvironment by activated satellite cells during hypertrophy."
The Journal of the Federation of American Societies for Experimental Biology. 2014 April.

These results provide evidence that satellite cells regulate the muscle environment during growth.

Kuang S, Kuroda K, Le Grand F, Rudnicki MA.
"Asymmetric self-renewal and commitment of satellite stem cells in muscle."
Cell. 2007 June.

We conclude that satellite cells are a heterogeneous population composed of stem cells and committed progenitors. These results provide critical insights into satellite cell biology and open new avenues for therapeutic treatment of neuromuscular diseases.

Stuelsatz P, Shearer A, Li Y, et. al.
"Extraocular muscle satellite cells are high performance myo-engines retaining efficient regenerative capacity in dystrophin deficiency."
Developmental Biology. 2015 January. Epub 2014 September.

> *Collectively, our study provides a comprehensive picture of [extraocular muscles] myogenic progenitors, showing that while these cells share common hallmarks with the prototypic [satellite cells] in somite-derived muscles, they distinctively feature robust growth and renewal capacities that warrant the title of high performance myo-engines and promote consideration of their properties for developing new approaches in cell-based therapy to combat skeletal muscle wasting.*

Farup J, Rahbek SK, Riis S, Vendelbo MH, Paoli Fd, Vissing K.
"Influence of exercise contraction mode and protein supplementation on human skeletal muscle satellite cell content and muscle fiber growth."
Journal of Applied Physiology. 2014 October.

> *Isolated concentric knee extensor resistance training appears to constitute a stronger driver of [satellite cell] content than eccentric resistance training while [fast and super fast twitch] fiber* hypertrophy *was accentuated when combining concentric resistance training with whey protein supplementation.*

Kvorning T, Kadi F, Schjerling P, et. al.
"The activity of satellite cells and myonuclei following 8 weeks of strength training in young men with suppressed testosterone levels."
Acta Physiologica (Oxford). 2015 March. Epub 2014 November.

> *Eight weeks of strength training enhances the myonuclear number in [fast and super fast twitch muscle] fibres...*

Day K, Shefer G, Shearer A, Yablonka-Reuveni Z.
"The depletion of skeletal muscle satellite cells with age is concomitant with reduced capacity of single progenitors to produce reserve progeny."
Developmental Biology. 2010 April.

> *Reserve cells emerge primarily within high-density colonies, and the number of clones that produce reserve cells is reduced with age. Thus, satellite cell depletion with age could be attributed to a reduced capacity to generate a reserve population.*

Molsted S, Andersen JL, Harrison AP, Eidemak I, Mackey AL.
"Fiber type-specific response of skeletal muscle satellite cells to high-intensity resistance training in dialysis patients."
Muscle & Nerve. 2015 November.

> *Increased myonuclear content of [fast and super fast twitch] muscle fibers of dialysis patients who perform resistance training suggests that [satellite cell] dysfunction is not the limiting factor for muscle growth.*

Mackey AL, Andersen LL, Frandsen U, Sjøgaard G.
"Strength training increases the size of the satellite cell pool in [slow twitch and fast/super fast twitch] fibres of chronically painful trapezius muscle in females."
Journal of Physiology. 2011 November.

Beltrami AP, Barlucchi L, Torella D, et. al.
"Adult cardiac stem cells are multipotent and support myocardial regeneration."
Cell. 2003 Sep 19.

Zhang Y, Sivakumaran P, Newcomb AE, et. al.
"Cardiac Repair With a Novel Population of Mesenchymal Stem Cells Resident in the HumanHeart."
Stem Cells. 2015 October. Epub 2015 Jul 29.

Sultana N, Zhang L, Yan J, et. al.
"Resident c-kit(+) cells in the heart are not cardiac stem cells."
Nature Communications. 2015 Oct 30.

Patsch C, Challet-Meylan L, Thoma EC, et.al.
"Generation of vascular endothelial and smooth muscle cells from human pluripotent stem cells."
Nature Cell Biology. 2015 August. Epub 2015 Jul 27.

Kennedy E, Mooney CJ, Hakimjavadi R, et. al.
"Adult vascular smooth muscle cells in culture express neural stem cell markers typical of resident multipotent vascular stem cells."
Cell and Tissue Research. 2014 October.

Yin H, Price F, Rudnicki MA.
"Satellite cells and the muscle stem cell niche."
Physiological Reviews. 2013 January. Review.

Snijders T, Nederveen JP, McKay BR, et al.
"Satellite cells in human skeletal muscle plasticity."
Frontiers in Physiology. 2015.

Seniors and Elderly: Targeted Studies

Fazelzadeh P, Hangelbroek RW, Tieland M, et. al.

"The Muscle Metabolome Differs between Healthy and Frail Older Adults."

Journal of Proteome Research. 2016 February. Epub 2016 Jan 22.

> *Age-related loss of physiological functions negatively affects quality of life. A major contributor to the frailty syndrome of aging is loss of skeletal muscle . . . Prolonged resistance-type exercise training resulted in an adaptive response of amino acid metabolism, especially reflected in branched chain amino acids and genes related to tissue remodeling. The effect of exercise training on branched-chain amino acid-derived acylcarnitines in older subjects points to a downward shift in branched-chain amino acid catabolism upon training.*

Walker S, Peltonen H, Häkkinen K.

'Medium-intensity, high-volume "hypertrophic" resistance training did not induce improvements in rapid force production in healthy older men."

Age (Dordr). 2015 June.

> *It is recommendable that resistance training programs for older individuals integrate protocols emphasizing maximum force/muscle* hypertrophy *and rapid force production in order to induce comprehensive health-related and functionally important improvements in this population.*

Unhjem R, Lundestad R, Fimland MS, Mosti MP, Wang E.

"Strength training-induced responses in older adults: attenuation of descending neural drive with age."

Age (Dordr). 2015 June.

> *These findings suggest that changes in supraspinal activation play a significant role in the age-related changes in muscle strength. Furthermore, motor system impairment can to some extent be improved by heavy resistance training.*

Melov S., Tarnopolsky Mark A,Beckman K, Felkey C, Hubbard A.

"Resistance Exercise Reverses Aging in Human Skeletal Muscle"

Public Library of Science.(2007, May).

Retrieved from http://journals.plos.org/plosone/article?id=10.1371/journal.pone.0000465.

> *Following exercise training the transcriptional signature of aging was markedly reversed back to that of younger levels for most genes that were affected by both age and exercise. We conclude that healthy older adults show evidence of mitochondrial impairment and muscle weakness, but that this can be partially reversed at the phenotypic level, and substantially reversed at the transcriptome level, following six months of resistance exercise training.*

Kalapotharakos VI, Diamantopoulos K, Tokmakidis SP.
"Effects of resistance training and detraining on muscle strength and functional performance of older adults aged 80 to 88 years."
Aging Clinical and Experimental Research. 2010 April.

Results indicate that a resistance exercise program induces favorable muscular and functional adaptations in very old adults. However, a significant part of the favorable adaptations obtained after resistance exercise may be lost within 6 weeks of detraining. Therefore, very old adults should follow a long-term and systematic routine of exercise throughout life, in order to improve and maintain their physical functions and to ameliorate their life status.

Rabelo HT, Bezerra LA, Terra DF, et. al.
"Effects of 24 weeks of progressive resistance training on knee extensors peak torque and fat-free mass in older women."
Journal of Strength and Conditioning Research. 2011 August.

Consistent with the literature, it is concluded that a progressive [resistance training] program promotes not only increases in muscle strength, as evaluated by an isokinetic dynamometer, but also in [fat free mass] as evaluated by the [dual energy X-ray absorptiometry], in elderly women.

Borde R, Hortobágyi T, Granacher U.
"Dose-Response Relationships of Resistance Training *in Healthy Old Adults: A Systematic Review and Meta-Analysis.*
Sports Medicine. 2015 December.

Training period, intensity, time under tension, and rest in between sets play an important role in improving muscle strength and morphology and should be implemented in exercise training programs targeting healthy old adults.

Gschwind YJ, Kressig RW, Lacroix A, Muehlbauer T, Pfenninger B, Granacher U.
"A best practice fall prevention exercise program to improve balance, strength / power, and psychosocial health in older adults: study protocol for a randomized controlled trial."
BMC Geriatrics. 2013 October.

It is expected that particularly the supervised combination of balance and strength / power training will improve performance in variables of balance, strength / power, body composition, cognitive function, psychosocial well-being, and falls self-efficacy of older adults.

Kalapotharakos V, Smilios I, Parlavatzas A, Tokmakidis SP.
"The effect of moderate resistance strength training and detraining on muscle strength and power in older men."
Journal of Geriatric Physical Therapy. 2007.

Muscle strength and vertical jump performance improved after short-term moderate resistance strength training. A short-term detraining period affects the muscle strength and power in older adults [61-75 years], but the neuromuscular function does not return to pretraining levels. This suggests that the continuation of a strength training program is essential for the maintenance of muscle strength, functional performance, and independence in older adults.

Macaluso A, De Vito G. "Muscle strength, power and adaptations to resistance training in older people."

European Journal of Applied Physiology. 2004 April. Review.

The selective atrophy of fast-twitch fibres has been ascribed to the progressive loss of motoneurons in the spinal cord with initial denervation of fast-twitch fibres, which is often accompanied by reinnervation of these fibres by axonal sprouting from adjacent slow-twitch motor units (MUs). In addition, single fibres of older muscles containing myosin heavy chains of both [slow and fast twitch fibers] show lower tension and shortening velocity with respect to the fibres of young muscles . . . the older muscle seems to be more resistant to isometric fatigue (fatigue-paradox), which can be ascribed to the selective atrophy of fast-twitch fibres...

Anton MM, Spirduso WW, Tanaka H.

"Age-related declines in anaerobic muscular performance: weightlifting and powerlifting."

Medicine and Science in Sports and Exercise. 2004 January.

Peak anaerobic muscular power, as assessed by peak lifting performance, decreases progressively even from earlier ages than previously thought; 2) the overall magnitude of decline in peak muscular power appears to be greater in tasks requiring more complex and powerful movements; 3) the age-related rates of decline are greater in women than in men only in the events that require more complex and explosive power; and 4) upper- and lower-body muscular power demonstrate similar rate of decline with age.

Martel GF, Roth SM, Ivey FM, et. al.

"Age and sex affect human muscle fibre adaptations to heavy-resistance strength training."

Experimental Physiology. 2006 March.

[Heavy resistance strength training] resulted in increased [cross-sectional area] of [all types of] muscle fibres in the trained leg of young men, [slow and fast twitch] fibres in young women, [fast twitch fibers] in older men, and [super fast twitch] fibres in older women... [Heavy resistance strength training] led to significant increases in [one-repetition maximum] and [fast twitch fiber cross-sectional area] in all groups; however, age and sex influence specific muscle fibre subtype responses to [heavy resistance strength training].

Häkkinen K, Kraemer WJ, Newton RU, Alen M.

"Changes in electromyographic activity, muscle fibre and force production characteristics during heavy resistance/power strength training in middle-aged and older men and women."

Acta Physiologica Scandanavica. 2001 January.

The findings support the concept of the important role of neural adaptations in strength and power development in middle-aged and older men and women. The muscle fibre distribution (percentage [fast twitch] fibres) seems to be an important contributor on muscle strength in older people, especially older women.

Kirkendall DT, Garrett WE Jr.

"The effects of aging and training on skeletal muscle."

The American Journal of Sports Medicine. 1998 July. Review.

Neither reduced muscle demand nor the subsequent loss of function is inevitable with aging. These losses can be minimized or even reversed with training.

Lambert CP, Evans WJ.

"Effects of aging and resistance exercise on determinants of muscle strength."

Journal of the American Aging Association. 2002 April.

Muscle co-activation appears to be substantially and similarly reduced (improved) in young and elderly individuals as a result of resistance training.

Kiilerich K, Ringholm S, Biensø RS, et. al.

"Exercise-induced pyruvate dehydrogenase activation is not affected by 7 days of bed rest." *Journal of Applied Physiology.* 2011 September.

Thompson LV.

"Effects of age and training on skeletal muscle physiology and performance."

Physical Therapy. 1994 January. Review.

Basu R, Basu A, Nair KS.

"Muscle changes in aging."

Journal of Nutrition, Health, and Aging. 2002.

Kalapotharakos VI, Tokmakidis SP, Smilios I, Michalopoulos M, Gliatis J, Godolias G.

"Resistance training in older women: effect on vertical jump and functional performance."

Journal of Sports Medicine and Physical Fitness. 2005 December.

Taaffe DR, Duret C, Wheeler S, Marcus R.

"Once-weekly resistance exercise improves muscle strength and neuromuscular performance in older adults."

*Journal of the American Geriatrics Society.*1999 October.

Foley A, Hillier S, Barnard R.

"Effectiveness of once-weekly gym-based exercise programmes for older adults post discharge from day rehabilitation: a randomised controlled trial."

British Journal of Sports Medicine. 2011 September.

Ogawa M, Yasuda T, Abe T.

"Component characteristics of thigh muscle volume in young and older healthy men."

Clinical Physiology and Functional Imaging. 2012 March.

Be sure to get your FREE BioLogic Workout Mobile App for iPhone and Android at the App Store and Google Play

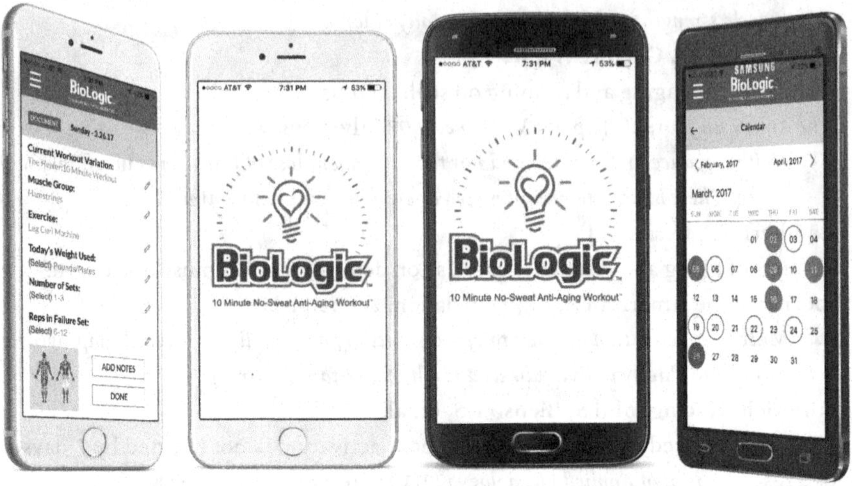

When prompted, enter **The Healer** *to activate the app, and visit us at BioLogicWorkout.com for tutorials*

COMING SOON! The BioLogic Workout Demonstration Sessions on Blue Ray, DVD, or Full HD through instant download

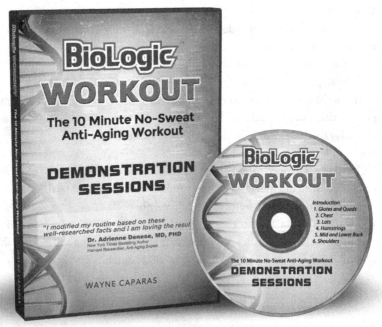

Go to BioLogicWorkout.com to get on the notification list, and when prompted, enter **The Healer** *as your promo code*

Printed in the United States
By Bookmasters

Printed in the United States
By Bookmasters